DERMATOPATHOLOGY HANDBOOK 2026

A Clinical Textbook Covering Reaction Pattern Recognition, Histologic Diagnosis, and Clinical Correlation for Pathology Residents

Ramon C. Henson, MD

Trademark Disclaimer

All brand names, product names, drug names, certification names, and registered trademarks mentioned in this textbook are the property of their respective owners. Their use in this publication does not imply endorsement, affiliation, or sponsorship by the trademark owner, nor does it imply that the trademark owner has reviewed, approved, or is in any way associated with this work. All trademarked names and registered marks appearing in this textbook are used solely for purposes of identification and educational reference, without any intent of trademark infringement.

Medical Disclaimer

This textbook is intended solely for educational and informational purposes and is designed to support the continuing professional development of licensed healthcare providers. The clinical content presented herein reflects information believed to be accurate and current at the time of publication; however, medicine evolves rapidly, and readers are advised that new research findings, updated clinical practice guidelines, and revised regulatory approvals may alter or supersede information contained in this work after its publication date.

Nothing in this publication constitutes medical advice, clinical guidance specific to any individual patient, or a substitute for the independent professional judgment of a licensed and qualified healthcare provider. No clinician-patient relationship is established, implied, or intended by the use of this textbook or any portion thereof. All clinical decisions, including but not limited to diagnosis, therapeutic selection, drug dosing, and patient monitoring, must be individualized based on thorough and direct assessment of the patient, the totality of current published evidence, applicable clinical practice guidelines, institutional protocols, and the informed professional judgment of the responsible clinician.

Drug information, dosages, treatment protocols, and therapeutic recommendations presented in this publication are offered for educational reference only and must be independently verified against current prescribing information, pharmacopeial references, and applicable regulatory approvals prior to clinical application. The author and publisher have made every reasonable effort to ensure the accuracy and completeness of the information presented; nevertheless, they expressly disclaim all liability for any adverse outcomes, clinical errors, patient harm, loss, or injury alleged to arise, directly or indirectly, from the use, misuse, or application of any information, recommendation, protocol, or clinical guidance contained in this publication.

TABLE OF CONTENT

PREFACE

Dermatopathology occupies a narrow but demanding seam between two specialties. The dermatologist arrives at the microscope already holding a clinical impression; the surgical pathologist arrives holding a lifetime of pattern recognition trained on organs that do not behave like skin. The dermatopathologist has to hold both at once, and do it quickly, because a skin biopsy report is rarely the end of a diagnostic process. It is usually the fulcrum on which a treatment decision turns within days.

This handbook was written for the resident or fellow standing at that fulcrum for the first hundred times: the pathology resident rotating through a busy dermatopathology service, the dermatology resident learning to read the slide behind the biopsy result, the newly independent dermatopathology fellow signing out alone for the first time, and the general surgical pathologist who reads skin specimens without a subspecialist down the hall. Each of these readers needs the same underlying skill, even though they arrive at it from different training pathways: the ability to look at a piece of tissue, recognize its reaction pattern, and move systematically from that pattern to a defensible diagnosis while ruling out the mimickers that make dermatopathology one of the more treacherous corners of anatomic pathology.

Why a Pattern-First Structure

Every major dermatopathology reference of the last half-century has converged on the same insight, usually credited to the algorithmic method popularized in the mid-twentieth century: skin disease is more tractable when it is first sorted by histologic reaction pattern (spongiotic, psoriasiform, lichenoid, vesiculobullous, granulomatous, vasculopathic, panniculitic) and only then narrowed to a specific diagnosis. This handbook is organized around that same logic, not as an afterthought but as the architecture of the book itself. Chapters follow reaction pattern for inflammatory disease and lineage for neoplastic disease, in the sequence a trainee actually encounters them: foundational histology and technique first, then the inflammatory reaction patterns in the order they are most commonly confused with one another, then the neoplastic categories organized by cell of origin.

The Reaction Pattern Recognition System

Built into every chapter is a five-part structural feature carried consistently throughout the book: the named reaction pattern, its histologic signature, the diagnostic decision it triggers, the trap logic that separates it from its most dangerous mimickers, and a single pattern anchor distilled to the one finding that should lock the diagnosis in memory. Each chapter closes with a Pattern Synthesis Recap that consolidates every pattern introduced in that chapter into a scannable reference, and the book closes with The Reaction Pattern Master Atlas, a fully indexed, cross-referenced consolidation of every pattern in the book, organized for the reader who needs an answer during sign-out rather than a chapter to read at leisure.

How This Book Is Organized

Part I establishes the histologic foundation: normal skin anatomy as it appears under the microscope, the technical apparatus of special stains and immunohistochemistry that supports every diagnosis in the chapters that follow, and the pattern-based method itself. Part II works through the inflammatory reaction patterns in turn, each chapter following the same internal architecture so that the reader's eye learns where to look for what. Part III addresses neoplastic dermatopathology, from melanocytic lesions and melanoma through epidermal, adnexal, mesenchymal, and lymphoproliferative disease. Part IV closes with special topics that do not fit neatly into either category: genodermatoses and pediatric disease, and the special diagnostic considerations of nail, mucosal, and genital skin.

A Note on Scope

This handbook is a clinical reference, not an examination workbook. It contains no practice questions, review questions, or self-assessment items of any kind. Its value is delivered entirely through clinical decision content: patterns, trap logic, diagnostic anchors, and the indexed atlas that consolidates them. Clinical cases throughout the book are narrative scenarios that walk through diagnostic reasoning from presentation to resolution; they are not multiple-choice exercises. The intent throughout is to build the reader's independent diagnostic judgment, not to test it.

CHAPTER 1: NORMAL SKIN HISTOLOGY AND THE APPROACH TO THE SKIN BIOPSY

Learning Objectives

1. Describe the histologic organization of normal epidermis, dermis, and subcutaneous fat, and relate each layer to the diagnostic questions it is used to answer.
2. Identify the major cutaneous adnexal structures and recognize their normal histologic appearance across anatomic sites.
3. Explain how site-specific and age-related histologic variation alters the interpretation of an otherwise unremarkable biopsy.
4. Select an appropriate biopsy technique for a given clinical scenario and assess a specimen for diagnostic adequacy.
5. Apply a systematic, low-power-to-high-power scanning approach to generate an initial histologic differential diagnosis.

Skin as a Diagnostic Organ

The Skin as a Three-Layered Diagnostic System

Skin is unusual among the organs a pathologist is asked to interpret because its normal architecture is itself the diagnostic scaffold. In most organs, the pathologist first establishes that an abnormality exists and then characterizes it; in skin, the three-layered structure of epidermis, dermis, and subcutaneous fat is so consistently reproducible from one healthy person to the next that any deviation from that expected architecture becomes immediately informative. A biopsy that shows intact basket-weave stratum corneum, a preserved granular layer, an unremarkable dermal-epidermal junction, and a papillary dermis free of inflammatory infiltrate is not merely unremarkable; it actively excludes an entire category of disease, because the reaction patterns that define most inflammatory dermatoses each leave a specific, recognizable signature on this same basic architecture.

This is why dermatopathology teaching begins with normal histology rather than with disease. Every reaction pattern discussed later in this book, whether spongiotic, psoriasiform, lichenoid, vesiculobullous, granulomatous, vasculopathic, or panniculitic, is defined as a departure from a specific baseline: spongiosis is intercellular edema superimposed on the normal keratinocyte lattice, psoriasiform hyperplasia is regularized elongation of the normal rete ridge pattern, lichenoid change is destruction of the normal basal layer by an unusually dense band of lymphocytes hugging the dermal-epidermal junction. A reader who has not internalized what normal looks like at each of these levels will struggle to recognize when a pattern departs from it, because the departure is defined entirely in relation to the baseline.

Why Skin Pathology Differs From Other Organ Systems

Two features of skin distinguish its pathology from that of other organs and justify the pattern-based method that structures this book. First, skin disease is compartmentalized: the same insult produces different histologic pictures depending on which compartment it predominantly affects, so that the diagnostic task is as much about localizing the process as characterizing it. A lymphocytic infiltrate that hugs the dermal-epidermal junction behaves diagnostically very differently from a lymphocytic infiltrate that fills the papillary dermis without touching the epidermis, even though both might be described in isolation simply as a dermal lymphocytic infiltrate. Second, skin disease is frequently systemic disease made visible: a biopsy of a leg ulcer, a purpuric papule, or an urticarial plaque is often a proxy for a process occurring simultaneously in the kidney, the lung, or the joint, so that histologic pattern recognition in skin carries diagnostic weight that extends well beyond the skin itself.

KEY POINT: The reaction pattern is not an abstraction layered on top of skin histology; it is the organizing principle of skin histology itself. Learning to recognize the seven or eight major reaction patterns is functionally equivalent to learning the histologic vocabulary of the entire specialty.

This organizing logic also explains why dermatopathology is taught and practiced differently from most other subspecialties within surgical pathology, where organ-specific tumor classification dominates the curriculum and inflammatory disease receives comparatively little dedicated attention. In skin, inflammatory disease is not a minor category alongside neoplasia; it is at least as large a share of routine sign-out volume, and the reaction-pattern method exists specifically because that volume of inflammatory disease could not be taught efficiently any other way. A trainee who internalizes the handful of reaction patterns early acquires a transferable skill that compounds across the rest of training, since every subsequent inflammatory chapter in this book, and a substantial portion of the neoplastic chapters as well, builds directly on the compartmental and pattern-recognition vocabulary introduced here.

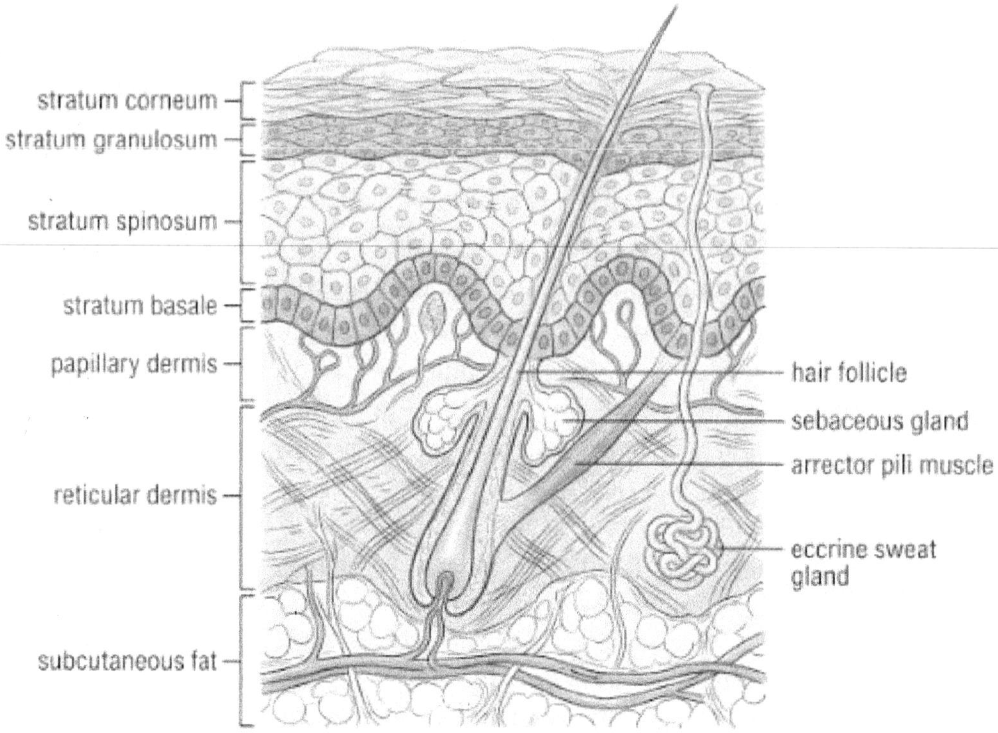

Epidermal, Dermal, and Subcutaneous Histology

Epidermal Architecture and Keratinocyte Maturation

The epidermis is a self-renewing, stratified squamous epithelium organized around a single unidirectional maturation program: keratinocytes are born in the stratum basale, flatten and accumulate keratohyalin granules as they ascend through the stratum spinosum and stratum granulosum, and are finally shed as anucleate corneocytes from the stratum corneum. Under normal conditions this transit takes approximately four weeks, and the epidermis at any moment contains a full cross-section of that timeline, which is why a single biopsy can capture the entire maturation sequence. Basal keratinocytes are cuboidal to columnar, sit on the basement membrane, and show a comparatively high nuclear-to-cytoplasmic ratio reflecting their proliferative role; they are interspersed with melanocytes, roughly one melanocyte for every ten basal keratinocytes in most body sites, and with Merkel cells and the dendritic processes of Langerhans cells that are more readily appreciated by immunohistochemistry than by routine hematoxylin and eosin staining.

The stratum spinosum owes its name to the intercellular bridges, formed by desmosomes, that appear as spine-like connections between adjacent keratinocytes on standard processing; these desmosomal attachments are the structural target of the pemphigus group of autoimmune blistering diseases discussed in Chapter 7, and their disruption is what produces the intraepidermal, suprabasal or subcorneal clefts characteristic of that group. The stratum granulosum is defined by basophilic keratohyalin granules within flattening keratinocytes and thins or disappears in several important pathologic states, most notably in the parakeratotic overlying epidermis of psoriasis, where retained nuclei in the stratum corneum reflect an accelerated maturation program that outpaces normal granular layer formation.

The Dermal-Epidermal Junction

The dermal-epidermal junction is a specialized basement membrane zone, anchoring the epidermis to the underlying dermis through hemidesmosomes, anchoring filaments, and anchoring fibrils built substantially from type VII collagen. Because this junction is the structural target of several distinct disease processes, its integrity or disruption carries specific diagnostic implications. In lichenoid interface dermatitis, a band-like lymphocytic infiltrate obscures and damages the basal layer, producing vacuolar change, individual keratinocyte necrosis, and eventually junctional clefting (a Max Joseph space) that can be mistaken for a primary blistering disease if the inflammatory band itself is not appreciated. In subepidermal immunobullous disease, by contrast, the split occurs cleanly at or just below this junction with comparatively little associated basal keratinocyte damage, and direct immunofluorescence is frequently required to distinguish the specific target antigen involved.

Dermal Composition and the Papillary-Reticular Distinction

The dermis is conventionally divided into a superficial papillary dermis and a deeper reticular dermis, a distinction that is more than descriptive convenience because many reaction patterns are defined by which compartment they predominantly involve. The papillary dermis contains thin, loosely arranged collagen bundles, a rich capillary plexus, and, normally, only a sparse population of resident lymphocytes, histiocytes, and mast cells clustered around the superficial vascular plexus. The reticular dermis contains thick, densely packed collagen bundles arranged roughly parallel to the skin surface, along with the deeper vascular plexus, eccrine coils, and the bulk of the pilosebaceous apparatus. A superficial perivascular lymphocytic infiltrate confined to the papillary dermis carries a very different differential diagnosis from a superficial and deep perivascular infiltrate extending into the reticular dermis, and recognizing which compartment is involved is one of the first branch points in pattern-based reasoning.

Subcutaneous Fat and the Panniculus

The subcutaneous fat, or panniculus, is organized into lobules of mature adipocytes separated by fibrous septa carrying the deep vascular supply. This lobular-septal architecture is the anatomic basis for the classification of panniculitis discussed in Chapter 10: processes that predominantly damage the septa (septal panniculitis, exemplified by erythema nodosum) produce a different clinical and histologic picture from processes that predominantly damage the fat lobules themselves (lobular panniculitis, exemplified by pancreatic panniculitis or lupus panniculitis), and correctly localizing the process to septum or lobule at scanning power is often the single most useful step in narrowing a panniculitis differential.

Cutaneous Vasculature and Neural Elements

The dermal vasculature is organized into two horizontally oriented plexuses connected by ascending and descending vessels: a superficial plexus at the papillary-reticular dermal junction, which sends individual capillary loops up into each dermal papilla, and a deep plexus at the dermal-subcutaneous junction. This two-plexus architecture is the anatomic basis for the superficial-versus-superficial-and-deep distinction used throughout the pattern-based classification of both inflammatory dermatoses and vasculitis: a process confined to the superficial plexus produces a different clinical lesion (typically smaller, more localized) than one also involving the deep plexus (typically larger, capable of ulceration or nodule formation), and the depth of vascular involvement identified on a biopsy is one of the most clinically actionable pieces of information a dermatopathology report can convey. Cutaneous nerves accompany the vasculature at both plexus levels and are generally inconspicuous on routine hematoxylin and eosin staining unless specifically sought, though specialized structures such as Meissner corpuscles in the dermal papillae of glabrous skin and Pacinian corpuscles in the deep dermis and subcutis of the palms and soles are occasionally encountered incidentally and should be recognized as normal structures rather than neoplasms.

Epidermal Layer	Location	Key Histologic Features	Diagnostic Relevance
Stratum basale	Deepest epidermal layer, on basement membrane	Cuboidal to columnar keratinocytes, melanocytes interspersed	Target of lichenoid interface damage; site of most cutaneous melanocytic proliferations
Stratum spinosum	Mid-epidermis	Polygonal keratinocytes with visible intercellular bridges	Site of acantholysis in pemphigus group disease
Stratum granulosum	Superficial to spinosum	Flattened keratinocytes with basophilic keratohyalin granules	Thinned or absent in psoriasiform and parakeratotic processes
Stratum corneum	Outermost layer	Anucleate, compacted corneocytes in basket-weave pattern	Parakeratosis, hyperkeratosis, and scale-crust patterns are read here

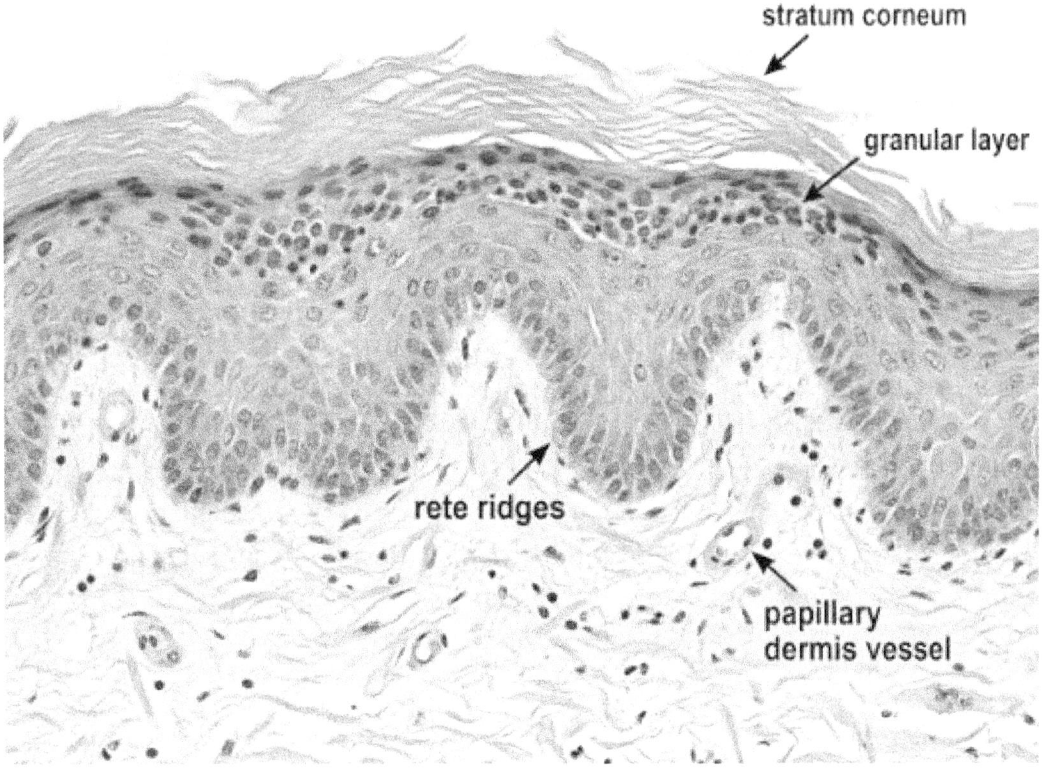

Adnexal Structure Histology

The Hair Follicle Unit

The hair follicle is the most structurally complex adnexal unit in skin and is conventionally divided, from superficial to deep, into the infundibulum, isthmus, and inferior segment (stem and bulb). The infundibulum extends from the skin surface to the entry of the sebaceous duct and is lined by epithelium continuous with, and histologically identical to, surface epidermis, which is why infundibular cysts fill with the same lamellated keratin seen in the stratum corneum. The isthmus extends from the sebaceous duct to the insertion of the arrector pili muscle and lacks a granular layer, keratinizing instead by a trichilemmal pathway that becomes diagnostically important when it is recapitulated in trichilemmal cysts and several adnexal neoplasms discussed in Chapter 16. The inferior segment, present only during the anagen growth phase, surrounds the dermal papilla and is the site of the follicular miniaturization changes that define androgenetic alopecia and the abrupt catagen-phase involution that characterizes alopecia areata.

The hair cycle itself carries diagnostic weight independent of any structural abnormality. Anagen, the active growth phase, occupies the great majority of a normal follicle's cycle and is characterized by a large, deeply pigmented bulb tightly encasing the dermal papilla. Catagen is a brief, tightly regulated involutional phase marked by apoptosis of the lower follicular epithelium and upward retraction of the follicle. Telogen is a quiescent resting phase in which the follicle is reduced to a small, club-shaped structure lacking a bulb or dermal papilla investment, sitting at a comparatively superficial dermal level before eventual shedding. A normal scalp biopsy shows the great majority of follicles in anagen, with telogen follicles representing a small minority; a shift in this ratio toward telogen, or the appearance of miniaturized vellus-like follicles in place of terminal follicles, is itself a histologic finding rather than merely the absence of one, and is discussed in the context of alopecia in later special-topics coverage.

Sebaceous and Apocrine Glands

Sebaceous glands are holocrine glands, meaning the entire cell disintegrates to release its lipid-rich contents into the follicular canal, producing the characteristic multilobular architecture of foamy, lipid-vacuolated cells with scalloped nuclei arranged around a central duct. They are concentrated on the face, scalp, and upper trunk and are essentially absent from palms and soles, a distribution that becomes relevant when sebaceous neoplasms and sebaceous hyperplasia are considered in their expected anatomic context. Apocrine glands, by contrast, are largely restricted to the axillae, anogenital region, and a scattering of modified apocrine structures such as the ceruminous glands of the external auditory canal and the mammary-like glands of the anogenital area; they show a distinctive decapitation secretion pattern in which a portion of apical cytoplasm pinches off into the gland lumen, a feature that is diagnostically useful in distinguishing apocrine from eccrine differentiation in adnexal neoplasms.

Eccrine Glands

Eccrine glands are distributed across nearly the entire skin surface, with particular density on palms, soles, and the axillae, and are organized into a deep coiled secretory portion in the lower dermis or upper subcutis and a straight, then spiraled, ductal portion that ascends to the skin surface. The secretory coil contains two cell populations, a larger pale-staining clear cell responsible for fluid and electrolyte secretion and a smaller darker mucin-containing cell, surrounded by a discontinuous layer of myoepithelial cells that is readily highlighted with smooth muscle actin or calponin immunohistochemistry when a neoplasm of eccrine origin is being characterized.

Nail Unit Histology

The nail unit is structurally distinct enough from the rest of the integument that it merits separate mention here and dedicated treatment in Chapter 20. The nail matrix, the proliferative epithelium beneath the proximal nail fold, produces the nail plate through a keratinization program that, unlike surface epidermis, occurs without a granular layer under normal conditions; the presence of a granular layer in the nail matrix or plate is consequently a pathologic finding rather than a normal variant, and is seen in several inflammatory and neoplastic nail unit conditions. The nail bed, extending from the distal matrix to the hyponychium, is firmly adherent to the underlying periosteum through a specialized dermis lacking a subcutaneous fat layer, which explains both the tight adherence of the nail plate and the tendency of nail bed pathology to produce onycholysis when that adherence is disrupted. Longitudinal biopsies that capture matrix, bed, and the proximal nail fold together are generally the most diagnostically informative specimen for nail unit disease, though they require particular technical care given the small and structurally delicate nature of the tissue involved.

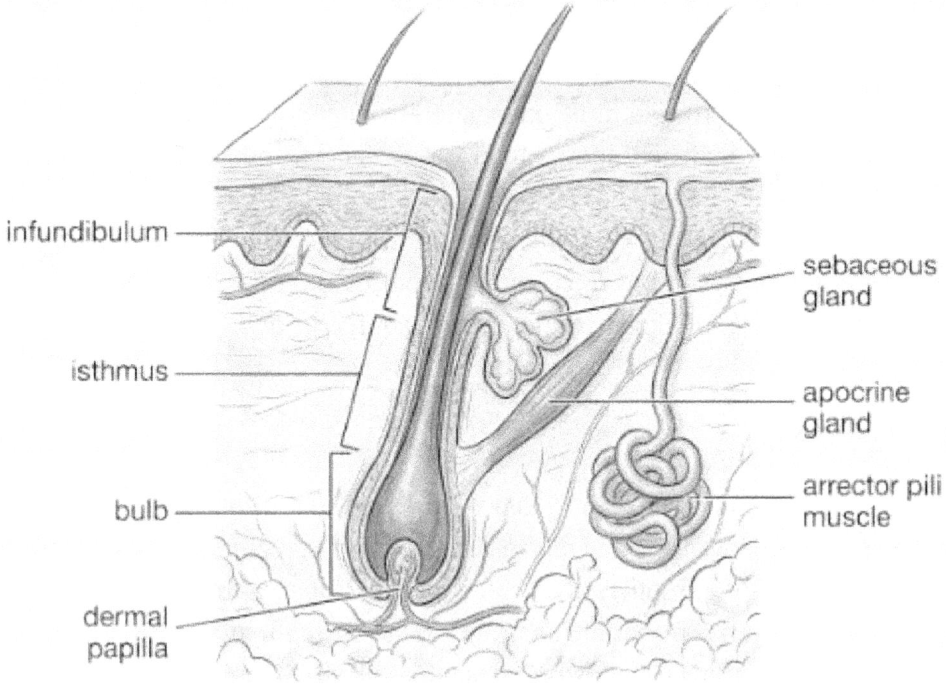

THE REACTION PATTERN RECOGNITION SYSTEM — Foundations of Adnexal Recognition

The Pattern: Normal Anagen Follicular Density Mistaken for a Pathologic Infiltrate

Histologic Signature: A transverse (horizontal) biopsy section through hair-bearing scalp shows numerous closely packed anagen follicular units with their surrounding fibrous tracts, which at low power can resemble a dense inflammatory infiltrate to an inexperienced reader unfamiliar with horizontal sectioning.

The Decision: Recognize the transverse plane of section, identify individual follicular epithelial structures with their concentric fibrous sheaths rather than diffuse inflammatory cells, and confirm a normal anagen-to-telogen ratio before considering a diagnosis of alopecia.

Trap Logic: The mimicker is a genuinely inflammatory cicatricial alopecia. The discriminating feature is architecture: normal anagen follicles retain a full complement of follicular units with intact sebaceous glands and no perifollicular fibrosis or interface change at the follicular epithelium, whereas cicatricial alopecia shows follicular dropout, perifollicular lymphocytic infiltrate targeting the isthmus and infundibulum, and eventual replacement of follicular units by fibrous tracts.

Pattern Anchor: Count follicular units and assess sebaceous gland preservation before diagnosing alopecia on a transverse section; loss of sebaceous glands is one of the earliest and most reliable indicators of scarring follicular injury.

Regional and Site-Specific Histologic Variation

Acral Skin

Palmar and plantar skin differs from skin at other sites in ways that directly affect interpretation. The stratum corneum is markedly thickened, the granular layer is correspondingly prominent, eccrine glands are present in high density, and hair follicles and sebaceous glands are entirely absent. A biopsy from acral skin therefore shows a compact hyperkeratotic stratum corneum that would be flagged as pathologic hyperkeratosis at any other body site but represents normal palmoplantar architecture; failure to account for site when interpreting keratin thickness is a recurring source of overcalled hyperkeratotic disorders in acral specimens.

Scalp and Hair-Bearing Skin

Scalp biopsies are frequently processed as horizontal (transverse) sections specifically to permit counting of follicular units and assessment of the anagen-to-telogen ratio, a technique that differs from the vertical sectioning used for essentially all other skin biopsies and that a reader must recognize to avoid misinterpreting normal transverse follicular anatomy as an inflammatory process, as illustrated in the Rhythm block above. Terminal hair follicles on the scalp normally extend into the subcutaneous fat, so a biopsy that fails to sample to an adequate depth may appear to show follicular miniaturization or loss simply because the deep bulbar portion of the follicle was not included in the specimen, a technical pitfall rather than a pathologic finding.

Mucosal and Genital Skin

Mucosal epithelium, including the labial and buccal mucosa and the glans penis, characteristically lacks a granular layer and stratum corneum under non-keratinizing conditions, so that parakeratosis and reduced granular layer thickness, which would be abnormal on trunk skin, are expected findings at these sites and must not be misread as evidence of a psoriasiform or lichenoid process. Genital skin, particularly vulvar and penile skin, shows a thinner epidermis with less prominent rete ridges than trunk skin and a dermis richer in vascular and neural elements, features that affect the appearance of otherwise familiar inflammatory and neoplastic processes when they occur at these sites, a theme developed further in Chapter 20.

Flexural and Intertriginous Skin

Flexural sites, including the axillae, groin, and inframammary folds, are subject to chronic friction, occlusion, and a warm, moist microenvironment that alters both normal histology and disease presentation. The stratum corneum at these sites is comparatively thin and may show mild compact hyperkeratosis or a subtle degree of spongiosis even in clinically unaffected skin, reflecting low-grade mechanical irritation rather than primary disease, and this baseline should be distinguished from the more pronounced spongiotic change of a true intertriginous dermatitis. Because flexural skin is disproportionately affected by intertrigo, inverse psoriasis, and Hailey-Hailey disease, all of which can show overlapping acantholytic or spongiotic features at this site, correlating the biopsy with the specific flexural location and its known baseline variation is a necessary step before applying the reaction-pattern framework developed in the following chapters.

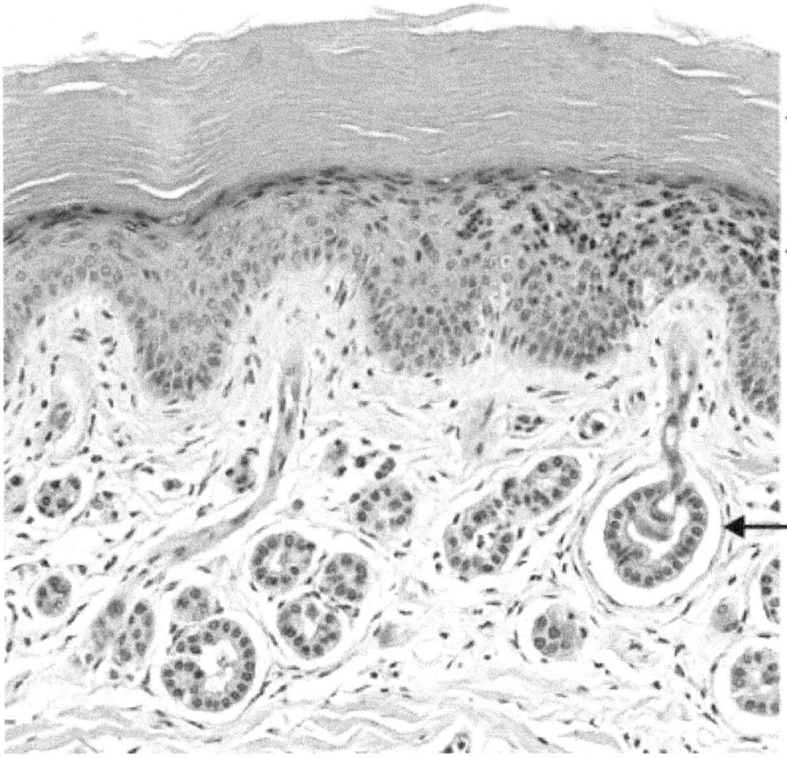

Neonatal and Pediatric Skin

Neonatal skin differs from adult skin in ways that affect both baseline interpretation and disease susceptibility. The epidermis is thinner, the dermal-epidermal junction is less securely anchored owing to a relative paucity of mature anchoring fibrils, and the dermis contains a higher proportion of ground substance relative to mature collagen, giving pediatric skin a greater propensity toward subepidermal separation under mechanical stress. Eccrine glands are present at birth in adult density but functionally immature, and sebaceous glands, stimulated by residual maternal androgens, may be transiently prominent in the neonatal period before regressing until the hormonal changes of adolescence reactivate them. These features matter diagnostically because several of the more severe pediatric blistering conditions, and the differential for neonatal vesiculopustular eruptions more broadly, depend on correctly distinguishing structurally normal but immature skin from a primary blistering disease.

Geriatric Skin and Photoaging

Aged and chronically photodamaged skin shows a set of changes that are near-universal in sun-exposed sites and must be distinguished from disease. The epidermis thins and the rete ridge pattern flattens, reducing the surface area of the dermal-epidermal junction and contributing to the increased shear fragility and easy bruising characteristic of aged skin. The papillary dermis develops solar elastosis, a basophilic degeneration of dermal collagen and elastic tissue that appears as amorphous, faintly basophilic material replacing the normal fibrillar collagen pattern and is one of the most reliable histologic indicators of chronic ultraviolet exposure. Solar elastosis is not itself a disease process, but its presence or absence is diagnostically informative: its presence confirms that a biopsy is from chronically sun-exposed skin, relevant to the differential of many neoplastic and some inflammatory processes, while its absence in a lesion clinically attributed to sun damage should prompt reconsideration of that clinical impression.

Skin of Color Considerations

Histologic principles apply consistently across all skin pigmentation, but several normal findings vary in prominence with constitutive pigmentation and should not be misread as pathologic. Basal layer pigmentation is more pronounced in darkly pigmentedskin, and melanophages, pigment-laden dermal macrophages, may be present in modest numbers in normal or minimally inflamed papillary dermis in patients with deeply pigmented skin, a finding that would be more strongly suggestive of an active inflammatory or postinflammatory process in lightly pigmented skin. Follicular and perifollicular pigment incontinence is similarly more commonly encountered as an isolated, non-specific finding. These variations do not change the underlying reaction-pattern framework, but they do shift the threshold at which a given finding should be considered diagnostically significant, and calibrating that threshold to the patient's baseline pigmentation is part of accurate interpretation rather than a separate diagnostic system.

CLINICAL PEARL: Solar elastosis, follicular pigment incontinence, and mild flexural spongiosis are common findings that describe the patient's baseline biology, not necessarily the disease process under investigation. Report them when present, but do not let them substitute for, or be mistaken as, the primary diagnostic finding.

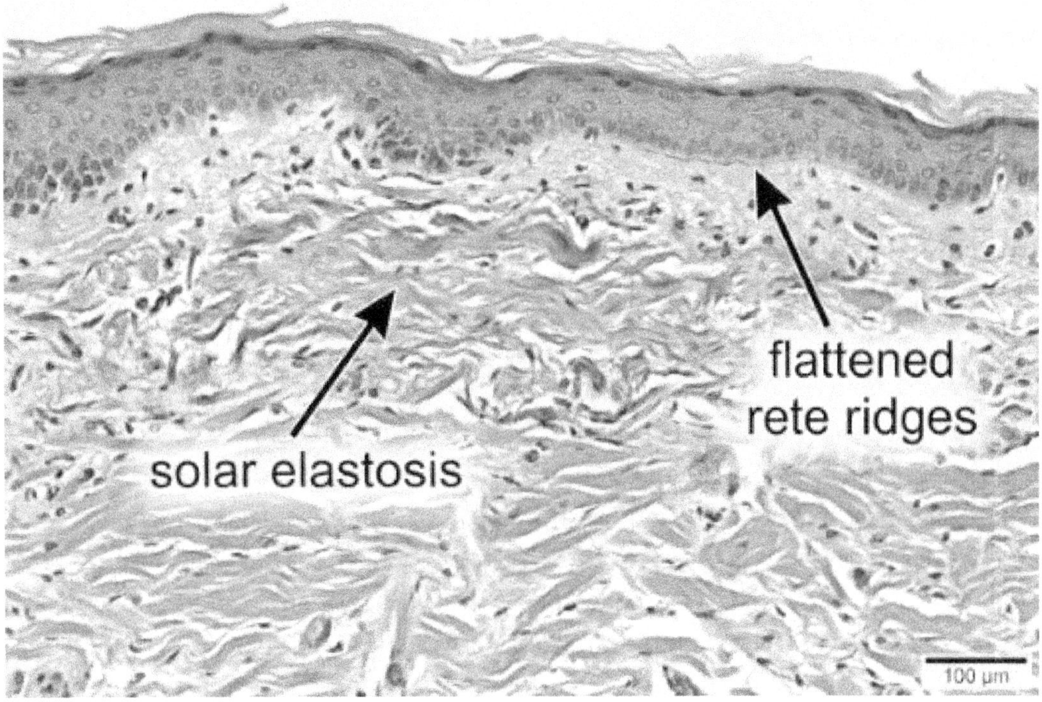

The Skin Biopsy: Type, Orientation, and Adequacy

Punch, Shave, and Excisional Biopsy: Choosing the Right Tool

The choice of biopsy technique determines, before the tissue ever reaches the laboratory, which reaction patterns can be reliably diagnosed. A punch biopsy samples a full-thickness cylindrical core extending through epidermis, dermis, and typically into subcutaneous fat, and is the preferred technique whenever a process involving the deep dermis or panniculus is suspected, since a shave biopsy that fails to sample fat cannot diagnose panniculitis regardless of how carefully the available tissue is examined. A shave biopsy removes only the epidermis and superficial to mid dermis and is well suited to predominantly epidermal or superficial dermal processes, such as most epidermal neoplasms and many inflammatory dermatoses confined to the papillary dermis, but is inadequate for evaluating depth of invasion in a pigmented lesion or for diagnosing a deep or panniculitic process. An excisional biopsy removes the full lesion with a margin of surrounding tissue and is preferred when a melanocytic lesion is being evaluated for possible melanoma, since accurate Breslow depth measurement requires that the base of the lesion be included in the specimen.

Specimen Orientation and Processing

Correct orientation during processing preserves the vertical relationship between epidermis, dermis, and subcutis that pattern-based diagnosis depends on. Punch and excisional specimens are conventionally bisected and embedded on their cut edge so that all three compartments are visualized in a single vertical section; a specimen embedded on its flat face instead produces a tangential section that can distort the apparent architecture and mimic epidermal hyperplasia or basal layer disease that is not actually present. Scalp specimens, as discussed above, are a deliberate exception, processed transversely to permit follicular counting, and the pathology report or requisition should specify when this technique has been used so that the reader interprets the section in the correct plane.

Handling and Labeling Considerations

Diagnostic accuracy depends on specimen integrity well before the tissue reaches the microtome, and several handling steps deserve explicit attention because their failure is difficult or impossible to correct retrospectively. Fixation in adequate volume and duration of neutral buffered formalin (generally a ten-to-one ratio of fixative to tissue volume) prevents the autolytic artifact that can obscure interface change and cellular detail; a specimen fixed in an inadequate volume of formalin, common when a large excision is placed in a container sized for a punch biopsy, may show central autolysis that renders the deepest and most clinically important portion of the specimen uninterpretable. When multiple biopsies are obtained from different sites in the same patient, for example paired lesional and perilesional biopsies for a suspected immunobullous disease, accurate site labeling and separate containers are essential, since a mislabeled or combined specimen can produce a direct immunofluorescence result that is technically valid but clinically uninterpretable because the site of origin is uncertain. Orientation sutures or ink marking, when clinically indicated for margin assessment, should be documented on the requisition in a manner that survives transcription into the laboratory information system, since orientation information that exists only on a hand-drawn diagram attached to a paper requisition is easily lost in transit.

Assessing Adequacy

1. Confirm that the biopsy technique matches the clinical question: full-thickness punch or incisional/excisional sampling for suspected panniculitis, deep infiltrates, or invasive neoplasia.
2. Confirm that subcutaneous fat is present in the section when a panniculitic or deeply infiltrative process is in the clinical differential.
3. Confirm that the specimen is oriented on its cut edge, with epidermis, dermis, and (when present) subcutis visualized in continuity in a single plane.
4. For pigmented lesions, confirm that the base and lateral margins of the lesion are represented so that depth and margin status can be assessed if required.
5. When adequacy cannot be confirmed, state the limitation explicitly in the report rather than rendering a diagnosis that exceeds what the tissue can support.

Biopsy Type	Typical Indication	Key Limitation
Punch biopsy	Inflammatory dermatoses, suspected panniculitis, deep infiltrates	Small diameter may undersample a heterogeneous or patchy process
Shave biopsy	Superficial epidermal lesions, most benign neoplasms	Cannot assess depth of invasion or sample subcutaneous fat
Excisional biopsy	Suspected melanoma, lesions requiring margin assessment	Larger procedure with more tissue processing and turnaround time

CAUTION: A superficial shave biopsy submitted with a clinical question of panniculitis or deep vasculitis cannot answer that question. The correct response is not to strain the available tissue for a diagnosis it cannot support, but to communicate the sampling limitation to the clinician and recommend a full-thickness punch or incisional biopsy if the clinical concern remains active.

Special Techniques: Frozen Sections and Immunobullous Sampling

Two circumstances call for handling that departs from the routine formalin-fixed, paraffin-embedded workflow described above, and recognizing them at the time of biopsy avoids the need for a repeat procedure. Frozen section processing is used intraoperatively during Mohs micrographic surgery and, less commonly, for rapid margin assessment of aggressive non-melanoma skin cancers; the technique trades a degree of cytologic and architectural clarity, since ice crystal artifact distorts nuclear detail and can thicken or fragment thin structures such as the dermal-epidermal junction, for the speed required to guide same-session surgical decisions. A frozen section diagnosis of a melanocytic lesion should be approached with particular caution, since the artifact introduced by freezing can obscure precisely the nuclear and architectural features that distinguish a nevus from melanoma, and most dermatopathology practices defer definitive melanocytic diagnosis to permanent sections even when a frozen section was performed for an unrelated margin question.

Suspected immunobullous disease requires a specifically bifurcated sampling strategy rather than a single biopsy. A lesional biopsy, ideally of an early, intact vesicle or bulla, is submitted in formalin for routine histology to characterize the level of the split and the associated inflammatory infiltrate. A separate perilesional biopsy, taken from clinically normal-appearing skin immediately adjacent to an active lesion, is submitted fresh or in a specialized transport medium (commonly Michel's medium, since formalin destroys the immunoreactivity direct immunofluorescence depends on) for direct immunofluorescence, which localizes the specific immunoreactant and staining pattern that distinguishes, for example, pemphigus vulgaris from bullous pemphigoid or dermatitis herpetiformis. Submitting only a single, formalin-fixed lesional biopsy for a case with a genuine immunobullous concern is one of the more consequential technical errors in dermatopathology practice, because it forecloses the direct immunofluorescence correlation that is frequently the deciding piece of evidence, a theme returned to in full in Chapter 7.

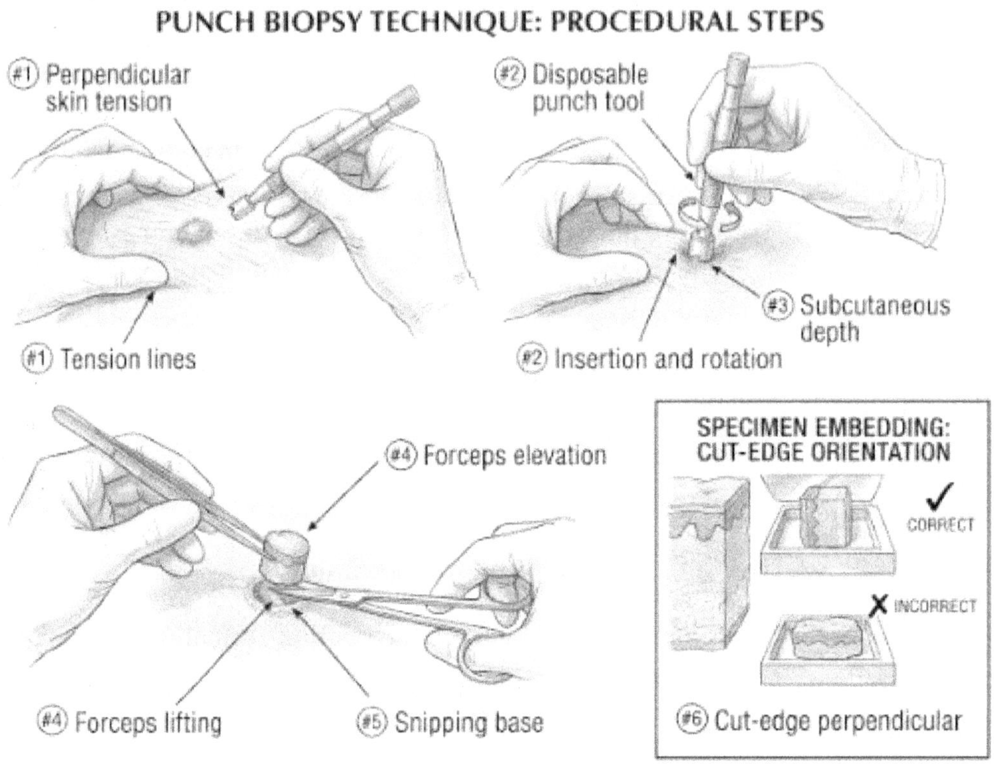

Special Considerations in Biopsy of Suspected Neoplasms

Neoplastic lesions place additional demands on biopsy planning that differ from those of inflammatory dermatoses. For a pigmented lesion in which melanoma is a genuine clinical concern, a narrow-margin excisional biopsy encompassing the entire lesion is preferred whenever anatomically and cosmetically feasible, because accurate assessment of symmetry, circumscription, and the depth of any invasive component, all central to distinguishing a benign nevus from melanoma and to staging melanoma once diagnosed, depends on visualizing the lesion in its entirety rather than a partial sample. When a partial biopsy of a pigmented lesion is unavoidable, for example because of lesion size or anatomic location, the report should explicitly acknowledge that grading and staging are limited to the tissue sampled and that a more definitive assessment may require complete excision, a limitation discussed further in the melanoma-specific staging considerations of Chapter 14. For suspected cutaneous lymphoma, by contrast, a larger punch or incisional biopsy is generally preferred over a small punch or shave, because architectural pattern (band-like, nodular, diffuse, or angiocentric) and adequate tissue for immunophenotypic and molecular studies are frequently decisive, and a superficial or fragmented specimen can be insufficient to resolve the distinction between a reactive infiltrate and an early lymphoproliferative process, a distinction developed in full in Chapter 18.

For suspected cutaneous soft tissue or adnexal neoplasms arising in the deep dermis or subcutis, an incisional or excisional biopsy that reaches an adequate depth is similarly important, since a shave biopsy that samples only the superficial portion of a deeper lesion may capture unrepresentative or entrapped overlying structures rather than the neoplasm itself, leading to a falsely reassuring or simply uninterpretable result. In each of these neoplastic scenarios, communication between the biopsying clinician and the interpreting pathologist about the specific diagnostic question at hand, rather than a generic requisition, meaningfully improves the likelihood that the technique chosen will actually answer that question.

Building the Histologic Differential

From Low Power to High Power: A Systematic Scanning Approach

Experienced dermatopathologists follow a remarkably consistent scanning sequence that novices benefit from adopting deliberately before it becomes automatic. At scanning magnification, the reader first establishes the overall silhouette of the process: is it confined to the epidermis, does it involve the superficial dermis, does it extend to the reticular dermis or subcutis, and is the distribution diffuse, patchy, perivascular, periadnexal, or nodular. This silhouette alone eliminates large categories of diagnosis before a single cell is examined at high power. At low power, the reader next localizes the principal abnormality to a specific compartment (epidermis, dermal-epidermal junction, papillary dermis, reticular dermis, vasculature, adnexa, or subcutis) and characterizes the dominant cell type of any infiltrate present. Only after this localization is complete does the reader move to high power to confirm specific cytologic features, such as the presence of eosinophilic cytoplasmic keratohyalin granules, nuclear atypia, or organism forms, that refine the diagnosis within the category already identified.

A Worked Example: From Low Power to Diagnosis

A 34-year-old patient presents with a several-week history of an itchy, poorly demarcated eruption on the volar forearms, and a punch biopsy is submitted with a clinical differential of eczematous dermatitis versus early psoriasis. At scanning power, the epidermis shows mild acanthosis without the regular, elongated rete ridge pattern that would suggest a psoriasiform process; instead, the epidermis appears loosely textured, and pale intercellular spaces are visible between keratinocytes even before higher magnification is applied. Localizing to the epidermal compartment at low power, the reader notes that this loosened, pale appearance corresponds to intercellular edema, spongiosis, most pronounced in the mid and lower spinous layer, accompanied by a superficial perivascular lymphocytic infiltrate with scattered eosinophils in the papillary dermis. Moving to high power confirms widened intercellular spaces with visible, stretched desmosomal connections between separating keratinocytes, without frank vesicle formation, and confirms that the perivascular infiltrate is composed predominantly of lymphocytes without atypia.

This sequence, silhouette first, then compartmental localization, then high-power confirmation, arrives at a diagnosis of a spongiotic dermatitis (the specific reaction pattern developed fully in Chapter 4) well before any single cytologic feature is examined in isolation. The scanning approach also structures what the report should and should not claim: the histologic pattern of spongiotic dermatitis is shared by several clinical entities, including allergic contact dermatitis, atopic dermatitis, and nummular dermatitis, and the biopsy alone, in the absence of the additional clinical and morphologic detail supplied by the treating clinician, cannot reliably distinguish among them. The value of the systematic approach is therefore not only diagnostic accuracy but also diagnostic honesty about what the tissue can and cannot resolve.

The report generated from this biopsy should therefore state the reaction pattern and its most likely clinical correlates rather than force a single named diagnosis the tissue cannot uniquely support: a descriptive diagnosis of spongiotic dermatitis, with a comment noting that the pattern is compatible with allergic contact dermatitis, atopic dermatitis, or nummular dermatitis and that clinicopathologic correlation is recommended, gives the treating clinician exactly the information the tissue can responsibly provide. This is a deliberately different posture from forcing the report toward the single diagnosis listed on the requisition, and it reflects a broader principle that recurs throughout this book: a dermatopathology report is most useful when it communicates the level of diagnostic certainty the tissue actually supports, distinguishing a pattern that narrows the differential to one specific entity from a pattern that narrows it to a small family of clinically similar conditions requiring the treating clinician's own correlation to resolve further.

Integrating Clinical Information

Histologic pattern recognition operates most reliably when paired with the clinical context in which the biopsy was obtained: lesion morphology, distribution, duration, and any relevant systemic findings. A superficial perivascular lymphocytic infiltrate with mild spongiosis carries a different most-likely diagnosis in a patient with a pruritic, poorly demarcated eruption of recent onset (favoring an eczematous process) than in a patient with a well-demarcated, chronic, minimally symptomatic plaque (favoring an early or resolving psoriasiform process). This is the essence of clinicopathologic correlation, and it is why the clinical information accompanying a specimen should be read before the slide, not treated as an afterthought consulted only if the histology proves ambiguous.

CLINICAL PEARL: When histology and clinical impression genuinely conflict, resist the instinct to force one into agreement with the other. A brief, specific request for additional clinical information, or a recommendation for repeat biopsy of a more representative area, is a more defensible response than a diagnosis manufactured to fit an incomplete picture.

Common Pitfalls for the Beginning Reader

Several errors recur predictably in early dermatopathology training and are worth naming explicitly rather than left to be learned by trial. The first is over-interpreting artifact: crush artifact from forceps handling, cautery artifact from electrosurgical shave technique, and folding or tangential sectioning artifact from processing can each mimic features of genuine pathology, and the beginning reader benefits from a deliberate habit of asking whether a finding is confined to a small, geometrically irregular area consistent with mechanical distortion before accepting it as a genuine histologic feature. The second is compartment confusion: attributing a finding to the wrong dermal level, for example describing a process as involving the papillary dermis when it is in fact confined to a periadnexal location in the mid dermis, propagates through the entire differential diagnosis because compartment is often the first and most powerful discriminator in pattern-based reasoning. The third is premature pattern closure: settling on the first plausible reaction pattern before systematically confirming that the full constellation of expected features is present, which is particularly hazardous when two patterns share a superficial resemblance at low power, such as early psoriasiform hyperplasia and a resolving spongiotic process, but diverge in specific features visible only on careful high-power review.

The fourth recurring error is treating a single high-power finding as sufficient for diagnosis without first establishing the low-power context that gives that finding its meaning. An eosinophil, for instance, is compatible with an extraordinarily broad range of processes, from a drug eruption to an arthropod bite reaction to a bullous pemphigoid, and its diagnostic weight depends almost entirely on the compartment, pattern, and company it is found in rather than its presence alone. The corrective habit, reinforced throughout this book's Rhythm Layer, is to always work from pattern to specific finding rather than the reverse: identify the reaction pattern first using the low-power and compartmental approach described above, and only then ask which specific high-power features, within that pattern, discriminate among the entities that produce it.

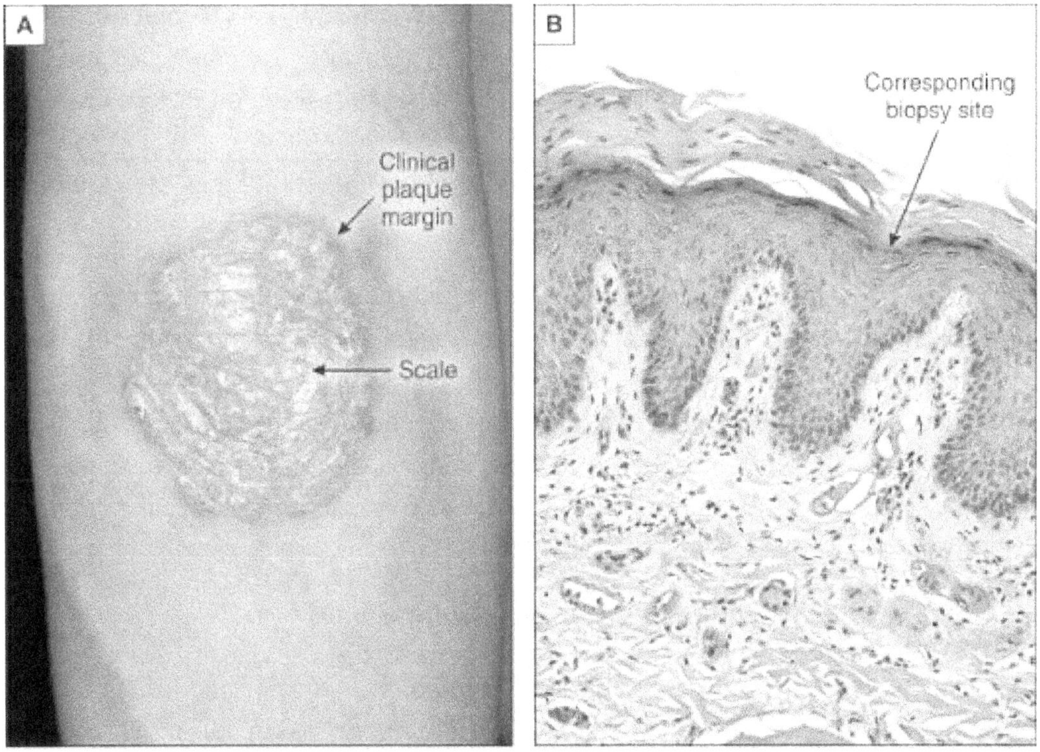

Plaque Psoriasis: Clinical and Histologic Correlation

Introducing the Reaction Pattern Recognition System

Why Pattern-First Reasoning Works

The chapters that follow are built around a single recurring structure, introduced here so that its logic is transparent before it is encountered dozens of times throughout the book. Every major diagnosis discussed in this text is presented through a five-part sequence that mirrors the actual cognitive steps of expert diagnostic reasoning: name the reaction pattern, describe the histologic signature that identifies it, state the diagnostic decision the pattern triggers, work through the trap logic that separates it from its most dangerous mimickers, and distill the whole sequence into a single pattern anchor, the one finding most likely to be remembered and applied correctly under time pressure.

How to Use This Book's Rhythm Layer

1. The Pattern: the named reaction pattern or specific entity under discussion, stated explicitly rather than implied.
2. Histologic Signature: the combination of findings that, taken together, identify the pattern reliably.
3. The Decision: the specific diagnostic conclusion or diagnostic pivot the pattern should trigger in practice.
4. Trap Logic: the histologic mimickers most likely to be confused with the pattern, and the specific feature that discriminates between them.
5. Pattern Anchor: a single high-yield finding, threshold, or rule that locks the pattern into memory for rapid recall at the microscope.

Each chapter closes with a Pattern Synthesis Recap that gathers every pattern introduced in that chapter into one consolidated, scannable reference, and the book as a whole closes with The Reaction Pattern Master Atlas, which indexes every pattern across every chapter by reaction-pattern category for rapid lookup during sign-out. This structure is a teaching and reference tool, not an assessment; nothing in this book asks the reader to select among lettered answer choices. Its purpose is to make the pattern-first reasoning that experienced dermatopathologists already use, explicit, repeatable, and available for lookup at the moment it is needed.

The Origins and Limits of Algorithmic Pattern Recognition

The pattern-first method is not a novel invention of this book; it formalizes a diagnostic tradition that dermatopathology developed specifically because inflammatory skin disease resisted the purely descriptive, disease-by-disease organization that worked reasonably well in other areas of surgical pathology. Mid-twentieth-century dermatopathologists observed that the same handful of tissue reactions, spongiosis, psoriasiform hyperplasia, interface change, vesiculation, granuloma formation, vasculitis, and panniculitis, recurred across dozens of clinically distinct diseases, and that trainees who tried to memorize each disease as an independent entity struggled far more than trainees who first learned to recognize the reaction pattern and then learned the differential diagnosis that pattern implied. This algorithmic tradition, developed most explicitly in the inflammatory dermatoses, has since proven durable enough to influence how neoplastic dermatopathology is taught as well, organized in this book by lineage (melanocytic, epidermal, adnexal, mesenchymal, lymphoid) in a structurally analogous way: identify the cell of origin and growth pattern first, then narrow within that category using specific cytologic and architectural criteria.

The method has real limits that a careful reader should hold in mind rather than discover through error. Reaction patterns are not mutually exclusive; a single biopsy can legitimately show overlapping features of two patterns, most commonly at the boundary between spongiotic and psoriasiform change or between lichenoid and vacuolar interface change, and forcing a specimen into a single pattern category when the tissue genuinely shows a mixed or transitional picture produces a falsely precise diagnosis. Patterns also evolve over the natural history of a single disease, so that a biopsy obtained early in the course of a condition may show a different pattern than a biopsy of the same disease obtained weeks later, which is one of the reasons lesion duration and evolution are essential clinical data points rather than incidental detail. The pattern-first method is best understood as a highly effective organizing strategy for generating and narrowing a differential diagnosis rapidly, not as a rigid taxonomy that every biopsy is obligated to fit cleanly, and the trap logic built into every Rhythm block in this book is designed specifically to flag the situations in which the obvious pattern assignment is the wrong one.

THE REACTION PATTERN RECOGNITION SYSTEM — Foundations of Histologic Pattern Recognition

---

The Pattern: Normal three-compartment skin architecture (epidermis, dermis, subcutis) as the baseline against which every reaction pattern in this book is defined.

Histologic Signature: Intact basket-weave stratum corneum, preserved granular layer, regular rete ridge pattern, unremarkable dermal-epidermal junction, sparse superficial perivascular infiltrate, normal adnexal density and hair cycle distribution appropriate to anatomic site and age.

The Decision: Establish site- and age-appropriate normal architecture before assessing any process for pathologic deviation; anatomic site, patient age, and constitutive pigmentation all change what counts as normal.

Trap Logic: Normal site-specific and age-related variation (acral hyperkeratosis, transverse follicular density, mucosal parakeratosis, solar elastosis, follicular pigment incontinence in skin of color) is mistaken for pathology when biopsy site, patient age, and skin type are not accounted for; the discriminating step is always confirming these variables before interpreting keratin thickness, follicular density, dermal collagen quality, or pigment distribution.

Pattern Anchor: Before diagnosing any epidermal, dermal, or follicular abnormality, confirm biopsy site, patient age, and baseline pigmentation; site- and age-appropriate normal variation is the most common source of false-positive overcalls in foundational dermatopathology.

Summary and Key Concepts

Normal skin architecture, organized into epidermis, dermis, and subcutis, is the diagnostic scaffold against which every reaction pattern in this book is defined.

Adnexal structures (hair follicle, sebaceous gland, apocrine gland, eccrine gland, and nail unit) each have a distinct normal histology that becomes the template for the adnexal neoplasms discussed in Chapter 16 and the special-site coverage in Chapter 20.

Site-specific variation, particularly at acral, scalp, flexural, and mucosal sites, alters what constitutes normal histology and is a recurring source of diagnostic error when not accounted for.

Age and constitutive pigmentation further shift the baseline: neonatal skin is structurally immature, photoaged skin shows solar elastosis, and skin of color shows more prominent basal pigmentation and melanophage presence at baseline.

Biopsy technique determines which reaction patterns can be diagnosed; matching technique to clinical question, careful specimen handling, and confirming adequacy before signing out are prerequisites to accurate diagnosis.

A systematic low-power-to-high-power scanning approach, integrated with clinical information, generates a reliable initial histologic differential and is the practical foundation of the Reaction Pattern Recognition System introduced in this chapter.

CHAPTER 2: SPECIMEN PROCESSING, SPECIAL STAINS, AND IMMUNOHISTOCHEMISTRY IN DERMATOPATHOLOGY

Learning Objectives

1. Describe the tissue processing pathway from fixation through sectioning and identify how deviations at each step produce recognizable artifact.
2. Select the appropriate histochemical special stain for a given diagnostic question and interpret its result correctly.
3. Apply immunohistochemical panels systematically to melanocytic, epithelial, lymphoid, and mesenchymal diagnostic problems.
4. Explain the technique, immunoreactant patterns, and interpretive pitfalls of direct immunofluorescence.
5. Describe the role of molecular and ancillary diagnostics, including fluorescence in situ hybridization and clonality studies, in dermatopathologic diagnosis.

Fixation, Processing, and Sectioning

Formalin Fixation and Tissue Processing

Every subsequent diagnostic step in dermatopathology, from routine hematoxylin and eosin interpretation through the most sophisticated molecular assay, depends on adequate initial fixation. Ten percent neutral buffered formalin, used at a fixative-to-tissue volume ratio of approximately ten to one, cross-links tissue proteins at a rate of roughly one millimeter of penetration per hour, which is why a large excision specimen submitted in an undersized container can remain inadequately fixed at its center for the entire standard processing interval even after an apparently sufficient total fixation time has elapsed. Underfixation produces a specific and recognizable artifact: autolytic change with nuclear smudging, cytoplasmic vacuolation, and epidermal separation from the underlying dermis that can closely mimic a genuine subepidermal blistering process, a distinction discussed further in the trap logic below. Overfixation, by contrast, is a less common but real problem, particularly for specimens intended for immunohistochemistry or molecular studies, since prolonged formalin exposure progressively masks epitopes and degrades nucleic acid, and most laboratories cap routine fixation at twenty-four to seventy-two hours for this reason.

After fixation, tissue is processed through a graded series of alcohols to remove water, cleared in a hydrophobic intermediate solvent such as xylene to remove the alcohol, and infiltrated with paraffin wax, a sequence that together prepares the tissue for embedding in a solid paraffin block from which thin sections can be cut. Automated tissue processors carry out this sequence overnight for routine specimens, and the total processing time, together with fixation time, is the principal determinant of turnaround time between biopsy and the initial slide review, a practical consideration that shapes how urgently a clinician can expect a diagnosis for a given specimen.

Embedding and Sectioning Technique

Embedding orientation, introduced in Chapter 1 as a determinant of whether a specimen is visualized in true cross-section or tangentially, is executed at this processing stage by the histotechnologist placing the tissue on its cut edge within the embedding mold before the paraffin solidifies around it. The resulting paraffin block is sectioned on a microtome at a standard thickness of four to six microns, thin enough that a single cell layer is not doubled upon itself yet thick enough to retain adequate tinctorial detail, and the ribbon of sections produced is floated on a warm water bath to remove folds before being mounted on a glass slide. Multiple step levels are frequently cut through a single block, particularly for melanocytic lesions and specimens in which the diagnostic focus (an isolated focus of invasion, a small vessel with intraluminal fibrin, an early follicular abnormality) may be present in only a fraction of the total tissue volume, and the decision to request additional levels is one of the most common and most useful ancillary steps available to a dermatopathologist before reaching for a special stain or immunohistochemical panel.

Common Processing Artifacts

Several artifacts recur across dermatopathology practice and merit specific recognition because they can each mimic genuine pathology. Crush artifact, produced by forceps compression during specimen handling, distorts nuclear morphology into elongated, hyperchromatic streaks that can be mistaken for a high-grade neoplastic process if the geometrically confined, non-anatomic distribution of the distortion is not appreciated. Cautery artifact from electrosurgical shave biopsy technique produces peripheral epithelial smudging, nuclear elongation in a palisaded pattern at the specimen edge, and coagulative change that can obscure margin assessment and, in more severe cases, mimic an infiltrative growth pattern at the periphery of a lesion. Freezing artifact, discussed in Chapter 1 in the context of intraoperative Mohs sections, produces intracellular and intercellular ice crystal vacuolation that widens the apparent intercellular space in a pattern that can be confused with genuine spongiosis if the frozen origin of the section is not communicated to the interpreting pathologist.

Processing Considerations for Immunohistochemistry and Molecular Studies

The standard fixation and processing pathway described above was optimized historically for routine morphologic assessment, and several of its steps require modification, or at minimum careful attention, when the specimen is anticipated to require immunohistochemistry or molecular testing. Formalin fixation cross-links proteins in a way that masks many antigenic epitopes, which is why nearly all immunohistochemical protocols begin with a heat-induced or, less commonly, enzymatic antigen retrieval step designed to reverse this masking before primary antibody application; the specific retrieval buffer, temperature, and duration are antibody-specific, and using an inappropriate retrieval protocol for a given marker is a recognized cause of false-negative immunohistochemical results that can be mistaken for a genuine biological absence of the target antigen. Extended formalin fixation beyond the standard twenty-four to seventy-two hour window compounds this epitope masking and, more consequentially for molecular studies, progressively fragments nucleic acid, so that a specimen fixed for an unusually prolonged interval, for example over a long holiday weekend without intermediate processing, may yield degraded DNA or RNA unsuitable for downstream sequencing even though its morphology on routine hematoxylin and eosin remains entirely satisfactory.

Because these downstream needs are not always apparent at the time of initial grossing, many practices adopt a policy of retaining a portion of larger specimens, when tissue volume allows, specifically to preserve the option of later molecular testing without requiring a second procedure. This forward-looking allocation, discussed further in the tissue stewardship considerations addressed later in this chapter, is a small addition to the grossing workflow that can materially affect whether a subsequently identified diagnostic question, for example a request for fluorescence in situ hybridization after an initially ambiguous melanocytic diagnosis, can be answered from the original specimen or requires a repeat biopsy.

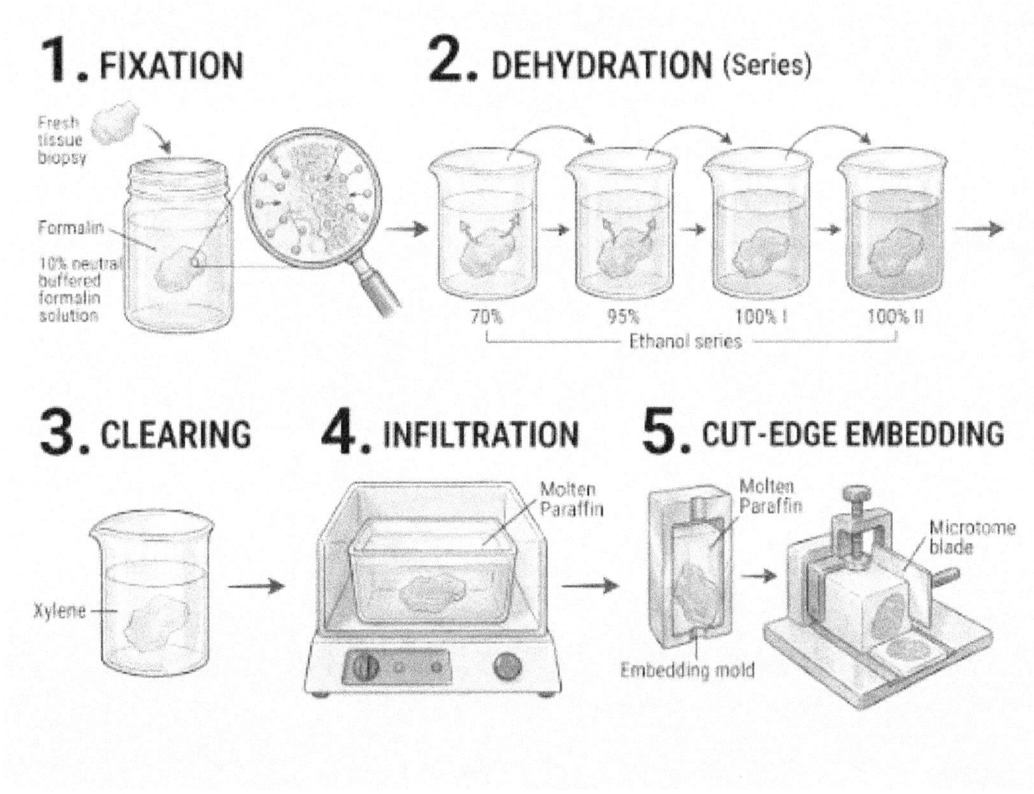

Decalcification and Special Processing Circumstances

Most dermatopathology specimens require no processing beyond the standard fixation-to-embedding pathway, but two circumstances call for a modified approach that a reader should recognize. Specimens containing bone or heavily calcified tissue, encountered occasionally in deep soft tissue tumors that abut periosteum or in longstanding calcinosis cutis, require decalcification, typically using a mild acid or chelating agent, before the tissue is soft enough to section without shattering or dulling the microtome blade; decalcification, like extended formalin fixation, can degrade nucleic acid and epitope integrity, so the duration should be limited to the minimum required and communicated to downstream interpreters if molecular testing is later requested. Nail unit specimens, discussed in Chapter 1 and developed fully in Chapter 20, contain a keratinized nail plate of variable hardness that similarly benefits from a brief softening step, commonly using a dilute potassium hydroxide or specialized nail-softening solution, before sectioning; omitting this step risks fragmenting the nail plate away from the underlying matrix and bed during microtomy, separating structures whose spatial relationship is often the central diagnostic question.

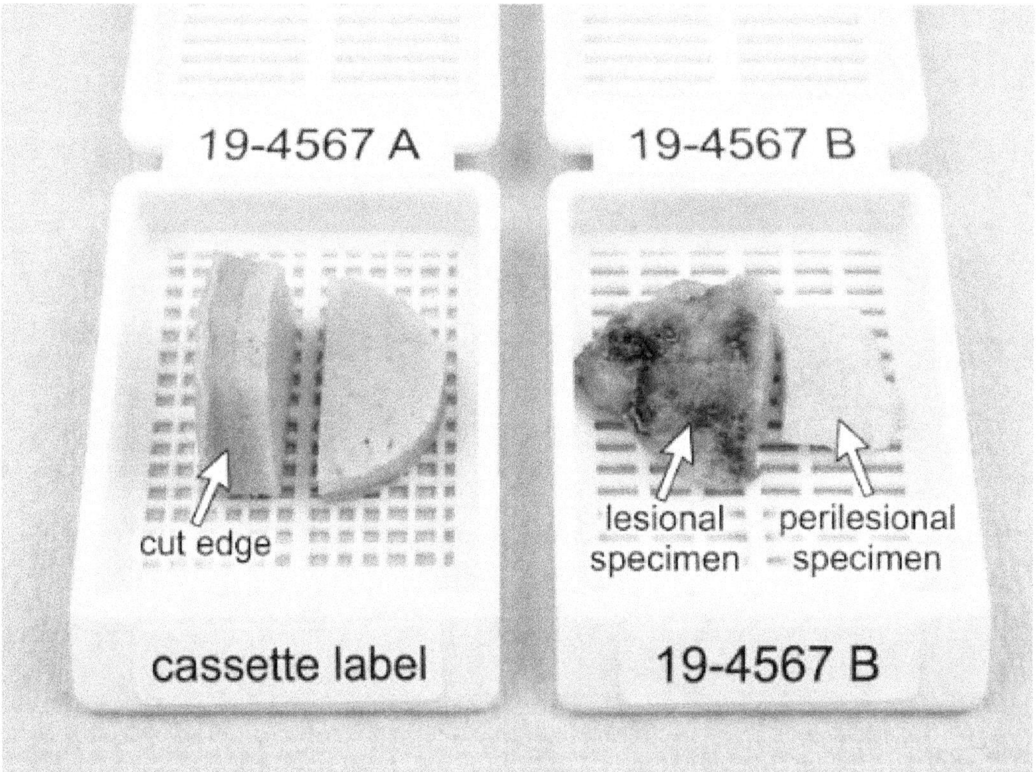

Histochemical Special Stains and Their Indications

Periodic Acid-Schiff and Fungal Organism Identification

Periodic acid-Schiff staining, most often used with diastase digestion (PAS-D) to eliminate confounding glycogen staining, highlights the polysaccharide-rich cell walls of fungal organisms as well as basement membrane material, making it useful both for identifying dermatophytes and other fungi in the stratum corneum and for assessing basement membrane thickening in conditions such as lupus erythematosus and porphyria cutanea tarda. Dermatophyte hyphae appear as PAS-D positive, magenta-staining septate structures typically confined to the stratum corneum, and a systematic scanning habit, examining the full thickness of the stratum corneum at the specimen edges where hyphae are often most concentrated, meaningfully improves detection sensitivity over a cursory review limited to the central portion of the section.

Grocott Methenamine Silver and Deep Fungal Infection

Grocott methenamine silver staining offers superior sensitivity for fungal organisms relative to PAS-D, particularly in deep or invasive fungal infections in which organism burden may be low, and stains fungal cell walls black against a green counterstained background, a high-contrast combination that facilitates detection of sparse organisms. Grocott methenamine silver is the preferred stain when a deep or angioinvasive fungal process such as mucormycosis or aspergillosis is a clinical concern, since these organisms are frequently present in low numbers within areas of necrosis where PAS-D positivity can be more difficult to distinguish from background tissue debris.

Elastic, Connective Tissue, and Melanin Stains

The Verhoeff-Van Gieson stain highlights elastic fibers in black against collagen counterstained red, and is used to assess elastic tissue integrity in conditions ranging from anetoderma and pseudoxanthoma elasticum, in which elastic fibers are fragmented or absent, to elastofibroma and connective tissue nevi, in which elastic tissue architecture is altered in a distinct pattern. The Fontana-Masson stain identifies melanin directly through its argentaffin reducing property, independent of the cytologic features used to identify melanocytes, and is particularly useful in distinguishing melanin pigment from hemosiderin in lesions with mixed brown pigmentation, since melanin stains black with Fontana-Masson while hemosiderin does not, a distinction that Perls Prussian blue staining resolves in the opposite direction by specifically identifying iron.

Congo Red, Giemsa, and Additional Targeted Stains

Congo red staining identifies amyloid deposits, which appear salmon-pink on standard light microscopy and, critically, display apple-green birefringence under polarized light, a finding required to confirm true amyloid rather than other Congo red-reactive material and essential to the diagnosis of primary cutaneous amyloidosis and cutaneous involvement by systemic amyloidosis. Giemsa staining highlights mast cell granules and is used both to confirm mastocytosis, in which an increased dermal mast cell population may be subtle on hematoxylin and eosin alone, and to identify certain infectious organisms, including

Leishmania amastigotes, that show characteristic morphology on Giemsa preparation. Acid-fast stains (Ziehl-Neelsen or Fite) identify mycobacteria, with the modified Fite stain preferred for Mycobacterium leprae given its comparatively fragile cell wall, and Alcian blue or colloidal iron staining identifies dermal mucin, useful in confirming the increased interstitial mucin characteristic of lupus erythematosus, granuloma annulare, and myxedema.

Additional Targeted Stains and Their Niche Applications

Beyond the frequently used stains detailed above, several additional histochemical techniques serve narrower but clinically important roles. Masson trichrome staining differentiates collagen (blue or green, depending on the specific trichrome variant) from smooth muscle and other cellular elements (red), and is useful in characterizing dermal fibrosis in morphea and scleroderma, where the pattern and depth of collagen thickening and entrapment of adnexal structures carry diagnostic and prognostic weight, as well as in confirming smooth muscle differentiation in leiomyoma and related smooth muscle neoplasms when immunohistochemical confirmation is not readily available. Toluidine blue, a metachromatic stain, highlights mast cell granules with a purple-red color against a blue background and offers a rapid, technically simple alternative to Giemsa for confirming mastocytosis, though Giemsa is generally preferred when organism identification is simultaneously in question. Von Kossa staining identifies calcium deposits directly through a silver-based reaction and is used to confirm and characterize the pattern of mineralization in calcinosis cutis, distinguishing dystrophic calcification associated with underlying tissue damage from metastatic calcification associated with abnormal calcium-phosphate metabolism.

Selecting among this expanded stain repertoire again follows the hypothesis-driven principle introduced above: a sclerotic dermal process with a differential spanning morphea, lichen sclerosus, and a scar generates a specific reason to reach for trichrome staining to assess the depth and pattern of collagen involvement, while a dermal nodule with a differential spanning smooth muscle and fibrohistiocytic origin generates a specific reason to reach for either trichrome or an appropriate immunohistochemical marker, but neither stain is a reasonable first step in a case that has not yet been narrowed to a differential these techniques are actually positioned to resolve.

Special Stain	Primary Target	Key Clinical Indication
PAS with diastase (PAS-D)	Fungal cell walls, basement membrane	Superficial dermatophyte infection; basement membrane thickening assessment
Grocott methenamine silver (GMS)	Fungal cell walls	Deep or angioinvasive fungal infection with low organism burden
Verhoeff-Van Gieson	Elastic fibers (black), collagen (red)	Anetoderma, pseudoxanthoma elasticum, connective tissue nevi

Fontana-Masson	Melanin	Distinguishing melanin from hemosiderin in pigmented lesions
Congo red (with polarization)	Amyloid	Primary cutaneous or systemic amyloidosis
Giemsa	Mast cell granules, Leishmania amastigotes	Mastocytosis; leishmaniasis
Fite (modified acid-fast)	Mycobacterium leprae and related organisms	Suspected leprosy or atypical mycobacterial infection
Alcian blue / colloidal iron	Dermal mucin	Lupus erythematosus, granuloma annulare, myxedema

A Practical Approach to Special Stain Selection

The special stains described in this section are most useful when selected to answer a specific hypothesis generated from routine histology rather than ordered as an undifferentiated panel. A biopsy showing a granulomatous infiltrate, for example, generates a specific short list of hypotheses (mycobacterial infection, deep fungal infection, a foreign body reaction, or a non-infectious granulomatous process such as sarcoidosis or granuloma annulare), and the special stain workup should be tailored to that list: PAS-D and Grocott methenamine silver to address the fungal possibilities, a Fite stain to address mycobacterial infection, and polarization of the routine hematoxylin and eosin section to identify birefringent foreign material, reserving Alcian blue or colloidal iron for the specific circumstance in which granuloma annulare or a related mucin-rich process remains in the differential after infectious causes have been reasonably excluded. Ordering the full battery of special stains reflexively on every granulomatous specimen, without first narrowing the differential using architectural and cytologic clues from the routine section (well-formed versus poorly formed granulomas, presence or absence of necrosis, palisading pattern, involvement of vessel walls), is inefficient, delays turnaround time, and can produce misleading incidental positivity that complicates rather than clarifies the diagnostic picture.

This same hypothesis-driven principle applies to the workup of a mucin-rich or amyloid-suspicious dermal infiltrate. A subtle increase in interstitial mucin on routine sections, most confidently confirmed with Alcian blue, narrows a differential that includes lupus erythematosus, granuloma annulare, and myxedema largely on the basis of the accompanying architectural context (an interface reaction pattern favors lupus, a palisaded or interstitial histiocytic infiltrate favors granuloma annulare, and a bland increase in mucin without significant inflammation favors myxedema), so that the special stain confirms a suspicion generated by pattern recognition rather than generating that suspicion on its own. Congo red staining, similarly, is reserved for lesions in which amyloid is already suspected on routine sections by the presence of amorphous, faintly eosinophilic to pale material in the papillary dermis or around vessels and adnexal structures, since Congo red performed reflexively on tissue without this preliminary suspicion carries a meaningful false-positive rate related to nonspecific staining of collagen and other extracellular material.

The Pattern: PAS-Positive Basement Membrane Material Mistaken for Fungal Hyphae

Histologic Signature: Thickened, PAS-D positive basement membrane at the dermal-epidermal junction and around superficial vessels in a biopsy from a patient with lupus erythematosus or porphyria cutanea tarda, which can superficially resemble the linear, magenta-staining structures of fungal hyphae to an inexperienced reader.

The Decision: Confirm true septate, branching hyphal morphology confined to the stratum corneum before diagnosing a dermatophyte infection; diffusely thickened basement membrane material at the dermal-epidermal junction or perivascularly is a distinct finding with different clinical significance.

Trap Logic: The mimicker is a genuine fungal infection. The discriminating feature is architecture and location: true hyphae are linear, septate, branching structures confined to the stratum corneum, while thickened basement membrane material is a continuous band at the dermal-epidermal junction or vessel walls without septation or branching.

Pattern Anchor: Hyphae live in the stratum corneum and branch; thickened basement membrane lives at the junction or vessel wall and does not. Location before morphology resolves the great majority of ambiguous PAS-D calls.

Immunohistochemical Panels in Skin Diagnosis

Melanocytic Markers

Melan-A (also known as MART-1) and SOX10 are the two most heavily relied upon melanocytic markers in routine dermatopathology practice, and they are frequently used together because each has distinct strengths. Melan-A shows strong, diffuse cytoplasmic staining in most melanocytic lesions and remains a reliable marker of both benign and malignant melanocytic proliferations, but it can show reduced sensitivity in desmoplastic melanoma, a subtype in which tumor cells assume a spindled, fibroblast-like morphology and frequently lose Melan-A expression. SOX10, a nuclear transcription factor marker, retains sensitivity in desmoplastic melanoma and is therefore the preferred first-line marker when this subtype is suspected, though it is not entirely melanocyte-specific and also stains Schwann cells and other neural crest-derived elements, a cross-reactivity that becomes diagnostically important when a spindle cell lesion is being evaluated for melanoma versus a neural sheath tumor, addressed in the Rhythm block below. S100 protein was the original melanocytic marker in widespread use and remains highly sensitive, though its lower specificity, given expression in Langerhans cells, neural elements, and some other cell types, has led most practices to favor Melan-A and SOX10 as primary markers with S100 retained as a sensitive screening or confirmatory adjunct.

Epithelial and Adnexal Markers

Pancytokeratin cocktails (such as AE1/AE3) confirm epithelial differentiation broadly and are useful in distinguishing a poorly differentiated epithelial neoplasm from a mesenchymal or lymphoid process when morphology alone is ambiguous. More specific keratin subtypes assist in refining adnexal differentiation: CK20, notably, shows a distinctive perinuclear dot-like positivity in Merkel cell carcinoma that is highly useful in distinguishing this aggressive neuroendocrine neoplasm from other small round blue cell tumors, while CK7 and CK15 patterns assist in characterizing follicular and sebaceous differentiation in adnexal neoplasms discussed fully in Chapter 16. Androgen receptor and adipophilin staining assist specifically in confirming sebaceous differentiation, relevant both to sebaceous neoplasm classification and to the workup of sebaceous carcinoma, which carries an association with Muir-Torre syndrome that has downstream implications for mismatch repair protein testing.

Lymphoid and Hematopoietic Markers

CD3 and CD5 identify T lymphocytes, the predominant infiltrate in most primary cutaneous lymphomas, while CD20 identifies B lymphocytes, relevant to the smaller subset of cutaneous B-cell lymphomas. Within the T-cell lineage, CD4 and CD8 subset markers, together with loss of pan-T-cell antigens such as CD7, assist in characterizing mycosis fungoides and related conditions, since aberrant antigen loss is one of several features used to distinguish a neoplastic T-cell infiltrate from a reactive one, a distinction developed fully in Chapter 18. CD30 identifies a specific subset of activated lymphocytes and is central to the diagnosis of lymphomatoid papulosis and primary cutaneous anaplastic large cell lymphoma, both of which show large, CD30-positive atypical cells despite substantial differences in clinical behavior. CD68 and CD163 identify histiocytic lineage, useful in confirming a granulomatous or histiocytic process, and CD1a and langerin (CD207) confirm Langerhans cell lineage in the workup of Langerhans cell histiocytosis.

Vascular, Mesenchymal, and Proliferation Markers

CD31 and ERG are highly sensitive endothelial markers used to confirm vascular differentiation in both benign and malignant vascular neoplasms, with ERG offering the practical advantage of nuclear rather than cytoplasmic staining, which simplifies interpretation in densely cellular lesions. CD34 identifies a broader range of mesenchymal and some epithelial structures, including dermatofibrosarcoma protuberans, in which diffuse CD34 positivity helps distinguish this locally aggressive neoplasm from dermatofibroma, which is typically CD34 negative and factor XIIIa positive, an inverse staining relationship that is one of the most practically useful immunohistochemical pairs in dermatopathology. Ki-67 provides a proliferation index that assists in distinguishing benign from malignant proliferations across multiple lineages, and BRAF V600E immunohistochemistry offers a rapid, tissue-conserving screen for this common activating mutation in melanoma, with a positive result supporting malignancy in an ambiguous melanocytic lesion, though a negative result does not exclude melanoma given the existence of BRAF-wild-type disease.

Building a Diagnostic Immunohistochemical Panel: A Systematic Approach

1. State the specific diagnostic question the panel is intended to answer (lineage confirmation, benign versus malignant distinction, or subtyping within an already-established lineage) before selecting individual markers.
2. Select at least one broad lineage marker (pancytokeratin for epithelial, S100 or SOX10 for melanocytic or neural, CD45 for hematolymphoid, CD31 or ERG for vascular) to establish the general category of differentiation.
3. Add lineage-specific markers within the category suggested by the broad marker to refine the diagnosis (for example, Melan-A and HMB45 following a positive SOX10 result to further characterize a melanocytic lesion).
4. Include at least one marker specifically chosen to exclude the leading mimicker in the differential diagnosis, rather than selecting markers only to confirm the favored diagnosis.
5. Interpret the completed panel as an integrated whole, weighing the pattern of positivity and negativity across all markers together with morphology, rather than anchoring the diagnosis to a single marker result.

This systematic construction matters because immunohistochemical panels are frequently ordered under diagnostic uncertainty, precisely the circumstance in which anchoring bias, weighting the first or most familiar marker result too heavily, is most likely to distort interpretation. A poorly differentiated dermal neoplasm of uncertain lineage illustrates the principle: rather than ordering a single presumptive marker based on the leading clinical impression, a broad screening panel spanning epithelial, melanocytic, lymphoid, and mesenchymal lineages is constructed first, and only after the broad category is established does the panel narrow to lineage-specific and mimicker-excluding markers within that category. This sequence costs additional tissue and turnaround time relative to a narrow, presumption-driven panel, but it substantially reduces the risk of a confidently wrong diagnosis built on a marker result that was never actually capable of distinguishing the entities genuinely in play.

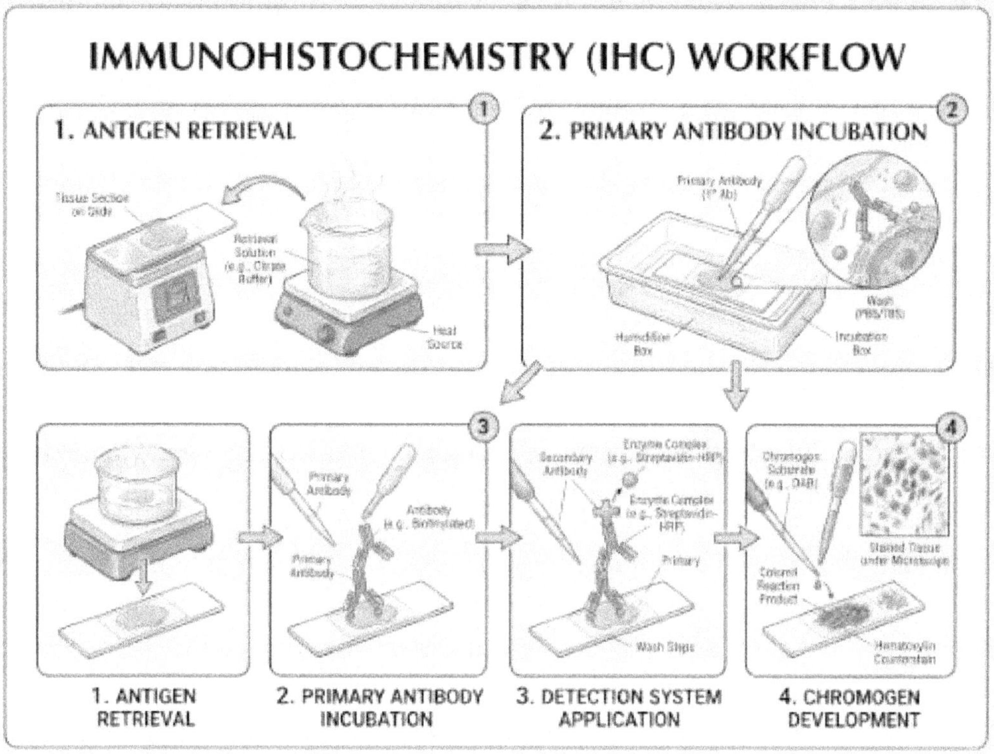
IMMUNOHISTOCHEMISTRY (IHC) WORKFLOW
1. ANTIGEN RETRIEVAL
2. PRIMARY ANTIBODY INCUBATION
1. ANTIGEN RETRIEVAL
2. PRIMARY ANTIBODY INCUBATION
3. DETECTION SYSTEM APPLICATION
4. CHROMOGEN DEVELOPMENT

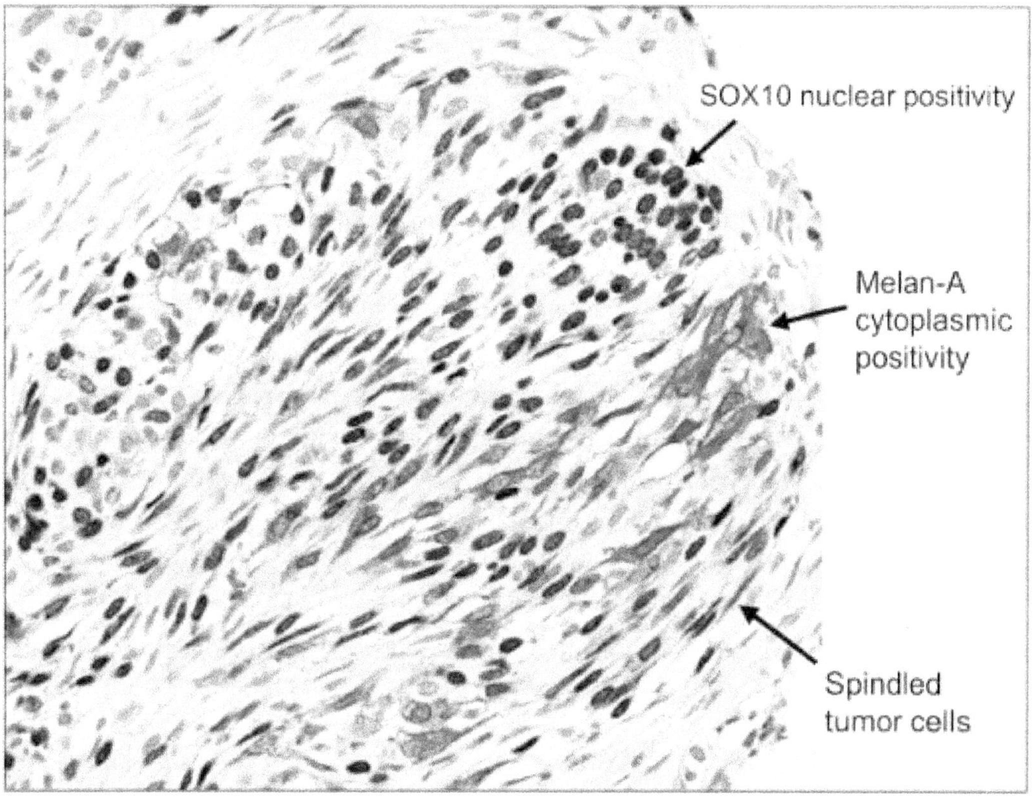
SOX10 nuclear positivity
Melan-A cytoplasmic positivity
Spindled tumor cells

THE REACTION PATTERN RECOGNITION SYSTEM — Immunohistochemical Marker Selection

The Pattern: SOX10 Positivity in a Dermal Spindle Cell Lesion — Desmoplastic Melanoma Versus Neural Sheath Tumor

Histologic Signature: A dermal spindle cell proliferation with fascicular or storiform architecture, SOX10 nuclear positivity, and variable S100 positivity, in which Melan-A staining is weak, patchy, or entirely negative.

The Decision: Do not treat SOX10 positivity alone as sufficient evidence of melanocytic differentiation in a spindle cell lesion; SOX10 also marks Schwann cells and other neural crest derivatives, so the diagnosis must integrate architectural pattern, cytologic atypia, and clinical context (a history of a preceding pigmented lesion favors melanoma) rather than resting on a single marker.

Trap Logic: The mimicker in each direction is the other diagnosis: a benign or malignant peripheral nerve sheath tumor can be SOX10 positive and closely mimic desmoplastic melanoma architecturally. The discriminating features are the presence of junctional melanocytic activity or a history of a prior pigmented lesion (favoring melanoma), versus a discrete encapsulated architecture, Antoni A and B areas, and Verocay bodies (favoring schwannoma), with the final distinction in ambiguous cases often requiring a broader panel and correlation with clinical history.

Pattern Anchor: SOX10 confirms neural crest lineage, not melanocytic lineage specifically; in a spindle cell lesion, SOX10 positivity is the beginning of the workup, not the end of it.

Antibody Panel Pitfalls and Cross-Reactivity

Immunohistochemical interpretation carries several recurring technical pitfalls beyond the marker-specific considerations already discussed. Background staining, resulting from inadequate blocking of endogenous peroxidase or biotin activity, can produce diffuse weak positivity that is mistaken for a genuine, if faint, positive result, and is distinguished from true positivity by its lack of the subcellular localization pattern (nuclear, cytoplasmic, or membranous) expected for the specific marker in use; a nuclear marker such as SOX10 showing diffuse cytoplasmic haze without discrete nuclear staining should be interpreted as background rather than true positivity. Edge artifact, in which tissue at the periphery of a section stains more intensely than the center due to uneven antibody or reagent distribution during the staining run, can similarly produce spuriously positive or spuriously negative results depending on where within the section the diagnostically relevant focus happens to lie, and is one of several reasons that appropriate positive and negative controls are run alongside every diagnostic immunohistochemical stain rather than relying on the case material alone to validate the technique.

Cross-reactivity, in which an antibody binds a target other than its intended antigen, is a further source of interpretive error, and awareness of the specific cross-reactivity patterns relevant to commonly used dermatopathology markers meaningfully reduces diagnostic mistakes. CD68, nominally a histiocytic marker, also stains some melanomas and a subset of other neoplasms, limiting its specificity when used as a sole marker of histiocytic lineage in a diagnostically ambiguous dermal infiltrate. Cytokeratin markers, particularly broad-spectrum cocktails, can show aberrant positivity in a minority of otherwise convincingly mesenchymal or melanocytic neoplasms, a phenomenon well documented in synovial sarcoma and some melanomas, which is why a single unexpected marker result is generally weighed against the full panel and morphology rather than treated as independently decisive. Recognizing these specific pitfalls, rather than treating every immunohistochemical result as an unambiguous binary output, is part of what distinguishes sophisticated ancillary test interpretation from mechanical panel reading.

Direct Immunofluorescence

Technique and Specimen Handling

Direct immunofluorescence requires fresh or specially transported tissue rather than formalin-fixed material, since formalin fixation destroys the antigenicity that fluorescently labeled antibodies depend on. As introduced in Chapter 1, the specimen is a perilesional biopsy of clinically uninvolved skin adjacent to an active lesion, submitted in Michel's transport medium (a specialized ammonium sulfate-based solution) or, when immediate processing is available, snap-frozen, and the laboratory then applies fluorescein-labeled antibodies against immunoglobulins (IgG, IgA, IgM) and complement components (C3) directly to cryostat sections, examining the result under a fluorescence microscope for the pattern and intensity of deposition.

Immunoreactant Patterns and Their Significance

The location and pattern of immunoreactant deposition, rather than the specific immunoglobulin class alone, carries the greatest diagnostic weight. Linear deposition of IgG and C3 along the dermal-epidermal junction is characteristic of the pemphigoid group of subepidermal blistering diseases, and salt-split skin technique, in which the specimen is incubated in sodium chloride to artificially separate the epidermis from the dermis along the lamina lucida, further localizes the deposition to the epidermal (roof) or dermal (floor) side of the split, distinguishing bullous pemphigoid (epidermal-side deposition) from epidermolysis bullosa acquisita and anti-p200 pemphigoid (dermal-side deposition). Intercellular, net-like deposition of IgG throughout the epidermis is characteristic of the pemphigus group, reflecting antibody binding to desmosomal cadherins between keratinocytes. Granular deposition of IgA at the dermal papillary tips is the defining finding of dermatitis herpetiformis, while granular deposition of IgG, IgM, and C3 in a band-like pattern at the dermal-epidermal junction, the so-called lupus band, supports a diagnosis of lupus erythematosus when present in lesional skin and, particularly, when present in sun-protected, clinically uninvolved skin, a finding with systemic diagnostic implications.

Two additional patterns extend this framework and are worth naming explicitly given their clinical severity. Linear IgA disease, distinct from both the pemphigoid group and dermatitis herpetiformis despite some clinical overlap with each, shows linear (rather than granular) IgA deposition along the dermal-epidermal junction, a pattern that underscores why immunoglobulin class and deposition geometry must both be assessed together rather than either alone; linear deposition of IgA specifically, rather than IgG, identifies this distinct entity with its own treatment implications. Paraneoplastic pemphigus, an uncommon but clinically severe variant occurring in association with an underlying neoplasm, most often lymphoproliferative, shows a combined direct immunofluorescence pattern with both intercellular epidermal deposition, as in conventional pemphigus, and, in a meaningful subset of cases, linear or granular junctional deposition as well, reflecting the broader and more heterogeneous autoantibody profile characteristic of this variant; recognizing this combined or atypical pattern, particularly in a patient with a known or suspected malignancy, should prompt specific consideration of paraneoplastic pemphigus rather than a routine pemphigus diagnosis.

Pitfalls in DIF Interpretation

1. Confirm that the biopsy was taken from perilesional, not lesional, skin; lesional skin frequently shows nonspecific or degraded immunoreactant deposition that can obscure the diagnostic pattern.
2. Distinguish true linear or granular immunoreactant deposition from nonspecific background fluorescence, which lacks the sharply localized distribution of a genuine positive result.
3. Recognize that a weakly positive or equivocal C3 deposition alone, without accompanying immunoglobulin deposition, has limited specificity and should be interpreted cautiously in isolation.
4. Correlate the DIF pattern with routine histology and clinical presentation before finalizing a diagnosis, since several immunobullous diseases show overlapping DIF patterns that are best resolved with the full clinical picture.

Indirect Immunofluorescence and Serologic Correlation

Indirect immunofluorescence complements direct immunofluorescence by detecting circulating autoantibodies in the patient's serum rather than immunoreactants already deposited in the patient's skin, and is performed by incubating diluted patient serum against a substrate, commonly monkey esophagus for pemphigus-group antibodies or salt-split normal human skin for pemphigoid-group antibodies, followed by a fluorescently labeled secondary antibody to visualize binding. A rising indirect immunofluorescence titer over the course of treatment correlates reasonably well with disease activity in pemphigus and is used clinically to help guide immunosuppressive therapy tapering, a correlation that is less consistently reliable in the pemphigoid group, where titer and clinical activity can diverge. Enzyme-linked immunosorbent assays targeting specific antigens, including desmoglein 1 and 3 in the pemphigus group and BP180 and BP230 in the pemphigoid group, have increasingly supplemented or in some laboratories replaced indirect immunofluorescence for antibody quantification, offering more precise titers though at the cost of the additional pattern information that immunofluorescence-based techniques can provide.

Direct immunofluorescence, indirect immunofluorescence, and antigen-specific serology are complementary rather than redundant, and the choice of which to pursue, or whether to pursue all three, depends on the specific clinical scenario. A patient with a classic clinical presentation and an unambiguous direct immunofluorescence pattern may not require indirect studies for diagnosis, while a patient with an atypical presentation, a discordant direct immunofluorescence result, or a need for objective disease-activity monitoring over time benefits from the additional information indirect immunofluorescence and serology provide. Communicating which of these studies has been performed, and which remain available if the initial results are inconclusive, is a practical service the dermatopathology report can provide to the treating clinician managing a diagnostically challenging immunobullous case.

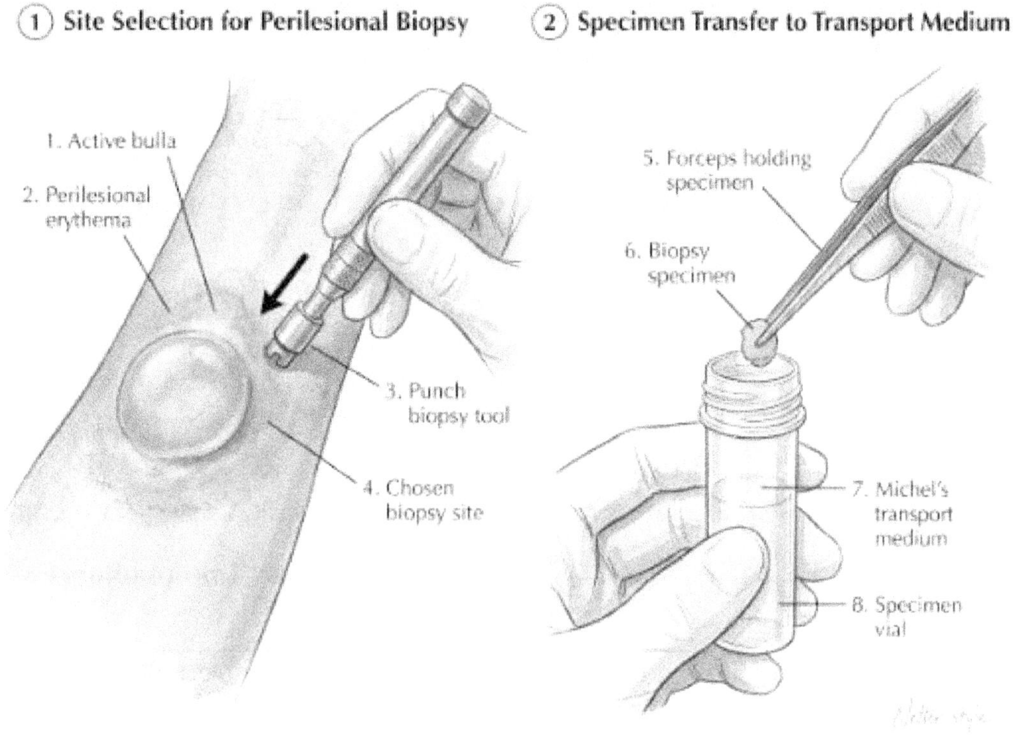

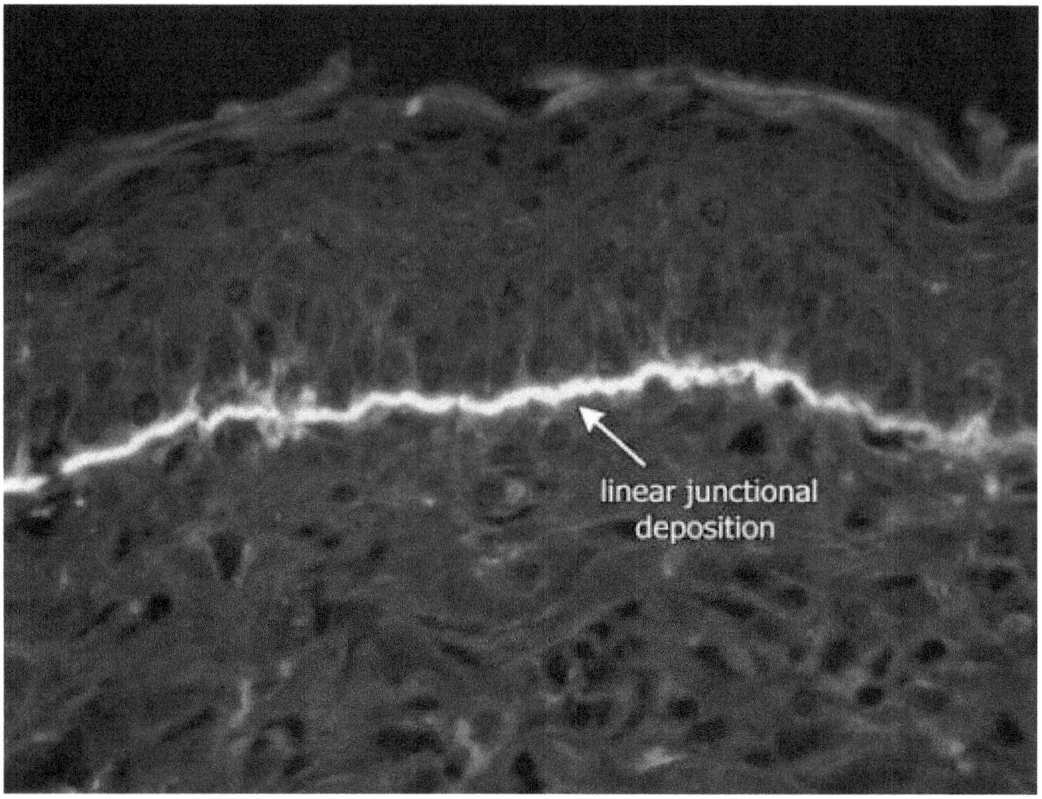

THE REACTION PATTERN RECOGNITION SYSTEM — Direct Immunofluorescence Pattern Recognition

The Pattern: Linear Versus Granular Immunoreactant Deposition at the Dermal-Epidermal Junction

Histologic Signature: Linear pattern: a smooth, continuous, ribbon-like band of fluorescence following the dermal-epidermal junction. Granular pattern: discontinuous, stippled clusters of fluorescence, often most prominent at the dermal papillary tips.

The Decision: Linear deposition of IgG and C3 supports the pemphigoid group; granular deposition of IgA at the papillary tips supports dermatitis herpetiformis; granular deposition of IgG, IgM, and C3 in a band distributed more broadly along the junction supports lupus erythematosus.

Trap Logic: The mimicker in each direction is misclassifying pattern under suboptimal technical conditions: a granular pattern can appear falsely linear if fluorescence intensity is very high and individual granules are not resolved, and a linear pattern can appear falsely granular if the section is thin or unevenly cut. The discriminating step is examining multiple fields at consistent exposure and, when genuinely ambiguous, correlating with salt-split skin results or routine histology.

Pattern Anchor: Linear equals pemphigoid-group biology (subepidermal, hemidesmosomal target); granular equals either dermatitis herpetiformis (papillary tip, IgA) or lupus (broader junctional band, multiple immunoreactants). Pattern first, then immunoglobulin class, resolves most DIF interpretations.

Molecular and Ancillary Diagnostics

Fluorescence In Situ Hybridization in Melanocytic Lesions

Fluorescence in situ hybridization panels targeting chromosomal loci frequently altered in melanoma (commonly including 6p25, 6q23, 11q13, and centromere 6) assist in distinguishing melanoma from a histologically ambiguous benign melanocytic proliferation such as a Spitz nevus or a nevus with atypical features, since melanoma more frequently shows the specific copy number gains and losses these probes are designed to detect. A positive result, defined by the number of nuclei showing the relevant abnormality exceeding a validated threshold, supports a malignant diagnosis, while a negative result is reassuring but not absolute, since a subset of melanomas, particularly Spitzoid melanoma, can show a normal fluorescence in situ hybridization pattern, meaning the test is best used as one contributory piece of evidence within the full morphologic and clinical context rather than as a standalone arbiter.

Clonality Studies in Cutaneous Lymphoma

Polymerase chain reaction-based clonality studies assess T-cell receptor gene rearrangement (or, less commonly in skin, immunoglobulin heavy chain rearrangement for B-cell processes) to determine whether a lymphocytic infiltrate represents a clonal, and therefore neoplastic, population or a polyclonal, reactive one. A clonal result supports but does not, by itself, establish a diagnosis of cutaneous lymphoma, since clonal populations can rarely be detected in some inflammatory dermatoses, and conversely early or partially treated mycosis fungoides can show a polyclonal or oligoclonal result despite genuine neoplastic disease, so clonality testing is interpreted alongside histology, immunophenotype, and clinical course rather than in isolation, a principle developed fully in Chapter 18.

Next-Generation Sequencing and Emerging Applications

Targeted next-generation sequencing panels are increasingly used to characterize the mutational landscape of ambiguous melanocytic lesions, distinguishing benign nevi, which typically show a single driver mutation (commonly BRAF or NRAS) without significant additional mutational burden, from melanoma, which typically accumulates additional mutations, including in the TERT promoter, as it progresses. These panels are also used in the workup of selected soft tissue and adnexal neoplasms to identify characteristic fusion events that support a specific diagnosis, and in confirming actionable mutations relevant to systemic therapy selection in advanced melanoma and other cutaneous malignancies. Access to these assays varies substantially by practice setting, and the decision to pursue molecular testing should weigh the specific diagnostic or therapeutic question at hand against the additional tissue requirement and turnaround time involved.

Practical Considerations: Test Selection and Tissue Stewardship

Molecular and ancillary diagnostics carry real costs, in tissue volume consumed, turnaround time incurred, and, in most health systems, direct financial expense, and their selection benefits from the same hypothesis-driven discipline recommended above for special stains. Fluorescence in situ hybridization and next-generation sequencing for an ambiguous melanocytic lesion are best reserved for cases in which routine morphology and standard immunohistochemistry have been fully exhausted and a genuine diagnostic ambiguity remains that the molecular result is likely to resolve, rather than ordered reflexively on every histologically atypical nevus, both because the tests are not infallible and because unnecessary testing depletes a tissue resource that may be needed for a subsequent diagnostic question, including staging studies if the lesion is ultimately confirmed malignant. Clonality testing in a suspected early cutaneous lymphoma is similarly most informative when the pretest suspicion, built from morphology and immunophenotype, is already at least moderate, since testing a low-suspicion case primarily returns polyclonal results that, while reassuring, add limited diagnostic value relative to their cost.

A useful working principle across this entire chapter is that special stains, immunohistochemistry, direct immunofluorescence, and molecular studies each answer a specific, narrow question generated by careful morphologic assessment, and each is most valuable when that question is articulated explicitly before the test is ordered. A dermatopathologist who can state precisely what a given ancillary result would need to show to change the working diagnosis, before that result is available, is applying these tools correctly; a dermatopathologist who orders a broad battery of studies hoping that something useful emerges is not, and the resulting reports tend to be longer without being more diagnostically useful.

Reporting Molecular Results in Context

How a molecular result is communicated in the final report matters nearly as much as the result itself, since a treating clinician without dermatopathology-specific training will act on the report's stated conclusion rather than independently reinterpreting a raw fluorescence in situ hybridization or sequencing readout. A report that states a positive fluorescence in situ hybridization result in isolation, without connecting it explicitly to the morphologic findings and the specific diagnostic question it was ordered to resolve, risks being read as more diagnostically absolute than the underlying test actually is; the more useful convention is to state the morphologic impression first, then report the molecular result as supporting or, when discordant, as requiring additional correlation, explicitly naming the limitation. This is particularly important for negative or equivocal molecular results in melanocytic lesions, where a negative fluorescence in situ hybridization result is reassuring but does not, by itself, exclude melanoma, and a report that fails to state this limitation risks a treating clinician incorrectly treating a negative molecular result as definitively benign in a lesion that other features still suggest warrants complete excision or clinical follow-up.

The same principle extends to clonality results in suspected cutaneous lymphoma, where a polyclonal result in a case with a high pretest suspicion based on morphology and immunophenotype should be reported as not excluding early or patch-stage disease, given the known limitations of clonality testing sensitivity at these stages, rather than reported in a way that could be read as ruling out lymphoma. Precise, appropriately hedged language in the molecular and ancillary study section of a dermatopathology report is not a matter of stylistic preference; it is a direct extension of the diagnostic honesty principle introduced in Chapter 1, applied specifically to results that carry a false sense of numerical or technological certainty relative to their actual, and often more limited, diagnostic weight.

KEY POINT: Ancillary studies refine and support a diagnosis built on careful morphologic assessment; they do not substitute for it. Every special stain, immunohistochemical panel, and molecular assay in this chapter is most reliably interpreted in the context of the reaction pattern and architecture already established at the microscope.

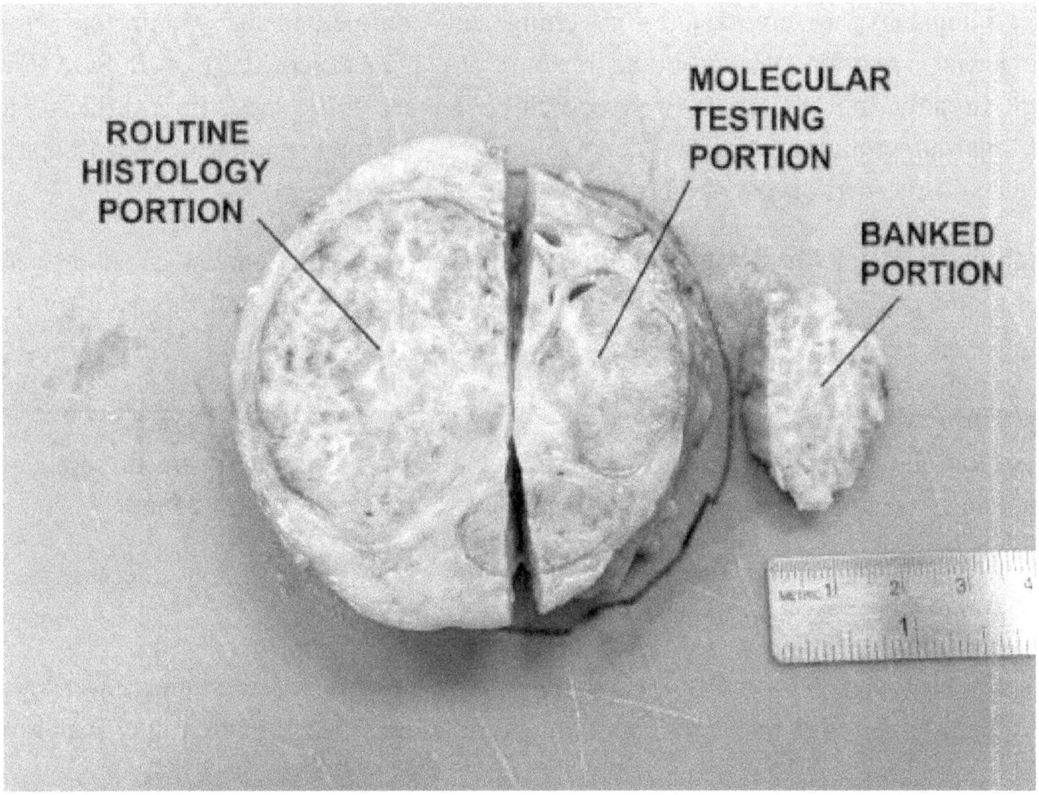

THE REACTION PATTERN RECOGNITION SYSTEM — Ancillary Study Decision Points

The Pattern: Three recurring ancillary-study decision points: special stain misinterpretation, melanocytic marker overreliance in spindle cell lesions, and direct immunofluorescence pattern confusion.

Histologic Signature: PAS-positive basement membrane material mistaken for fungal hyphae; SOX10 positivity treated as sufficient evidence of melanocytic lineage in a spindle cell lesion; linear and granular DIF patterns confused under suboptimal technical conditions.

The Decision: In each case, the ancillary result is integrated with architecture, location, and clinical context rather than read as a standalone answer.

Trap Logic: Fungal hyphae are septate, branching, and confined to the stratum corneum; basement membrane material is a continuous non-branching band at the junction or vessel wall. SOX10 marks neural crest lineage broadly, not melanocytes specifically. Linear DIF deposition reflects subepidermal, hemidesmosomal-target biology; granular deposition reflects immune complex deposition at the papillary tips (IgA, dermatitis herpetiformis) or a broader junctional band (lupus).

Pattern Anchor: Every ancillary test in this chapter answers a specific, narrow question; before ordering or interpreting one, state the question it is being asked to answer, and read the result only against that question.

Summary and Key Concepts

Adequate fixation and correct specimen orientation at the processing stage are prerequisites for every downstream diagnostic step, from routine histology through molecular testing.

Histochemical special stains each answer a specific, narrow diagnostic question; selecting the correct stain depends on first generating a specific hypothesis from routine histology.

Immunohistochemical panels for melanocytic, epithelial, lymphoid, vascular, and mesenchymal lineages are most reliably interpreted as one component of a broader diagnostic picture rather than as a standalone answer.

Direct immunofluorescence requires specifically handled perilesional tissue and is interpreted primarily by immunoreactant pattern and location rather than immunoglobulin class alone.

Molecular and ancillary diagnostics, including fluorescence in situ hybridization, clonality studies, and next-generation sequencing, refine diagnosis in ambiguous melanocytic and lymphoid proliferations but are interpreted within the full morphologic and clinical context established earlier in the workup.

CHAPTER 3: THE PATTERN-BASED APPROACH TO INFLAMMATORY SKIN DISEASE

Learning Objectives

1. Describe the historical development and cognitive rationale of the pattern-based (algorithmic) method in dermatopathology.
2. Define the major inflammatory reaction patterns and identify the anatomic compartment and defining histologic feature of each.
3. Apply a three-step sequence (pattern assignment, differential narrowing, diagnosis) to an inflammatory dermatosis biopsy.
4. Recognize the common pitfalls of pattern assignment, including anchoring, site- and stage-dependent variation, and overlapping or transitional patterns.

Origins of the Algorithmic Method

Historical Development of Pattern-Based Reasoning in Dermatopathology

The pattern-based method that structures this book was not designed in the abstract; it emerged from a specific pedagogical problem that dermatopathology confronted more acutely than most other areas of surgical pathology. Inflammatory skin disease comprises hundreds of clinically distinct named entities, and a purely disease-by-disease teaching approach, learn eczema, then learn psoriasis, then learn lichen planus, and so on as an unordered list, produced trainees who could recognize a textbook-perfect example of a disease they had specifically studied but who floundered when confronted with an unfamiliar or atypical presentation of a related condition. Mid-twentieth-century dermatopathologists, most influentially through the algorithmic teaching tradition that dominates the field's pedagogy to this day, observed that this same enormous list of diseases could be organized into a much smaller number of recurring tissue reaction patterns, and that teaching the pattern first, with the specific disease list nested underneath it as a differential diagnosis, produced trainees who could reason through unfamiliar presentations far more successfully than trainees taught disease-by-disease.

This reorganization did more than simplify teaching; it reflected a genuine biological insight. The skin has a limited structural repertoire for responding to injury, whether that injury is immunologic, infectious, physical, or metabolic in origin, and many different etiologic insults converge on the same handful of histologic responses. Spongiosis, the intercellular edema that defines the spongiotic pattern, is the skin's stereotyped response to a broad range of provoking antigens and irritants, whether the specific trigger is a topical allergen, an ingested drug, or an endogenous inflammatory process, and this convergence is precisely why the reaction pattern, rather than the specific etiologic agent, is the more tractable first-level organizing principle for histologic diagnosis.

This convergence principle also explains a feature of dermatopathology practice that can initially seem counterintuitive to trainees arriving from other areas of pathology: a definitive histologic diagnosis is not always the achievable or even the appropriate endpoint of an inflammatory dermatosis biopsy. Because multiple etiologically distinct diseases can produce histologically identical or near-identical spongiotic, psoriasiform, or interface patterns, the tissue itself sometimes reaches the limit of what it can distinguish, and the diagnostic task shifts from identifying a single named disease to characterizing the pattern precisely enough that the treating clinician, armed with clinical information the pathologist does not have, can complete the diagnosis. This is not a failure of the pattern-based method; it is an accurate reflection of the biological reality that skin has a finite number of ways to respond to injury, and the method's honesty about this limitation, formalized in the descriptive-diagnosis-with-differential reporting convention introduced in Chapter 1, is one of its genuine strengths relative to an approach that pressures every biopsy toward a single, potentially overconfident named diagnosis.

The Cognitive Structure of Expert Diagnostic Reasoning

Studies of expert diagnostic reasoning across medicine, not specific to dermatopathology, consistently describe a two-stage cognitive process: a rapid, largely unconscious pattern-recognition stage in which the expert's visual system matches the case at hand against a large internal library of previously seen patterns, followed by a slower, more deliberate analytical stage in which the expert consciously verifies that the pattern-matched impression is consistent with the specific features present and actively searches for evidence that would argue against it. Novices, lacking a well-developed pattern library, are forced to rely almost entirely on the slower analytical stage, working through features one at a time in a effortful and error-prone sequence, which is both slower and, counterintuitively, less accurate than expert pattern recognition, because the deliberate feature-by-feature approach is more vulnerable to being led astray by an early, salient but ultimately misleading finding.

The explicit, structured teaching of reaction patterns is an attempt to accelerate a trainee's progression from the novice's effortful analytical mode toward the expert's rapid pattern-recognition mode, by making the pattern library that experts have developed through years of case exposure available in codified form from the outset of training. This is also why the trap logic built into every Rhythm block in this book is not incidental; expert pattern recognition is powerful but not infallible, and the specific failure mode of expert pattern recognition, premature closure on a plausible but incorrect pattern match, is best countered not by abandoning pattern recognition in favor of laborious feature-by-feature analysis but by pairing pattern recognition with an explicit, rehearsed habit of checking the leading pattern against its most dangerous mimickers before finalizing a diagnosis.

Why Pattern Recognition Outperforms Disease-by-Disease Memorization

Three specific advantages make pattern-based reasoning more effective than disease-by-disease memorization for the specific diagnostic task dermatopathology presents. First, pattern-based reasoning is generative rather than purely recall-based: a trainee who has learned that a given reaction pattern implies a specific differential diagnosis can reason toward a plausible diagnosis for an unfamiliar or atypical case by first identifying the pattern and then applying the general differential associated with that pattern, whereas a trainee relying on disease-specific recall has no productive strategy when the case does not match a previously memorized example closely enough to trigger recall. Second, pattern-based reasoning is more efficient to teach and to apply because the number of patterns is small (seven to eight major categories, each covered in a dedicated chapter of this book) relative to the number of diseases nested within them, so that a fixed amount of learning effort invested in mastering the patterns yields disproportionate diagnostic coverage across the full range of inflammatory dermatoses. Third, pattern-based reasoning aligns with how reaction patterns are actually communicated in clinical practice and in the broader pathology literature, so that a dermatopathologist fluent in this vocabulary can communicate efficiently and precisely with colleagues and can navigate the specialty's reference literature, which is itself substantially organized along pattern-based lines, far more effectively than a colleague working from disease-specific recall alone.

Limitations and Ongoing Evolution of the Algorithmic Method

The algorithmic method, for all its pedagogical and diagnostic power, has never claimed to be a complete or static classification of skin disease, and understanding its limitations is as important as understanding its strengths. The method was developed primarily around inflammatory dermatoses and was subsequently extended, with reasonable but imperfect success, to organize neoplastic dermatopathology along an analogous lineage-based logic, as this book does in Part III. Some disease processes resist clean assignment to a single reaction pattern from the outset, either because they genuinely combine features of multiple patterns as a defining characteristic of the disease itself, rather than as an artifact of biopsy timing or site, or because they represent a distinct entity that the eight-pattern framework was never designed to capture cleanly, such as certain poikilodermatous processes that combine epidermal atrophy, basal vacuolar change, and dermal telangiectasia in a way that draws on interface pattern vocabulary without being a straightforward lichenoid or vacuolar interface process.

The method has also continued to evolve since its original development, incorporating refinements as immunohistochemistry, molecular diagnostics, and an expanding understanding of disease mechanism have revealed finer distinctions within categories that were once treated as histologically uniform. The interface pattern, for example, has been increasingly subdivided in the specialty literature according to the specific balance of vacuolar change, lymphocyte density, and associated findings such as dermal mucin or vascular changes, distinctions that carry increasing diagnostic and even therapeutic relevance as targeted treatments for specific interface-pattern diseases have become available. A reader should therefore treat the framework presented in this chapter, and elaborated throughout this book, as a living, evidence-responsive structure rather than a fixed taxonomy handed down unchanged, useful precisely because it has continued to absorb refinement rather than because it achieved a final, complete form at its inception.

KEY POINT: Pattern recognition and disease-specific knowledge are not competing strategies; pattern recognition is the organizing scaffold onto which disease-specific knowledge is hung. A trainee still needs to know the specific features of allergic contact dermatitis, but learning that entity as one member of the spongiotic pattern family, alongside its distinguishing features relative to atopic and nummular dermatitis, is far more durable than learning it in isolation.

How This Book's Rhythm Layer Operationalizes the Method

The Reaction Pattern Recognition System introduced in Chapter 1 is this book's direct implementation of the two-stage expert reasoning process described above, and understanding that connection explicitly makes the Rhythm Layer easier to use as intended rather than as a decorative feature layered on top of ordinary chapter text. The Pattern and Histologic Signature components of each Rhythm block correspond to the rapid pattern-recognition stage: they state, explicitly and by name, the pattern match a reader should be developing intuitively as they examine a comparable case at the microscope. The Decision, Trap Logic, and Pattern Anchor components correspond to the deliberate verification stage: they walk through the specific checking process an expert performs before finalizing that pattern match, naming the mimicker most likely to produce a false match and the specific feature that resolves the ambiguity. A trainee who works through Rhythm blocks not as isolated facts to memorize but as worked demonstrations of this two-stage reasoning process, applied repeatedly across dozens of specific diagnostic scenarios throughout this book, is building the same cognitive structure that produces genuine diagnostic expertise, simply on an accelerated and more explicit timeline than unstructured case-by-case clinical exposure alone would provide.

This is also why every Rhythm block in this book, including the two presented later in this chapter, follows the identical five-part structure regardless of which reaction pattern or specific diagnostic scenario it addresses. Structural consistency is a deliberate design choice: a reader who has internalized the five-part sequence as a repeatable habit, name the pattern, state its signature, commit to a decision, check the trap logic, anchor the takeaway, can apply that same habit unprompted at the microscope, long after this book's specific worked examples have been supplemented or superseded by the reader's own accumulated case experience. The goal of the Rhythm Layer, in other words, is ultimately to make itself unnecessary, by training a reasoning habit durable enough to operate without an external structural prompt once it has been sufficiently rehearsed.

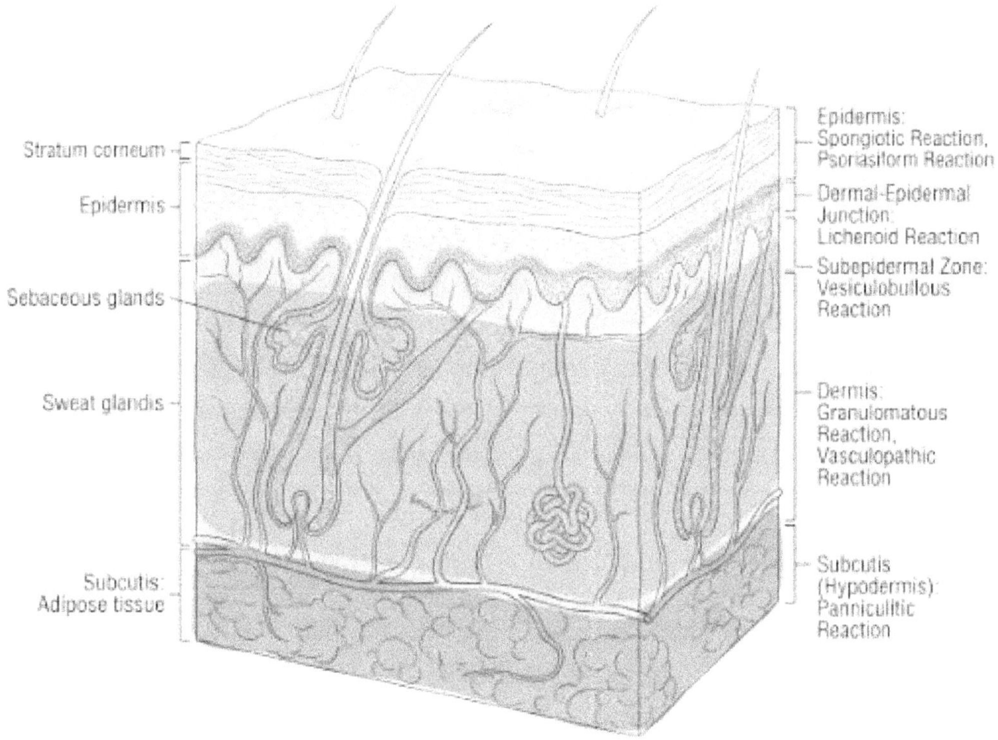

Defining the Major Reaction Patterns

Epidermal-Predominant Patterns: Spongiotic and Psoriasiform

The spongiotic pattern is defined by intercellular epidermal edema, visible as widened intercellular spaces with stretched but intact desmosomal connections between keratinocytes, progressing in more severe cases to intraepidermal vesicle formation as the edema mechanically separates keratinocytes beyond the point their desmosomal attachments can withstand. It is accompanied, in its acute form, by a superficial perivascular lymphocytic infiltrate, often with eosinophils, and evolves over time, with chronic or lichenified spongiotic dermatitis developing overlying epidermal hyperplasia that can begin to resemble the psoriasiform pattern, a transition developed further later in this chapter. The psoriasiform pattern is defined by regular, elongated epidermal hyperplasia (elongation of the rete ridges in a regular, test-tube-in-a-rack configuration) accompanied by thinning of the suprapapillary epidermis and, in its prototypical form, parakeratosis with an accompanying diminished or absent granular layer, reflecting the accelerated keratinocyte transit time characteristic of this pattern's prototype disease, psoriasis, discussed fully in Chapter 5.

Junctional Patterns: Lichenoid and Interface

The lichenoid and interface patterns share a common anatomic target, the dermal-epidermal junction and basal keratinocyte layer, but differ in the density and distribution of the associated inflammatory infiltrate. The lichenoid pattern is defined by a dense, band-like lymphocytic infiltrate that hugs the dermal-epidermal junction and obscures it, accompanied by basal keratinocyte vacuolar change, individual keratinocyte necrosis (Civatte bodies), and, in well-developed lesions, a sawtooth pattern of rete ridge configuration, prototypically exemplified by lichen planus and covered fully in Chapter 6. The vacuolar interface pattern shows the same basal layer damage, vacuolar change and individual keratinocyte necrosis, but with a comparatively sparse, patchy lymphocytic infiltrate that does not obscure the junction to the same degree, a pattern prototypically exemplified by lupus erythematosus and erythema multiforme, and the density and character of the infiltrate, dense and band-like versus sparse and patchy, is frequently the single most useful discriminator between these two related but clinically distinct pattern families.

The Blistering Pattern: Vesiculobullous and Vesiculopustular Disease

The vesiculobullous pattern is defined not by a single level but by the specific level at which epidermal or subepidermal separation occurs, since the level of split is the primary organizing axis for this entire disease category, developed fully in Chapter 7. Intraepidermal splits are further subdivided by mechanism, acantholytic (loss of keratinocyte cohesion, as in the pemphigus group), spongiotic (edema-driven, as in severe acute spongiotic dermatitis), or necrolytic (keratinocyte necrosis-driven), while subepidermal splits are subdivided by the specific target antigen and associated direct immunofluorescence pattern, as detailed in Chapter 2. The vesiculopustular subset specifically involves accumulation of neutrophils, either alone or admixed with eosinophils, within the intraepidermal or subcorneal blister cavity, and is relevant to a differential spanning infectious, autoimmune, and neutrophilic dermatosis etiologies.

Dermal Patterns: Granulomatous and Vasculopathic

The granulomatous pattern is defined by aggregates of activated histiocytes, often accompanied by multinucleated giant cells, organized into either well-formed granulomas with a discrete, compact architecture (prototypically infectious or sarcoidal) or poorly formed, interstitial granulomatous infiltrates dispersed between collagen bundles (prototypically granuloma annulare and related palisaded and interstitial granulomatous entities), a distinction developed fully in Chapter 8. The vasculopathic pattern encompasses both true vasculitis, defined by inflammatory cell infiltration of the vessel wall itself with associated fibrinoid necrosis, and vasculopathy without true inflammatory wall destruction, such as thrombotic or occlusive processes, and is further subdivided by the caliber of vessel predominantly involved (small vessel, as in leukocytoclastic vasculitis, versus medium vessel, as in polyarteritis nodosa), a distinction with direct implications for the associated systemic differential diagnosis, developed fully in Chapter 9.

Deep Patterns: Panniculitic and Sclerosing

The panniculitic pattern, as introduced in Chapter 1, is organized primarily along the septal-versus-lobular axis, with septal panniculitis (prototypically erythema nodosum) predominantly damaging the fibrous septa between fat lobules and lobular panniculitis (prototypically pancreatic panniculitis, lupus panniculitis, and subcutaneous panniculitis-like T-cell lymphoma) predominantly damaging the adipocytes within the lobules themselves, a distinction covered fully in Chapter 10. A related but histologically distinct sclerosing pattern, characterized by thickened, homogenized dermal collagen with progressive entrapment and eventual loss of adnexal structures, defines the connective tissue disease category covered in Chapter 11, including morphea and scleroderma, and shares some overlapping features with chronic lichen sclerosus, underscoring that the reaction-pattern framework, while organized around a comparatively small number of major categories, still requires attention to specific architectural and cytologic detail to resolve entities that share superficial pattern-level similarity.

Reaction Pattern	Primary Compartment	Defining Histologic Feature	Prototypical Disease	Full Coverage
Spongiotic	Epidermis	Intercellular edema	Allergic contact dermatitis	Chapter 4
Psoriasiform	Epidermis	Regular rete elongation, parakeratosis	Psoriasis	Chapter 5
Lichenoid / Interface	Dermal-epidermal junction	Basal vacuolar change, band-like or patchy infiltrate	Lichen planus, lupus erythematosus	Chapter 6
Vesiculobullous	Intraepidermal or subepidermal	Level and mechanism of split	Pemphigus, bullous pemphigoid	Chapter 7
Granulomatous	Dermis	Histiocytic aggregates, well- or poorly-formed	Granuloma annulare, sarcoidosis	Chapter 8
Vasculopathic	Dermal and subcutaneous vessels	Vessel wall inflammation or occlusion	Leukocytoclasti c vasculitis	Chapter 9
Panniculitic	Subcutis	Septal or lobular fat involvement	Erythema nodosum	Chapter 10
Sclerosing / Connective Tissue	Dermis	Thickened, homogenized collagen	Morphea, scleroderma	Chapter 11

Secondary Patterns and Findings Not Fully Captured by the Eight-Pattern Framework

A small number of recurring histologic findings sit alongside, rather than cleanly within, the eight major reaction patterns and deserve explicit mention so that a reader does not attempt to force them into a category they do not naturally fit. Atrophic changes, epidermal thinning with flattening of the rete ridge pattern, occur as a feature of several distinct processes, from the chronic endpoint of certain interface-pattern diseases such as longstanding lupus erythematosus and lichen sclerosus, to the physiologic changes of aged and photodamaged skin discussed in Chapter 1, to a component of specific atrophic variants of otherwise pattern-classifiable diseases such as atrophic lichen planus. Rather than constituting a ninth independent pattern, atrophy is better understood as a modifier that can be superimposed on several of the primary patterns, and its presence should prompt the reader to ask which underlying pattern, and which stage of that pattern's evolution, the atrophic change is occurring within.

Similarly, a poikilodermatous presentation, combining epidermal atrophy, mottled pigmentary change, telangiectasia, and a variable degree of basal vacuolar change and dermal lymphocytic infiltrate, is better understood as a clinical and histologic composite that draws primarily on interface pattern biology, occurring in conditions ranging from poikiloderma of Civatte to the poikilodermatous variant of mycosis fungoides discussed in Chapter 18, than as a pattern unto itself. The practical lesson from both of these examples is the same one introduced in the discussion of pattern overlap above: the eight-pattern framework is a highly effective organizing scaffold for the great majority of inflammatory dermatoses, but a small number of findings and presentations are better handled as modifiers or composites layered onto the primary framework than forced into an artificially expanded pattern list, and recognizing which situation applies is itself part of the diagnostic skill this book aims to build.

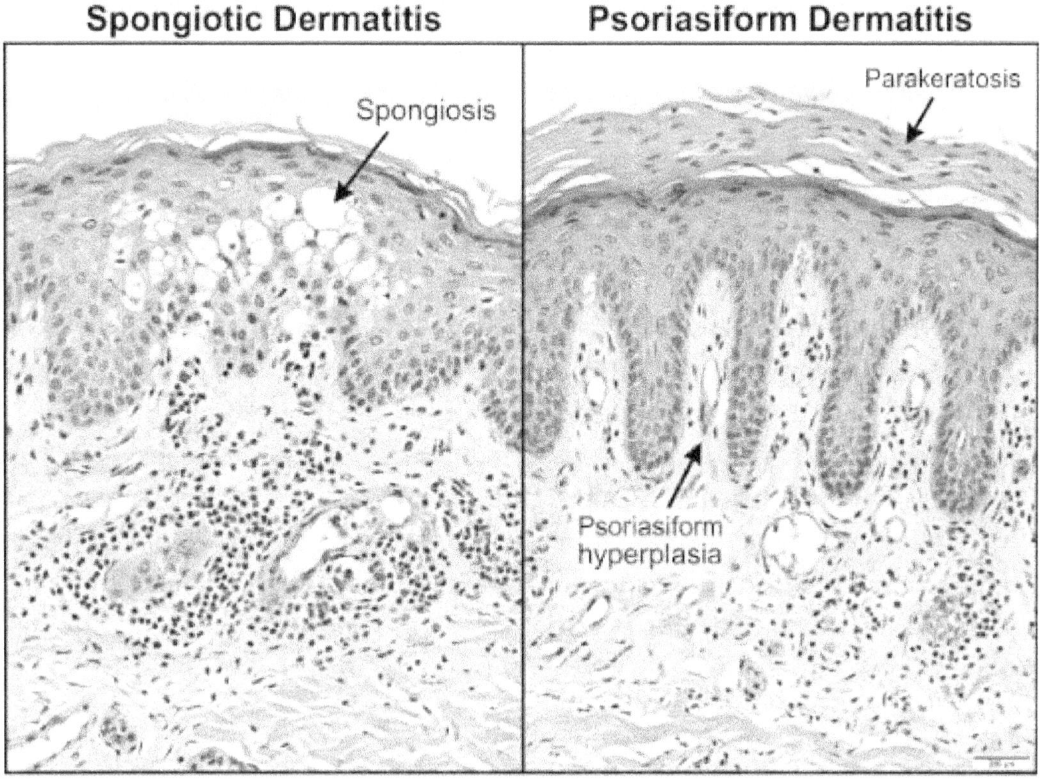

THE REACTION PATTERN RECOGNITION SYSTEM — Pattern Evolution Over Disease Course

---

The Pattern: Spongiotic Pattern Evolving Toward a Psoriasiform Pattern in Chronic Eczematous Dermatitis

Histologic Signature: A biopsy from a longstanding, repeatedly scratched or rubbed eczematous plaque shows compact hyperkeratosis, prominent epidermal hyperplasia with elongated rete ridges, and a diminished degree of spongiosis relative to what would be expected in an acute lesion, superimposed on a background of hypergranulosis rather than the parakeratosis and reduced granular layer typical of true psoriasis.

The Decision: Recognize that chronic mechanical trauma (lichenification) converts the histologic appearance of a spongiotic process toward a psoriasiform silhouette at low power, and specifically seek residual spongiosis, hypergranulosis rather than reduced granular layer, and a compatible clinical history of a pruritic, rubbed lesion before reclassifying the process as psoriasiform disease.

Trap Logic: The mimicker is true psoriasis. The discriminating features favoring chronic spongiotic (lichenified) dermatitis over psoriasis are hypergranulosis (versus diminished granular layer), residual foci of spongiosis, and a superficial perivascular infiltrate with occasional eosinophils (versus the more purely lymphocytic and neutrophilic infiltrate, often with intracorneal or subcorneal neutrophilic collections, of psoriasis).

Pattern Anchor: Hypergranulosis with residual spongiosis favors lichenified eczema; a diminished granular layer with parakeratosis and neutrophils favors psoriasis. When both are present, favor the diagnosis the clinical history most strongly supports and state the overlap explicitly in the report.

It is worth noting explicitly why this book organizes its inflammatory chapters (Chapters 4 through 11) in the specific sequence shown in the table above, since the ordering is itself pedagogically motivated rather than arbitrary. Spongiotic and psoriasiform disease are presented first because they are both epidermal-predominant and among the most frequently encountered patterns in routine practice, giving the reader early, high-volume exposure to the low-power scanning and compartmental localization skills introduced in Chapter 1. The lichenoid and interface pattern follows because it shares the epidermal proximity of the first two patterns while introducing the added complexity of basal layer damage and its immunologic underpinnings, building naturally toward the vesiculobullous pattern, in which basal and junctional damage can progress to frank blister formation. The granulomatous and vasculopathic patterns, both primarily dermal rather than epidermal, are grouped together next, and the panniculitic and sclerosing patterns close the section as the deepest and structurally most distinct categories, requiring the reader to extend the compartmental reasoning built in earlier chapters to the subcutis and to a primarily fibrotic, rather than inflammatory-cell-rich, dermal process.

From Pattern to Differential to Diagnosis

The Three-Step Diagnostic Sequence

The practical application of the pattern-based method proceeds through three sequential steps, each building on the one before it. The first step, pattern assignment, applies the low-power scanning approach introduced in Chapter 1 to assign the biopsy to one of the major reaction patterns based on its dominant architectural and compartmental features. The second step, differential narrowing, applies the specific secondary features associated with the assigned pattern, distribution of the infiltrate, presence or absence of specific cell types, associated epidermal or vascular changes, to narrow the broad differential diagnosis implied by the pattern down to a small number of specific candidate diagnoses. The third step, diagnosis, integrates this narrowed histologic differential with the clinical information accompanying the specimen, lesion morphology, distribution, duration, and relevant history, to arrive at a final diagnosis or, when the tissue and clinical information together cannot resolve the differential further, a descriptive diagnosis with a stated differential, as illustrated in the worked example in Chapter 1.

It is worth pausing on why this sequencing, pattern first, then differential, then diagnosis, rather than the reverse, produces more reliable results. A reader who instead begins by asking "which specific disease does this look like" is implicitly relying on holistic pattern matching against a mental library of remembered cases, a strategy that works reasonably well for classic presentations of common diseases but degrades rapidly for atypical presentations or less common entities that a reader may have limited direct experience with. The three-step sequence forces a more structured, and therefore more transferable, path through the same reasoning: pattern assignment relies only on recognizing one of a small, fixed number of compartmental and architectural configurations, a task with a much shorter learning curve than recognizing hundreds of individual diseases, and each subsequent step narrows a bounded, previously established differential rather than requiring the reader to generate a differential diagnosis from an unbounded list of possibilities. This is precisely the structural advantage described in the discussion of pattern-based reasoning earlier in this chapter, now made concrete as a specific, repeatable diagnostic procedure.

Using Secondary Features to Narrow Within a Pattern

Each reaction pattern implies a specific set of secondary features that experienced readers use systematically to narrow the differential once the primary pattern has been established. Within the spongiotic pattern, for example, the presence of numerous eosinophils favors allergic contact dermatitis or a drug reaction, while a paucity of eosinophils with a more purely lymphocytic infiltrate favors atopic or nummular dermatitis; the presence of parakeratosis with retained cornified layer nuclei in mounds favors a more chronic or evolving process; and follicular accentuation of the spongiotic change favors a specific subset of eczematous reactions localized to the follicular infundibulum. This same principle, using pattern-specific secondary features rather than a generic checklist, applies within every major pattern and is developed in full for each pattern in its dedicated chapter; the general skill introduced here, actively seeking the secondary features relevant to whichever pattern has been assigned, transfers across all of them.

When Patterns Overlap or Evolve

As the Rhythm block above illustrates, reaction patterns are not static, and a single disease process can present with different patterns at different points in its natural history, or with genuinely overlapping features of two patterns at a single point in time. Early bullous pemphigoid, before frank subepidermal blister formation, can show a predominantly eosinophilic spongiotic pattern (eosinophilic spongiosis) that only later evolves into the more diagnostic subepidermal blistering pattern; a biopsy obtained at this early stage should be interpreted with this evolution explicitly in mind rather than dismissed as a nonspecific eosinophilic dermatitis when the clinical picture (tense bullae developing over an urticarial background in an elderly patient) is suggestive. Recognizing genuine overlap, rather than forcing a single pattern assignment onto a biopsy that legitimately shows transitional or mixed features, is a mark of diagnostic sophistication rather than diagnostic failure, provided the report communicates the overlap and its implications clearly to the treating clinician.

A Second Worked Example: Applying the Three-Step Sequence to a Dermal Infiltrate

A 58-year-old patient with a several-month history of firm, asymptomatic annular plaques on the dorsal hands undergoes punch biopsy with a clinical differential of granuloma annulare versus a cutaneous lymphoma. Step one, pattern assignment, begins at low power: the epidermis is unremarkable and normal in architecture, ruling out the epidermal-predominant and junctional patterns as primary considerations, while the dermis shows scattered histiocytic aggregates dispersed interstitially between collagen bundles rather than organized into discrete, well-formed granulomas, establishing a granulomatous pattern of the poorly formed, interstitial subtype. Step two, differential narrowing, applies the secondary features specific to this pattern subtype: increased interstitial mucin, assessed with an Alcian blue special stain as discussed in Chapter 2, would favor granuloma annulare, while a monomorphous, atypical lymphocytic component admixed with the histiocytes, best assessed with an immunohistochemical panel including CD3, CD4, CD8, and CD30 as discussed in Chapter 2, would favor a cutaneous T-cell lymphoma with a granulomatous or histiocyte-rich pattern, a recognized though uncommon presentation.

Step three, diagnosis, integrates the histologic findings, in this hypothetical case a positive Alcian blue stain confirming increased interstitial mucin and a CD3/CD4/CD8 panel showing a polytypic, non-atypical T-cell population, with the clinical presentation of firm annular plaques, a morphology and distribution classically associated with granuloma annulare, to arrive at a final diagnosis of interstitial granuloma annulare. This worked example illustrates why the three-step sequence, rather than any single step in isolation, constitutes the diagnostic method: pattern assignment alone (poorly formed granulomatous pattern) narrows the differential substantially but does not resolve it, differential narrowing using ancillary studies further sharpens the distinction, and only the final integration with clinical morphology and distribution, itself informed by the specific pattern and ancillary findings, produces a diagnosis that the treating clinician can act on with confidence.

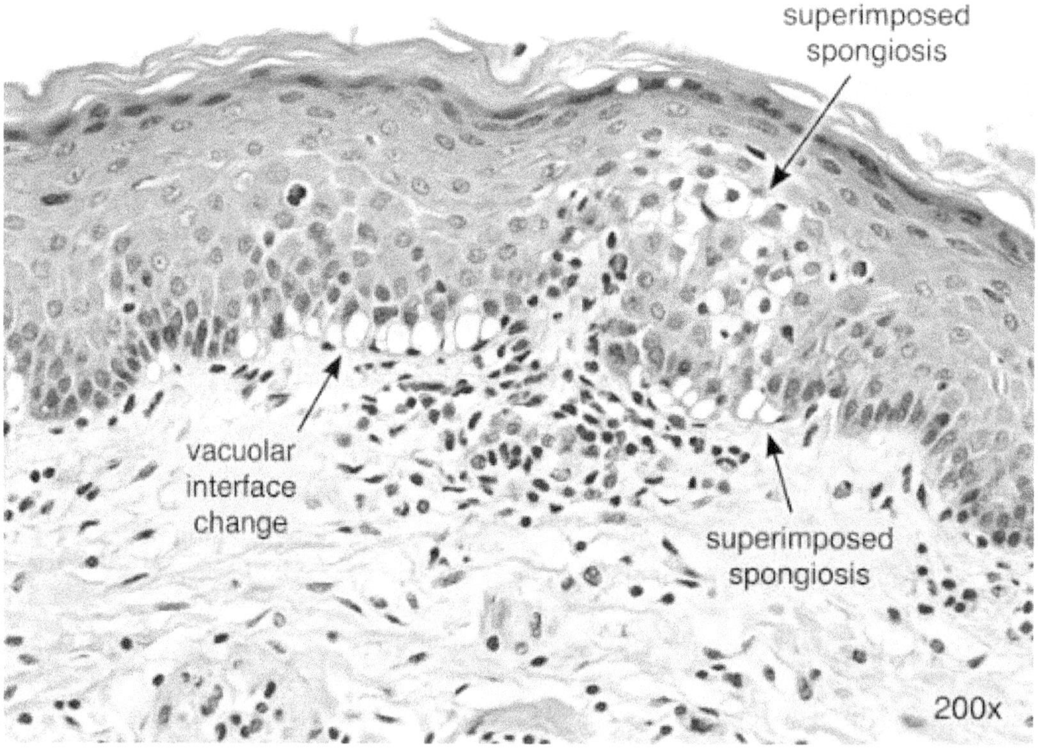

Common Pitfalls in Pattern Assignment

Pattern Anchoring and Premature Closure

The same rapid pattern-recognition process that makes expert diagnosis efficient also creates a specific vulnerability: once a pattern is provisionally assigned, there is a cognitive tendency to selectively notice features that confirm the assigned pattern and to discount or overlook features that would argue against it, a phenomenon well described in the general medical decision-making literature as anchoring bias. In dermatopathology, this manifests as, for example, assigning a psoriasiform pattern based on a prominent low-power impression of rete elongation and then failing to systematically assess the granular layer and stratum corneum for the parakeratosis expected in true psoriasis, features that, if genuinely absent, would argue for a different diagnosis such as chronic spongiotic dermatitis. The corrective habit, built into the Trap Logic component of every Rhythm block in this book, is to deliberately and explicitly check the assigned pattern against its known mimickers before finalizing a diagnosis, rather than treating pattern assignment as a single-step process that ends once an initial plausible match is found.

Site- and Stage-Dependent Pattern Variation

As developed in Chapter 1's discussion of site-specific normal histology, the same disease process can present with a modified histologic pattern depending on the anatomic site biopsied, and this site-dependence extends to reaction pattern assignment specifically. Psoriasis on palmar or plantar skin, for example, can show a less classically psoriasiform architecture than psoriasis on trunk or extremity skin, owing to the already thickened baseline stratum corneum and altered rete ridge pattern at these sites described in Chapter 1, and a reader unfamiliar with this site-specific variation risks under-recognizing psoriasiform change at acral sites or, conversely, over-calling a psoriasiform pattern based on baseline acral hyperkeratosis alone. Stage-dependent variation, the tendency of a single disease to show different patterns at different points in its evolution as illustrated above, compounds this challenge, and the practical corrective for both site- and stage-dependent variation is the same: always interpret the observed pattern in light of the specific biopsy site and the stated or inferred duration of the clinical lesion, rather than applying a single, context-free template for what a given pattern should look like.

Site- and stage-dependent variation compounds when they occur together, and the reader benefits from actively considering both dimensions rather than checking each in isolation. A biopsy of longstanding, repeatedly traumatized acral psoriasis, for example, combines the site-specific baseline hyperkeratosis discussed above with the lichenification-driven pattern shift toward a less classically psoriasiform architecture discussed earlier in this chapter, producing a biopsy that can be doubly removed from the textbook prototype of psoriasis a trainee first learns. The corrective is not a separate rule for combined site-and-stage variation, but the same underlying discipline applied more deliberately: explicitly asking, for any biopsy that does not match the expected prototype cleanly, whether site, stage, chronicity, or a combination of these factors could explain the deviation before concluding that the deviation instead reflects a different underlying disease altogether.

Combined and Transitional Patterns

A final recurring pitfall is the assumption that every biopsy must resolve cleanly into exactly one of the major reaction patterns. As discussed above, genuine combined and transitional patterns occur, and forcing such a biopsy into a single pattern category, discarding real findings that do not fit the chosen category, produces a diagnosis that is falsely precise and potentially misleading to the treating clinician. The appropriate response to a genuinely mixed or transitional picture is to report the combination explicitly, for example describing a biopsy as showing features of both a spongiotic and an early psoriasiform process with a comment on the differential this combination suggests, rather than to arbitrarily select one pattern and suppress mention of the other. This same principle, favoring accurate, appropriately qualified reporting over falsely precise categorization, recurs throughout this book and is one of the defining features of the pattern-based method as it is intended to be practiced rather than as it is sometimes reduced to in oversimplified teaching.

CLINICAL PEARL: A report that says "predominantly psoriasiform pattern with a component of spongiosis, differential includes evolving psoriasis and chronic spongiotic dermatitis" is more useful, and more honest, than a report that forces the same findings into a single, falsely confident diagnosis.

Institutional and Systems-Level Sources of Diagnostic Error

Not every source of pattern-assignment error originates at the microscope. Turnaround time pressure, particularly in high-volume practices where a large daily case count must be signed out within a fixed interval, can compress the deliberate verification stage of expert diagnostic reasoning discussed earlier in this chapter, pushing a reader toward accepting the first plausible pattern match without the systematic mimicker check that the trap logic framework is designed to enforce. Incomplete clinical information, whether because a requisition form was filled out cursorily, because the ordering clinician's own differential was itself incomplete, or because relevant history (a new medication, a recent travel history, an underlying systemic disease) was simply not communicated, removes one of the three legs of the diagnostic sequence described above and forces the dermatopathologist to rely more heavily, and less reliably, on histology alone.

Recognizing these systems-level contributors to diagnostic error is not an excuse for individual diagnostic lapses, but it does inform two practical countermeasures worth building into routine practice. First, a standardized personal habit of explicitly running through the trap logic for the assigned pattern before finalizing any inflammatory dermatosis diagnosis, regardless of caseload pressure, protects against the anchoring bias that time pressure otherwise amplifies. Second, a low threshold for requesting additional clinical information when the information provided is insufficient to complete the third step of the diagnostic sequence, rather than proceeding to a diagnosis that outruns the available data, shifts the systems-level problem of incomplete information back to the clinical team best positioned to supply it, and is a defensible and professionally expected response rather than an admission of diagnostic uncertainty to be avoided.

THE REACTION PATTERN RECOGNITION SYSTEM — Anchoring Bias in Pattern Assignment

---

The Pattern: Premature Pattern Closure on a Lichenoid Drug Eruption Misread as Lichen Planus

Histologic Signature: A dense, band-like lymphocytic infiltrate at the dermal-epidermal junction with basal vacuolar change and Civatte bodies, closely resembling classic lichen planus at low power, but with scattered eosinophils within the infiltrate and a somewhat more variable, less sharply sawtooth rete ridge pattern.

The Decision: Before finalizing a diagnosis of lichen planus, systematically assess for features that favor a lichenoid drug eruption instead: eosinophils within the infiltrate, parakeratosis (uncommon in classic lichen planus), and a less regular, more variable rete ridge configuration, and correlate with medication history.

Trap Logic: The mimicker is lichen planus itself, and the discriminating features run in both directions: eosinophils, parakeratosis, and a deeper or more perivascular extension of the infiltrate favor a drug eruption, while a purely lymphocytic infiltrate, hypergranulosis, and a sharply defined sawtooth rete pattern favor idiopathic lichen planus. A new or recently changed medication in the clinical history is the single most useful non-histologic discriminator.

Pattern Anchor: Eosinophils in an otherwise classic lichenoid infiltrate are a deliberate prompt to ask about medications before signing out lichen planus; the histologic overlap between these two entities is substantial enough that clinical correlation is often decisive.

THE REACTION PATTERN RECOGNITION SYSTEM — Site-Dependent Pattern Variation

---

The Pattern: Acral Psoriasis Under-Recognized Because of Baseline Site-Specific Hyperkeratosis

Histologic Signature: A biopsy from palmar or plantar psoriasis shows a less dramatically elongated, regular rete pattern than trunk psoriasis, set against the already thickened baseline stratum corneum of acral skin described in Chapter 1, so that the psoriasiform architecture is comparatively subtle and can be overshadowed by the prominent hyperkeratosis expected at this site regardless of disease.

The Decision: Assess rete ridge regularity and granular layer status relative to the specific acral baseline established in Chapter 1, rather than relative to the trunk-skin baseline a reader may default to reflexively, and specifically seek parakeratosis with an accompanying diminished granular layer, which remains a reliable discriminator even at acral sites.

Trap Logic: The mimicker is chronic mechanical hyperkeratosis of palmar or plantar skin unrelated to psoriasis (callus or chronic friction change), which shares the baseline thickened stratum corneum but lacks the parakeratosis, diminished granular layer, and regular rete elongation of true psoriasiform disease. The discriminating features are the same core psoriasiform criteria applied against the correct site-specific baseline, not a different set of criteria altogether.

Pattern Anchor: At acral sites, do not let baseline hyperkeratosis substitute for the specific psoriasiform criteria of parakeratosis and granular layer loss; anchor the assessment to what is abnormal for that site, not to hyperkeratosis in isolation.

THE REACTION PATTERN RECOGNITION SYSTEM — The Pattern-Based Method Itself

The Pattern: The eight major inflammatory reaction patterns (spongiotic, psoriasiform, lichenoid/interface, vesiculobullous, granulomatous, vasculopathic, panniculitic, sclerosing) as the organizing framework for the chapters that follow.

Histologic Signature: Each pattern is defined by a specific anatomic compartment and a specific defining histologic feature, summarized in the master comparison table in this chapter.

The Decision: Apply the three-step sequence, pattern assignment, differential narrowing using pattern-specific secondary features, and integration with clinical information, to every inflammatory dermatosis biopsy.

Trap Logic: Anchoring bias (premature closure on an initial pattern match), site- and stage-dependent pattern variation, and genuine combined or transitional patterns are the three recurring sources of pattern-assignment error; each is countered by deliberate, explicit checking rather than by abandoning pattern-based reasoning.

Pattern Anchor: A reaction pattern is a starting hypothesis to be actively tested against its mimickers, not a final answer reached the moment a plausible match is recognized.

Summary and Key Concepts

The pattern-based method organizes the hundreds of named inflammatory dermatoses into a small number of recurring tissue reaction patterns, reflecting the skin's limited structural repertoire for responding to diverse etiologic insults.

Expert diagnostic reasoning combines rapid pattern recognition with deliberate verification against mimickers; explicit trap logic is how this book operationalizes the verification step for trainees still building their own pattern library.

Eight major reaction patterns, spongiotic, psoriasiform, lichenoid/interface, vesiculobullous, granulomatous, vasculopathic, panniculitic, and sclerosing, each with a defining compartment and histologic feature, structure the chapters that follow.

A three-step sequence, pattern assignment, differential narrowing with pattern-specific secondary features, and integration with clinical information, is the practical application of the method to any inflammatory dermatosis biopsy.

Anchoring bias, site- and stage-dependent variation, and genuine pattern overlap are the three most common sources of diagnostic error in pattern assignment, and each is best countered by explicit, deliberate checking rather than avoided by abandoning the pattern-based approach.

CHAPTER 4: THE SPONGIOTIC REACTION PATTERN

Learning Objectives

1. Define the spongiotic reaction pattern and classify its major clinical subtypes.
2. Describe the etiologic mechanisms and clinical associations of the major spongiotic dermatoses.
3. Identify the histopathologic features and diagnostic criteria that distinguish the spongiotic subtypes from one another.
4. Correlate histologic findings with clinical presentation and apply clinicopathologic correlation to a spongiotic biopsy.
5. Construct a differential diagnosis for the spongiotic pattern and discriminate it from its major histologic mimickers.
6. Select appropriate ancillary studies and understand the management implications of a spongiotic diagnosis.

Definition and Classification

Defining the Spongiotic Pattern

The spongiotic reaction pattern, introduced conceptually in Chapters 1 and 3, is defined histologically by intercellular edema within the epidermis, most pronounced in the spinous layer, in which fluid accumulation widens the space between keratinocytes while their desmosomal attachments remain intact, producing a characteristic appearance of keratinocytes stretched apart but still tethered to one another by visible intercellular bridges. As fluid accumulation progresses, this widening can proceed to frank intraepidermal vesicle formation, in which pockets of fluid coalesce into discrete spaces still traversed by attenuated desmosomal connections, a feature that distinguishes spongiotic vesiculation from the acantholytic vesiculation of the pemphigus group discussed in Chapter 7, where desmosomal loss rather than fluid accumulation is the primary mechanism of keratinocyte separation.

The pattern is accompanied, in its typical form, by a superficial perivascular lymphocytic infiltrate within the papillary dermis, often admixed with eosinophils in proportions that vary meaningfully by etiology, and by exocytosis of lymphocytes into the spongiotic epidermis itself, visible as scattered individual lymphocytes migrating between keratinocytes toward the stratum corneum. The pattern is, as established in Chapter 3, shared across a family of clinically distinct diseases united by this common tissue response to a broad range of provoking stimuli, and the remainder of this chapter develops the specific features that allow the major spongiotic dermatoses to be distinguished from one another within this shared architectural framework.

Classification of the Major Spongiotic Subtypes

The spongiotic dermatoses are conventionally classified by presumed etiologic mechanism, a classification that, while imperfect, has genuine histologic correlates developed throughout this chapter. Allergic contact dermatitis results from a type IV, delayed-type hypersensitivity reaction to a specific external allergen following prior sensitization, and typically shows a comparatively brisk eosinophil-rich infiltrate. Irritant contact dermatitis results from direct chemical or physical injury to the epidermis without an immunologic sensitization step, and shows a pattern that can range from spongiotic to overtly necrotic depending on the severity and nature of the irritant, generally with fewer eosinophils than the allergic subtype. Atopic dermatitis, occurring in the context of the broader atopic diathesis, shows a comparatively lymphocyte-predominant infiltrate with a variable eosinophil component and, in chronic lesions, the lichenification changes discussed in Chapter 3. Nummular dermatitis presents as coin-shaped plaques with a histologic picture that overlaps substantially with both allergic contact and atopic dermatitis, and is frequently a descriptive rather than a mechanistically distinct diagnosis. Id reaction (autoeczematization) refers to a generalized spongiotic eruption occurring at a site distant from a primary inflammatory or infectious focus, believed to reflect a systemic immunologic response to that distant focus. Dyshidrotic (pompholyx) dermatitis, a site-specific variant occurring on the palms and soles, shows pronounced spongiosis and vesiculation modified by the thick acral stratum corneum discussed in Chapter 1, often producing deeper, more clinically apparent vesicles than spongiotic dermatitis at other sites.

Subtype	Presumed Mechanism	Typical Infiltrate Composition	Distinguishing Clinical Clue
Allergic contact dermatitis	Type IV hypersensitivity to external allergen	Eosinophil-rich	Geometric or linear distribution matching allergen contact
Irritant contact dermatitis	Direct chemical or physical injury	Variable, often fewer eosinophils	Distribution matches irritant exposure, no sensitization latency
Atopic dermatitis	Barrier dysfunction with immune dysregulation	Lymphocyte-predominant, variable eosinophils	Flexural distribution, personal or family atopic history
Nummular dermatitis	Overlapping with contact and atopic mechanisms	Variable	Coin-shaped, well-demarcated plaques
Id reaction	Systemic response to a distant inflammatory focus	Lymphocyte-predominant	Generalized eruption with an identifiable primary focus elsewhere
Dyshidrotic (pompholyx) dermatitis	Multifactorial, site-specific	Lymphocyte-predominant with vesiculation	Deep-seated vesicles confined to palms and soles

The Spectrum From Contact Reaction to Systemic Eruption

The classification presented above is organized along a spectrum from the most externally localized processes (contact dermatitis, in which the trigger is applied directly to the skin at a specific site) to the most internally driven and generalized processes (atopic dermatitis and id reaction, in which an endogenous predisposition or a distant inflammatory focus produces a widespread eruption without a localized external trigger). This spectrum is a genuinely useful organizing concept for the differential diagnosis of any individual spongiotic biopsy, because the clinical distribution pattern, localized and geometric versus widespread and symmetric, tracks reasonably well with position along this spectrum and is often available to the pathologist even when detailed exposure history is not. A biopsy accompanied by a clinical photograph or a clear distribution description showing a sharply demarcated patch corresponding to a watchband, earring, or article of clothing sits confidently at the contact end of the spectrum, while a biopsy accompanied by a description of widespread, symmetric involvement of flexural creases sits confidently at the atopic end, and this positioning, established before histologic review even begins, usefully primes the specific secondary features the reader should look for at the microscope.

Nummular dermatitis and dyshidrotic dermatitis occupy an intermediate position on this spectrum in a specific and clinically useful sense: both are defined primarily by their distinctive clinical morphology, coin-shaped plaques for nummular dermatitis and deep-seated acral vesicles for dyshidrotic dermatitis, rather than by a specific presumed external trigger or a specific systemic predisposition, and both can occur as an idiopathic process or as a morphologic variant superimposed on an underlying atopic or contact-related process. This intermediate positioning is a reminder that the classification scheme presented in this chapter, like the broader eight-pattern framework discussed in Chapter 3, is a highly useful organizing tool rather than a set of mutually exclusive, biologically airtight categories, and a biopsy showing nummular morphology in a patient with an established atopic history is reasonably interpreted as an atopic dermatitis variant rather than as a wholly separate diagnostic entity requiring independent workup.

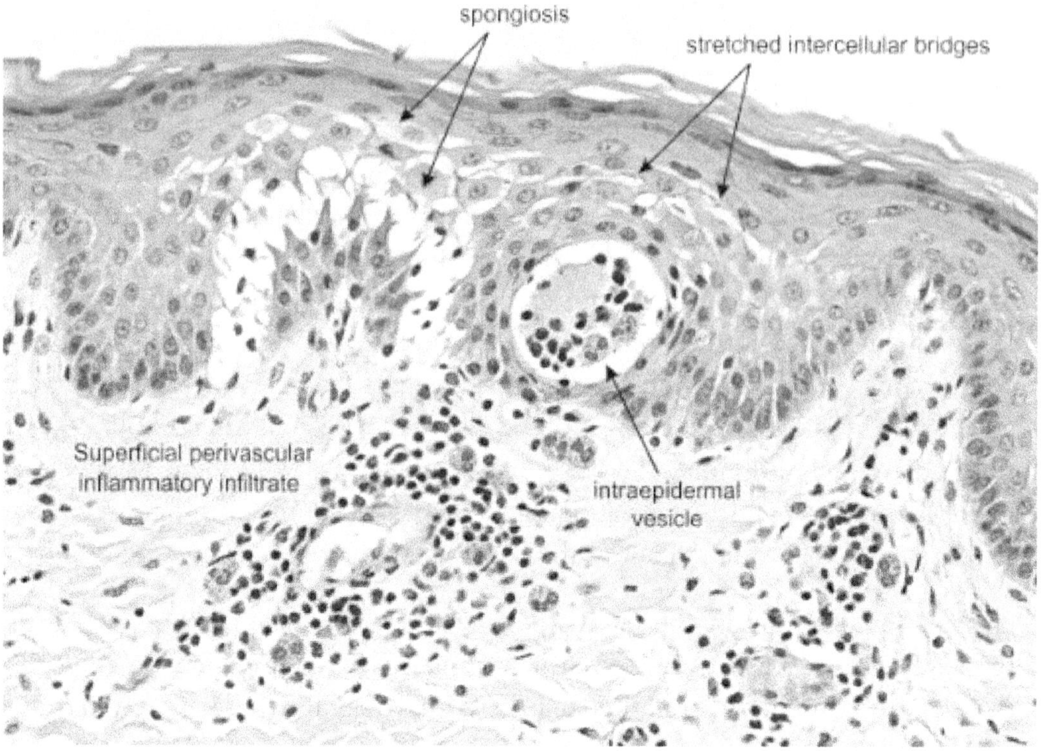

Etiology and Clinical Associations

Allergens, Irritants, and Sensitization

Allergic contact dermatitis requires a prior sensitization event, in which an external hapten binds cutaneous proteins and is processed by Langerhans cells to generate allergen-specific memory T cells, so that clinical disease manifests only on re-exposure, typically forty-eight to seventy-two hours after contact in a previously sensitized individual. Common allergens encountered in dermatopathology practice include nickel, fragrance and preservative components of topical products, rubber accelerators, and, increasingly, components of topical medications themselves, including topical corticosteroids and antibiotics, a circumstance in which the treatment for one dermatitis becomes the trigger for a superimposed contact dermatitis, a clinically important and sometimes underrecognized scenario. Patch testing, performed by the referring clinician rather than the dermatopathologist, remains the diagnostic gold standard for confirming a specific allergen, and the biopsy's role is primarily to confirm the spongiotic pattern and reasonably exclude alternative diagnoses rather than to identify the specific allergen itself, a limitation the report should state clearly.

The Atopic Diathesis and Barrier Dysfunction

Atopic dermatitis reflects a combination of epidermal barrier dysfunction, frequently related to filaggrin gene mutations that impair stratum corneum structural integrity, and a predisposition toward a T helper type 2-skewed immune response, together producing a chronic, relapsing spongiotic dermatitis with a strong tendency toward flexural distribution and a frequent personal or family history of atopy, including asthma and allergic rhinitis. The chronicity of atopic dermatitis means that biopsies obtained from longstanding lesions frequently show the lichenification changes discussed in Chapter 3, superimposing epidermal hyperplasia on a background of persistent, if diminished, spongiosis, and a biopsy obtained specifically to confirm atopic dermatitis in a patient with a classic clinical presentation is relatively uncommon in practice, since the diagnosis is usually made clinically; biopsy is more often obtained when the clinical picture is atypical or when a superimposed process (secondary infection, allergic contact dermatitis to a treatment, or, in the appropriate clinical context, early cutaneous lymphoma) is being specifically excluded.

Systemic and Drug-Related Associations

Systemic drug reactions can produce a spongiotic pattern as one of several possible morphologic presentations of cutaneous drug hypersensitivity, and a spongiotic drug eruption typically shows a somewhat more diffuse and symmetric distribution than allergic contact dermatitis, without the geometric or linear configuration that contact exposure often produces, alongside a comparatively prominent eosinophil-rich infiltrate. Id reactions, as introduced above, illustrate a distinct systemic association: a spongiotic eruption at a site remote from an active dermatophyte infection, venous stasis dermatitis, or other primary inflammatory focus reflects an immunologic response to that distant process rather than a direct local insult, and recognizing this association, primarily through the clinical history rather than the biopsy alone, is essential to directing treatment toward the primary focus rather than the secondary eruption.

Occupational and Environmental Exposure Patterns

Occupational allergic and irritant contact dermatitis together account for a substantial share of work-related skin disease and merit specific mention because the diagnostic and reporting considerations differ somewhat from sporadic, non-occupational contact dermatitis. Healthcare workers face frequent irritant exposure from hand hygiene products and, less commonly, allergic sensitization to rubber accelerators in gloves or to specific medications handled without adequate barrier protection; hairdressers and cosmetologists face sensitization risk from hair dye components, particularly para-phenylenediamine, and from persulfate bleaching agents; and construction and metalworking trades face both irritant exposure from cement and solvents and allergic sensitization to chromate and nickel. A biopsy in a patient with an occupational exposure history showing a spongiotic pattern with a distribution corresponding to areas of occupational contact (hands, forearms, or a site corresponding to protective equipment) should prompt the report to note this correlation explicitly, since a confirmed occupational allergic contact dermatitis carries workers' compensation and workplace modification implications beyond the immediate clinical management of the eruption itself.

Photoallergic and phototoxic contact dermatitis represent a further environmentally modified subset, in which a topically applied or, less commonly, systemically administered agent produces a spongiotic reaction only in combination with ultraviolet light exposure, typically confined to sun-exposed skin with relative sparing of covered areas such as the upper eyelids, the area under the chin, and skin covered by clothing or a wristwatch. Recognizing this photo-distributed pattern clinically, and correlating it with medication history (certain diuretics, tetracyclines, and nonsteroidal anti-inflammatory drugs are common phototoxic culprits) or topical product history (certain sunscreen ingredients and fragrance components are recognized photoallergens), is largely a clinical rather than histologic exercise, though the biopsy confirms the underlying spongiotic pattern and can help exclude alternative photodistributed processes such as polymorphous light eruption or cutaneous lupus erythematosus.

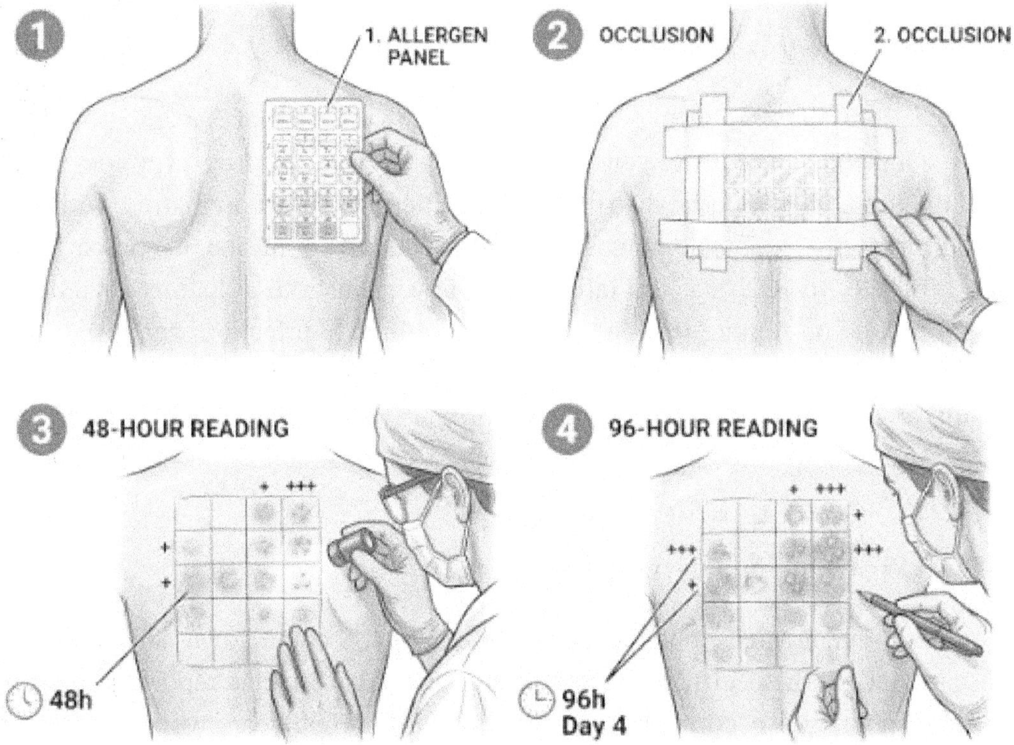

THE REACTION PATTERN RECOGNITION SYSTEM — Eosinophil-Rich Spongiotic Dermatitis

The Pattern: Eosinophil-Rich Spongiotic Dermatitis as an Early Clue to Allergic Contact Dermatitis or Drug Reaction

Histologic Signature: Spongiotic dermatitis with a superficial perivascular infiltrate in which eosinophils constitute a substantial proportion of the inflammatory cells, sometimes with eosinophils extending into the spongiotic epidermis itself.

The Decision: A prominent eosinophilic component should prompt specific consideration of allergic contact dermatitis or a drug reaction over atopic or irritant dermatitis, and should be explicitly noted in the report given its relevance to the clinician's subsequent allergen or medication investigation.

Trap Logic: The mimicker is early bullous pemphigoid, introduced in Chapter 3, which can present as eosinophilic spongiosis before frank subepidermal blister formation. The discriminating feature is clinical: an elderly patient with tense bullae developing over an urticarial background should prompt direct immunofluorescence to exclude early pemphigoid, even when the biopsy alone shows only a spongiotic pattern.

Pattern Anchor: Eosinophil-rich spongiosis in an elderly patient is eosinophilic spongiosis of bullous pemphigoid until proven otherwise; confirm with clinical correlation and, when appropriate, direct immunofluorescence before settling on a purely eczematous diagnosis.

Histopathologic Features and Diagnostic Criteria

Acute Spongiotic Dermatitis

The acute stage of spongiotic dermatitis, corresponding to a clinically recent eruption, shows the most pronounced degree of intercellular edema, often with microvesicle formation, minimal to absent parakeratosis, and a normal or only mildly thickened stratum corneum, since insufficient time has elapsed for the epidermal hyperplasia of chronic disease to develop. The papillary dermis shows edema in addition to the perivascular inflammatory infiltrate, occasionally prominent enough to produce dermal papillary widening visible at low power, and exocytosis of inflammatory cells, particularly eosinophils in the allergic and drug-related subtypes, into the epidermis is often most conspicuous at this stage.

Subacute and Chronic Spongiotic Dermatitis

As spongiotic dermatitis persists or recurs, the histologic picture evolves in a stereotyped direction: spongiosis becomes progressively less pronounced, parakeratosis develops and increases, and epidermal hyperplasia (acanthosis) with elongation of the rete ridges develops, producing the lichenification changes and psoriasiform overlap discussed in Chapter 3. This evolution means that the specific histologic stage of a spongiotic biopsy, acute, subacute, or chronic, correlates imperfectly but meaningfully with the clinical duration of the lesion, and stating the histologic stage explicitly in the report provides useful information to the treating clinician about how the observed histology relates to the clinical timeline, particularly when clinical duration and histologic stage appear discordant, a discrepancy that can itself carry diagnostic significance.

Follicular and Site-Specific Variants

Spongiosis can localize preferentially to the follicular infundibulum rather than the interfollicular epidermis, producing follicular spongiotic dermatitis (spongiotic folliculitis), a pattern seen in a subset of atopic dermatitis presentations, particularly in patients with a follicular-predominant clinical morphology, and in some drug eruptions. Palmoplantar dyshidrotic dermatitis, as introduced above, shows spongiosis modified by the markedly thickened acral stratum corneum discussed in Chapter 1, producing deeper, more clinically apparent vesicles that can require a somewhat different histologic threshold for recognition than spongiosis at thinner-skinned sites, underscoring again the general principle that site-appropriate baseline expectations must inform interpretation of any reaction pattern.

Quantifying and Communicating Severity

Beyond staging a spongiotic biopsy as acute, subacute, or chronic, several additional histologic features carry information about disease severity that is useful to communicate in the report. The extent of intraepidermal vesiculation, ranging from subtle intercellular widening to confluent microvesicle or frank vesicle formation, correlates reasonably well with the clinical severity of the acute eruption and can help the treating clinician gauge whether the biopsied lesion represents a mild or a more significant flare. The density of the dermal inflammatory infiltrate and the degree of papillary dermal edema similarly provide a rough severity gauge, and a biopsy showing unusually marked papillary dermal edema, sometimes progressing to subepidermal vesiculation from edema alone, should be distinguished from a primary subepidermal blistering process by the accompanying spongiotic epidermal changes and the absence of the specific direct immunofluorescence findings discussed in Chapter 2.

Secondary changes resulting from scratching or rubbing, excoriation with resultant epidermal erosion, superficial hemorrhage, and serum crust, are common in symptomatic spongiotic dermatoses given the pruritic nature of most entities in this category, and their presence or absence provides an indirect but clinically relevant indicator of symptom severity and duration. A biopsy showing extensive excoriation change should prompt consideration of whether the excoriation itself, rather than the underlying spongiotic process, is contributing meaningfully to the clinical picture, particularly in patients with an underlying psychodermatologic component to their pruritus, a consideration that falls outside the scope of the histologic diagnosis itself but that the report can appropriately flag when the excoriation change is disproportionate to the underlying inflammatory findings.

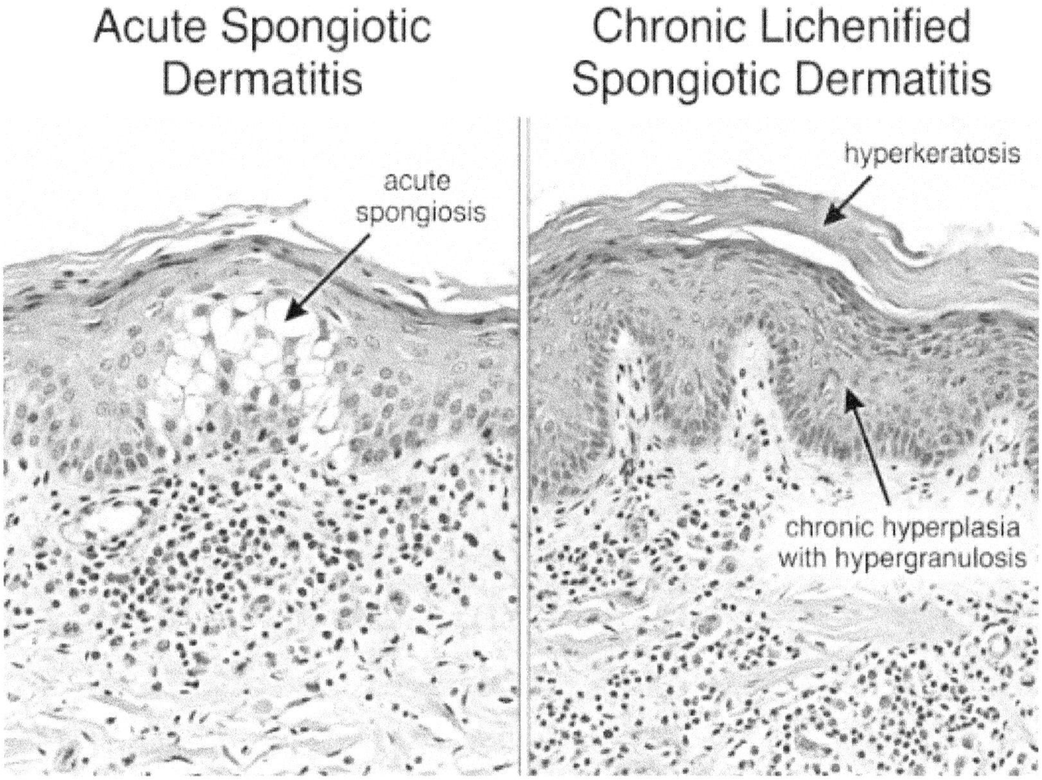

Clinical Presentation and Clinicopathologic Correlation

Morphology and Distribution as Diagnostic Clues

Clinical morphology and distribution carry substantial diagnostic weight in the spongiotic dermatoses precisely because, as established above, histology alone frequently cannot distinguish among the major subtypes with confidence. A geometric, linear, or otherwise non-anatomic distribution strongly favors an external contact exposure (allergic or irritant) over an endogenous process, since the human body does not spontaneously produce disease in a straight line, while a flexural distribution in a patient with an atopic history favors atopic dermatitis, and a generalized, symmetric distribution following an identifiable primary infectious or inflammatory focus favors an id reaction. This is the practical application of the clinicopathologic correlation principle introduced in Chapter 1: the biopsy establishes the reaction pattern and stage with confidence, while the specific clinical distribution and history most reliably resolve the differential among the pattern's constituent diagnoses.

The Role of the Pathology Report in Guiding Clinical Workup

Because definitive subtyping frequently requires clinical information the pathologist may not have at the time of interpretation, a well-constructed spongiotic dermatitis report actively guides the treating clinician's subsequent workup rather than simply naming a pattern. Noting the presence and degree of eosinophilia, the histologic stage (acute versus chronic), and any features favoring a specific subtype over others gives the clinician concrete information to weigh against the clinical presentation, and explicitly recommending patch testing when an eosinophil-rich pattern raises allergic contact dermatitis as a leading consideration is a direct, clinically actionable contribution the report can make beyond simply stating "spongiotic dermatitis, clinical correlation recommended."

CLINICAL PEARL: The single most useful piece of clinical information for a spongiotic dermatitis biopsy is often the simplest: what does the lesion look like, and where is it. A description of morphology and distribution, more than an extensive review of systems, most efficiently narrows the spongiotic differential.

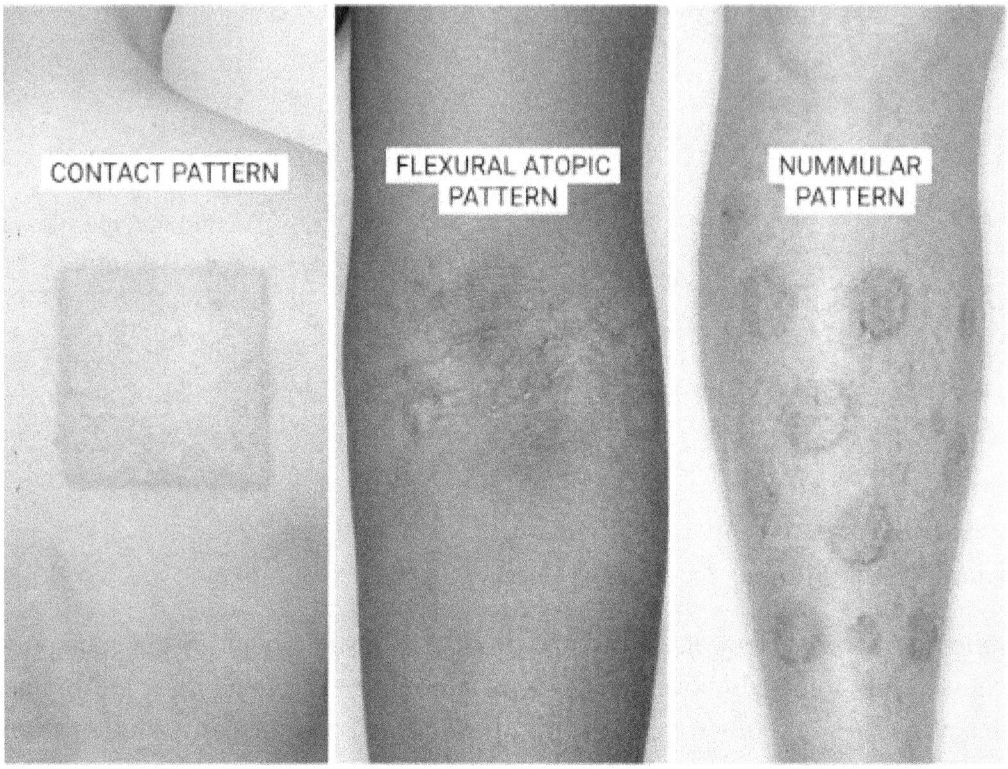

Age-Specific Presentations

The spongiotic dermatoses show meaningful age-dependent variation in both prevalence and typical distribution that further informs clinicopathologic correlation. Infantile atopic dermatitis characteristically involves the face, scalp, and extensor extremities, a distribution that shifts toward the classic flexural pattern (antecubital and popliteal fossae, neck, and wrists) by later childhood and adulthood, so that a spongiotic biopsy from an infant with facial or scalp involvement is entirely consistent with atopic dermatitis despite not showing the flexural distribution a clinician might otherwise expect from the adult-onset literature. Nummular dermatitis and dyshidrotic dermatitis both show a broader adult age distribution without the same infantile predominance, and irritant contact dermatitis of the hands shows an occupational-age predominance reflecting the working population most exposed to relevant irritants, considerations that together mean patient age itself, provided on the requisition, is a further useful piece of clinical context for narrowing the spongiotic differential alongside morphology and distribution.

Geriatric patients present a further specific consideration: asteatotic dermatitis (xerotic eczema), reflecting age-related and often environmentally exacerbated reduction in epidermal barrier lipid content, produces a spongiotic pattern that can be difficult to distinguish histologically from mild atopic or irritant dermatitis, and is most reliably identified through the clinical context of a shin- or trunk-predominant, dry, cracked ("crazy-paving") morphology in an older patient, often with a seasonal winter predominance related to low ambient humidity. Stasis dermatitis, occurring on the lower extremities of patients with chronic venous insufficiency, similarly produces a spongiotic pattern but is accompanied by the dermal changes of chronic venous hypertension, including dermal fibrosis, hemosiderin deposition, and often a proliferation of small thick-walled vessels, features that extend beyond the epidermal spongiotic pattern itself and that the report should note when present, since they support the venous etiology and distinguish the process from a primary idiopathic eczematous dermatitis.

Differential Diagnosis and Histologic Mimickers

A Worked Example: Resolving an Ambiguous Eosinophilic Spongiotic Biopsy

A 72-year-old patient presents with a two-week history of pruritic, erythematous patches on the trunk and proximal extremities, without clinically evident blisters, and a punch biopsy is submitted with a clinical differential of drug eruption versus atopic dermatitis. Applying the three-step sequence introduced in Chapter 3, pattern assignment at low power identifies a spongiotic pattern with a superficial perivascular infiltrate rich in eosinophils, some of which extend into the epidermis. Differential narrowing considers the specific secondary features relevant to this pattern: the patient's age (seventy-two), the eosinophil-predominant infiltrate, and the absence of a clear geometric or occupational contact history together shift the differential away from allergic contact dermatitis and toward either a drug reaction or early bullous pemphigoid, per the Rhythm block trap logic developed above.

The third step, diagnosis, requires clinical correlation that the biopsy alone cannot supply: has the patient started a new medication in the preceding weeks, and is there any history, even subtle, of tense blistering or an urticarial background to the eruption. In this hypothetical case, the treating clinician confirms that the patient started a new antihypertensive medication one month prior and has noted no blistering, favoring a drug-induced spongiotic eruption over bullous pemphigoid, though the report appropriately recommends clinical follow-up and, should any blistering subsequently develop, a repeat biopsy with direct immunofluorescence to definitively exclude evolving pemphigoid. This worked example illustrates a recurring principle of this chapter: the histologic pattern (eosinophil-rich spongiosis) narrows the differential substantially but does not, by itself, resolve the specific etiology in an elderly patient, where the stakes of missing early pemphigoid are clinically significant enough to warrant an explicitly stated safety-net recommendation even when the initial clinical correlation favors a more benign explanation.

Distinguishing Spongiotic Dermatitis From Psoriasiform Disease

As developed extensively in Chapter 3, chronic lichenified spongiotic dermatitis can closely mimic the psoriasiform pattern, and the discriminating features, hypergranulosis versus diminished granular layer, residual spongiosis versus its absence, and the composition of the inflammatory infiltrate, remain the primary tools for resolving this overlap when it occurs in the spongiotic dermatoses specifically. A biopsy showing genuinely ambiguous features between chronic spongiotic dermatitis and psoriasis should be reported with both possibilities explicitly named, per the diagnostic honesty principle established in Chapter 3, rather than forced toward one diagnosis based on a single dominant low-power impression.

Distinguishing Spongiotic Dermatitis From Early Immunobullous Disease

As illustrated in the Rhythm block above, eosinophilic spongiosis can represent an early or evolving stage of bullous pemphigoid rather than a primary eczematous process, and this distinction carries substantial clinical weight, since bullous pemphigoid requires a fundamentally different management approach than allergic contact or atopic dermatitis. Beyond the clinical clues discussed above (elderly patient, urticarial background, evolution toward tense bullae), a low threshold for correlating an eosinophil-rich spongiotic biopsy with the full clinical picture, and for pursuing direct immunofluorescence when that picture is even moderately suggestive of pemphigoid, is the most reliable safeguard against this specific and clinically consequential mimicker.

Distinguishing Spongiotic Dermatitis From Dermatophyte Infection

Superficial dermatophyte infection (tinea) can itself produce a spongiotic dermatitis in the epidermis underlying the infected stratum corneum, reflecting an inflammatory response to the fungal organisms and their metabolic products, so that a biopsy showing spongiotic dermatitis with a prominent neutrophilic component within the stratum corneum, or with a pattern described by the sandwich sign (parakeratosis both above and below a zone of more normal-appearing stratum corneum, reflecting episodic shedding and regrowth of infected keratin), should prompt a PAS-D special stain, as discussed in Chapter 2, to specifically exclude a fungal etiology before a purely eczematous diagnosis is finalized. This is a clinically important mimicker to exclude specifically because the treatment implications diverge sharply: topical corticosteroids, a mainstay of eczematous dermatitis management, can worsen an unrecognized dermatophyte infection.

Distinguishing Spongiotic Dermatitis From Miliaria and Other Sweat-Related Eruptions

Miliaria, resulting from eccrine duct obstruction and subsequent leakage of sweat into the surrounding epidermis or dermis, can produce a histologic picture that overlaps with spongiotic dermatitis, particularly miliaria rubra, in which duct obstruction at the level of the mid-epidermis produces spongiotic change and an accompanying inflammatory infiltrate concentrated around the obstructed eccrine duct rather than diffusely distributed as in a typical eczematous process. The distinguishing histologic feature is this periductal, rather than diffuse, distribution of both the spongiosis and the associated infiltrate, best appreciated by specifically tracing an eccrine duct through the section and assessing whether the epidermal changes are concentrated immediately around it; clinically, miliaria typically presents in the context of heat, occlusion, or fever, a history that further supports this diagnosis over a primary eczematous process.

Distinguishing Spongiotic Dermatitis From Early Pityriasis Rosea and Other Papulosquamous Mimickers

Pityriasis rosea, a self-limited papulosquamous eruption believed to follow a viral trigger, can show a histologic picture combining mild spongiosis with focal parakeratosis and a superficial perivascular lymphocytic infiltrate, occasionally with extravasated erythrocytes in the papillary dermis, a combination that can overlap with a mild or resolving spongiotic dermatitis. The clinical presentation, a herald patch followed by a generalized eruption of oval, scaly plaques with a characteristic "Christmas tree" distribution along skin cleavage lines on the trunk, is usually sufficiently distinctive to resolve the diagnosis even when the histologic findings alone are nonspecific, again illustrating the recurring theme of this chapter that the spongiotic pattern and its close mimickers are frequently better resolved through careful clinical correlation than through histology in isolation.

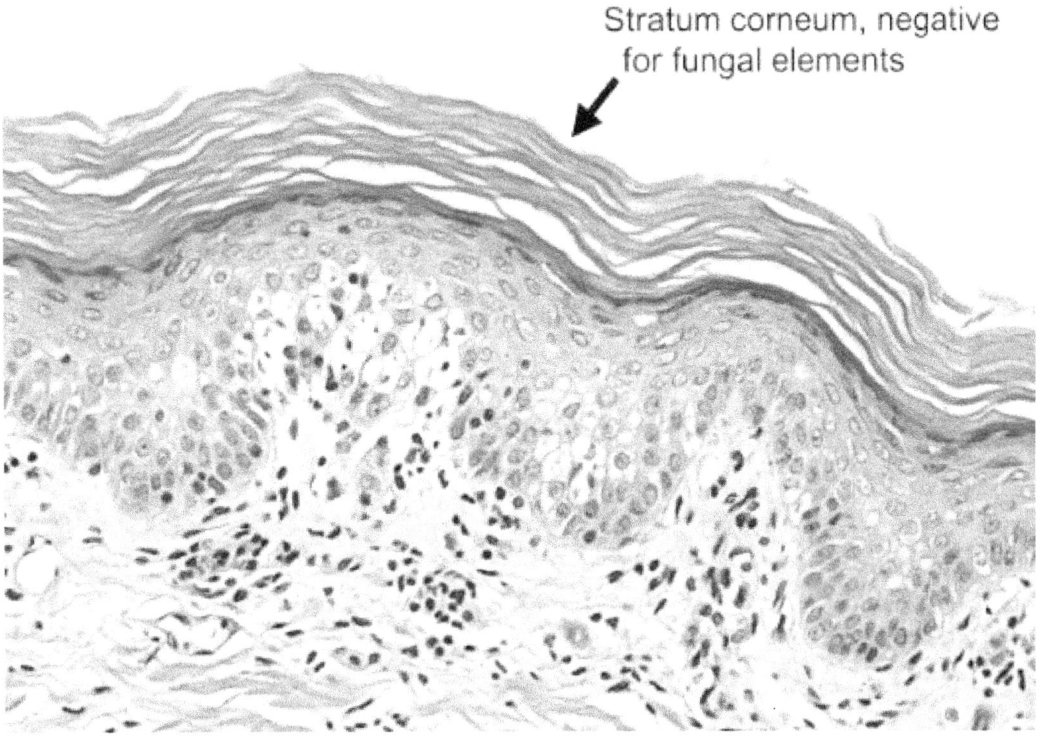

Ancillary Studies

Special Stains in the Spongiotic Workup

As discussed above, PAS-D staining is the primary ancillary study relevant to the spongiotic pattern, specifically to exclude dermatophyte infection when clinical or histologic features raise this possibility, including a neutrophil-rich component within the stratum corneum, a sandwich sign, or a clinical presentation with an annular, expanding morphology suggestive of tinea. Beyond this specific indication, special stains play a limited role in the routine workup of an otherwise typical spongiotic dermatitis, consistent with the hypothesis-driven approach to special stain ordering developed in Chapter 2.

The Limited Role of Immunohistochemistry

Immunohistochemistry is not routinely required for the diagnosis of spongiotic dermatitis, since the diagnosis rests on architectural and cytologic features assessable on routine hematoxylin and eosin staining. The principal circumstance in which immunohistochemistry becomes relevant is when a spongiotic-pattern biopsy raises concern for early or patch-stage mycosis fungoides, discussed fully in Chapter 18, in which case a T-cell immunophenotypic panel and, when appropriate, clonality studies as discussed in Chapter 2 may be pursued; this circumstance is more often prompted by an atypical or treatment-refractory clinical course than by the spongiotic pattern in isolation, since early mycosis fungoides can present with subtle findings that do not always meet the classic criteria (marked epidermotropism with disproportionately little spongiosis, atypical lymphocytes with cerebriform nuclei) that would immediately distinguish it from a routine eczematous process.

CAUTION: A treatment-refractory spongiotic dermatitis, particularly in an older adult, warrants specific consideration of early mycosis fungoides and, when clinically appropriate, a repeat biopsy with immunohistochemical and molecular workup rather than an assumption that the original diagnosis was simply undertreated.

Direct Immunofluorescence in the Spongiotic Workup

Direct immunofluorescence, discussed extensively in Chapter 2, is not a routine component of the spongiotic dermatitis workup but becomes directly relevant in the specific circumstance already discussed above: eosinophil-rich spongiosis in a clinical context suggestive of early bullous pemphigoid. In this scenario, a perilesional biopsy submitted specifically for direct immunofluorescence, in addition to the routine lesional biopsy showing the spongiotic pattern, can identify the linear IgG and C3 deposition at the dermal-epidermal junction that confirms pemphigoid before frank subepidermal blistering develops, allowing earlier initiation of appropriate immunosuppressive therapy than would be possible if the diagnosis were deferred until classic bullae appeared. Communicating this specific recommendation, rather than a generic suggestion for "further workup as clinically indicated," is a concrete way the report can add value in a diagnostically ambiguous eosinophilic spongiotic case.

Correlating Ancillary Findings With the Overall Clinical Picture

As with every ancillary study discussed in Chapter 2, the results of any special stain, immunohistochemical panel, or molecular test obtained in the spongiotic workup are most usefully interpreted as one component of an integrated diagnostic picture rather than as a standalone answer. A negative PAS-D stain in a clinically atypical, treatment-refractory eruption does not exclude all infectious or infestation-related etiologies (scabies, for example, requires a different diagnostic approach entirely, seeking the mite, ova, or fecal pellets rather than fungal organisms), and a negative T-cell clonality study does not exclude early mycosis fungoides given the sensitivity limitations discussed in Chapter 2. The consistent discipline of stating explicitly what a given ancillary result does and does not resolve, rather than allowing a negative result to be read as a blanket exclusion, protects both the accuracy of the report and the clinical decision-making that follows from it.

Management Implications

Connecting Diagnosis to Treatment Pathway

The specific spongiotic subtype identified, or the differential diagnosis stated when a single subtype cannot be confirmed, directly shapes the treating clinician's management approach. Allergic contact dermatitis management centers on allergen identification through patch testing and subsequent avoidance, an approach that differs fundamentally from the barrier repair and anti-inflammatory strategies that anchor atopic dermatitis management, and from the trigger-focused approach relevant to id reactions, in which treating the distant primary process is often necessary for the secondary eruption to resolve. A pathology report that clearly communicates the histologic findings most relevant to distinguishing among these pathways, rather than a generic diagnosis of spongiotic dermatitis alone, materially assists the treating clinician in selecting the most efficient management strategy for the individual patient.

When Histology Should Prompt Reconsideration of the Clinical Diagnosis

Occasionally, histologic findings diverge meaningfully from the clinical impression stated on the requisition, and the report should communicate this divergence directly rather than simply confirming a pattern consistent with, but not specific for, the submitted clinical diagnosis. A biopsy submitted with a clinical diagnosis of atopic dermatitis that instead shows a prominent eosinophil-rich infiltrate with a distribution history suggestive of a specific product exposure should prompt the report to explicitly raise allergic contact dermatitis as an alternative or additional consideration, since this specific redirection, communicated clearly rather than buried in a lengthy differential, is often what allows a patient with a longstanding, previously mismanaged eruption to finally receive an effective, correctly targeted treatment.

Longitudinal Management and the Role of Repeat Biopsy

Spongiotic dermatitis is, for most patients, a chronic or recurrent condition rather than a single self-limited episode, and this longitudinal course has specific implications for how repeat biopsies, when obtained, should be interpreted relative to a patient's prior biopsy history. A repeat biopsy obtained during a flare in a patient with an established diagnosis of atopic dermatitis is typically obtained not to reconfirm the underlying diagnosis but to specifically exclude a superimposed process, most commonly secondary infection (bacterial, viral, or fungal), a superimposed allergic contact dermatitis to a treatment being used, or, in a treatment-refractory or atypical case, early cutaneous lymphoma as discussed above. Framing the diagnostic question explicitly in the report, stating what specifically was and was not addressed by the current biopsy relative to the patient's known underlying diagnosis, is more useful to a treating clinician managing a chronic relapsing patient than a report that treats each biopsy as an isolated, context-free specimen.

Treatment response itself carries diagnostic information that can retrospectively inform the interpretation of an earlier biopsy, and dermatopathologists benefit from remaining open to this feedback loop when it is available, for example through a clinical note accompanying a subsequent specimen or a direct communication from the treating clinician. A spongiotic dermatitis that fails to respond to appropriate topical anti-inflammatory therapy and allergen avoidance should prompt reconsideration of the original differential, including the mimickers discussed throughout this chapter, rather than an assumption that the original diagnosis was correct and the treatment simply inadequate; this principle, treating diagnosis as provisional and open to revision in light of clinical course, is a recurring theme that will return throughout the inflammatory dermatoses covered in the chapters that follow.

THE REACTION PATTERN RECOGNITION SYSTEM — The Spongiotic Pattern Family

---

The Pattern: The spongiotic reaction pattern and its major clinical subtypes: allergic and irritant contact dermatitis, atopic dermatitis, nummular dermatitis, id reaction, and dyshidrotic dermatitis.

Histologic Signature: Intercellular epidermal edema with preserved desmosomal attachments, superficial perivascular lymphocytic infiltrate with variable eosinophils, and a stereotyped evolution from acute (marked spongiosis, minimal hyperplasia) to chronic (diminished spongiosis, hyperkeratosis, hypergranulosis, epidermal hyperplasia).

The Decision: Assign the spongiotic pattern and its histologic stage, characterize the inflammatory infiltrate composition, and integrate with clinical morphology and distribution to narrow the differential among the pattern's constituent diagnoses.

Trap Logic: Chronic lichenified spongiotic dermatitis can mimic the psoriasiform pattern; eosinophil-rich spongiosis can represent early bullous pemphigoid; dermatophyte infection can produce a secondary spongiotic pattern. Each mimicker is resolved by a specific discriminating step: assessing granular layer status and residual spongiosis, correlating with clinical bullous disease features, and performing a PAS-D stain, respectively.

Pattern Anchor: Eosinophil-rich spongiosis in an elderly patient is pemphigoid until clinically excluded; treatment-refractory spongiotic dermatitis warrants consideration of mycosis fungoides; a neutrophil-rich or sandwich-sign spongiotic pattern warrants a PAS-D stain before an eczematous diagnosis is finalized.

Summary and Key Concepts

The spongiotic reaction pattern is defined by intercellular epidermal edema with preserved desmosomal attachments, and encompasses allergic and irritant contact dermatitis, atopic dermatitis, nummular dermatitis, id reaction, and dyshidrotic dermatitis as its major clinical subtypes.

The pattern evolves in a stereotyped way from acute (marked spongiosis, minimal hyperplasia) to chronic (diminished spongiosis, hyperkeratosis, hypergranulosis, epidermal hyperplasia), and the histologic stage should be stated explicitly in the report.

Clinical morphology and distribution, rather than histology alone, most reliably distinguish among the spongiotic subtypes, reflecting the shared tissue response that defines the pattern.

Eosinophil-rich spongiosis, chronic lichenified spongiotic dermatitis, and dermatophyte-associated spongiotic change are the three most important mimickers to actively exclude, corresponding respectively to early bullous pemphigoid, psoriasiform disease, and tinea infection.

The pathology report's specific characterization of infiltrate composition, histologic stage, and features favoring a specific subtype directly and materially guides the treating clinician's subsequent workup and management pathway.

CHAPTER 5: THE PSORIASIFORM REACTION PATTERN

Learning Objectives

1. Define the psoriasiform reaction pattern and classify its major clinical subtypes and mimickers.
2. Describe the immunopathogenesis of psoriasis and the mechanisms underlying non-psoriatic psoriasiform conditions.
3. Identify the histopathologic features and diagnostic criteria of psoriasis and distinguish evolving from fully developed lesions.
4. Correlate histologic findings with clinical morphology, distribution, and systemic associations including psoriatic arthritis.
5. Construct a differential diagnosis for the psoriasiform pattern and discriminate psoriasis from its major histologic mimickers.
6. Select appropriate ancillary studies and understand how histologic findings inform the psoriasis management pathway.

Definition and Classification

Defining the Psoriasiform Pattern

The psoriasiform reaction pattern, introduced in Chapters 1 and 3, is defined by regular, elongated epidermal hyperplasia in which the rete ridges extend downward in a uniform, test-tube-in-a-rack configuration, accompanied by thinning of the suprapapillary epidermal plate directly overlying the tips of the dermal papillae. This regularity of rete elongation distinguishes the psoriasiform pattern from the irregular epidermal hyperplasia seen in other contexts, such as a verrucous or papillomatous neoplasm, and reflects a specific, accelerated keratinocyte proliferation program rather than a nonspecific reactive thickening of the epidermis.

The pattern is further defined by its characteristic cornification abnormality: parakeratosis, the retention of nuclei within the stratum corneum, reflecting a keratinocyte transit time so accelerated that the normal several-week maturation program compresses to a matter of days, insufficient for complete nuclear degradation before the cell reaches the skin surface. This accelerated transit is also responsible for the diminished or absent granular layer characteristic of the pattern, since the keratohyalin granule synthesis that defines the stratum granulosum requires more time than the compressed psoriasiform maturation program allows, a mechanistic link between the pattern's two most visually distinctive features, parakeratosis and granular layer loss, that is worth holding explicitly in mind rather than treating as two independent, coincidentally co-occurring findings.

Classification of Psoriasiform Diseases

Psoriasis vulgaris, the prototype and most common member of this pattern family, presents as well-demarcated, erythematous plaques with silvery scale, typically favoring extensor surfaces, the scalp, and the gluteal cleft, and accounts for the great majority of psoriasiform biopsies encountered in routine practice. Guttate psoriasis presents as numerous small, drop-like papules and plaques, often erupting abruptly following a streptococcal pharyngeal infection, and shows a histologic picture that can be less fully developed than chronic plaque psoriasis given its typically more acute onset. Pustular psoriasis, encompassing both localized (palmoplantar) and generalized (von Zumbusch) forms, adds a prominent neutrophilic component to the psoriasiform architecture, with subcorneal pustules that can be substantial enough to dominate the histologic picture. Erythrodermic psoriasis, a generalized, severe variant potentially complicated by significant systemic morbidity including fluid and electrolyte disturbance, can show a somewhat less specific psoriasiform picture given the diffuse, confluent nature of the process.

Beyond psoriasis itself, the psoriasiform pattern encompasses a family of related conditions united by the shared architectural response but distinguished by specific etiologic and histologic features developed throughout this chapter. Pityriasis rubra pilaris, a distinct papulosquamous disorder with a characteristic islands-of-sparing clinical pattern, produces a psoriasiform histology with several specific discriminating features from true psoriasis. Chronic dermatophytosis (tinea) can produce a psoriasiform pattern through prolonged low-grade epidermal irritation by fungal organisms, and, as discussed in Chapter 4 in the context of the spongiotic pattern, requires special stain exclusion before a purely inflammatory psoriasiform diagnosis is finalized. Psoriasiform drug eruptions, seborrheic dermatitis in its more chronic and hyperplastic presentations, and, in the appropriate clinical context, early or patch-stage mycosis fungoides with a psoriasiform architecture round out the differential this chapter develops.

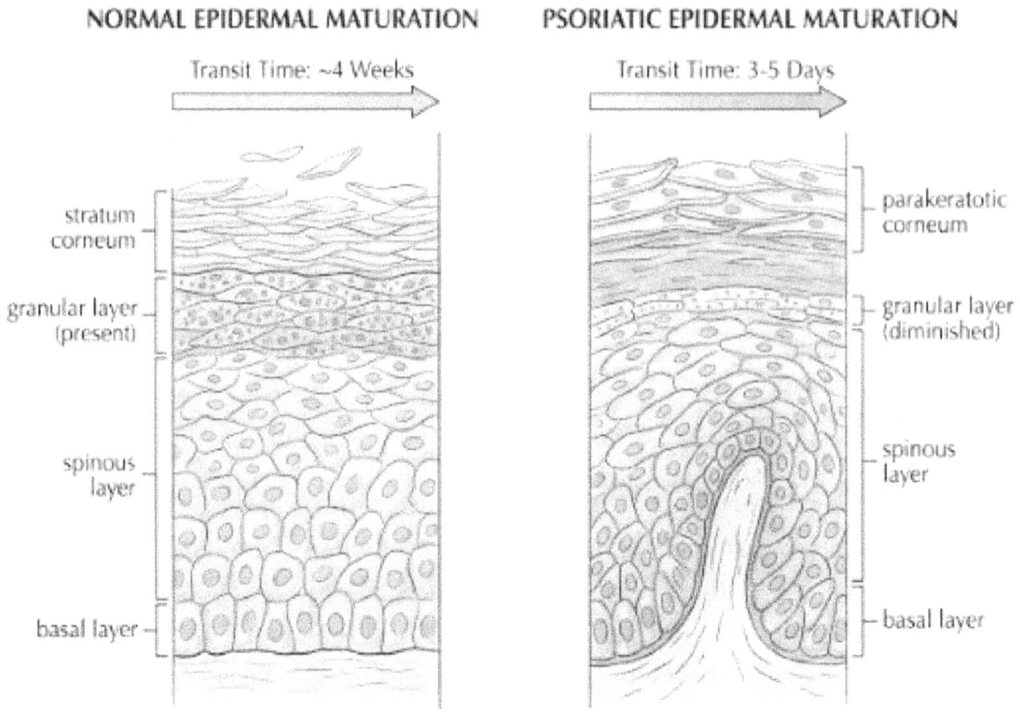

Psoriasiform Entity	Key Distinguishing Histologic Feature	Key Clinical Clue
Psoriasis vulgaris	Regular rete elongation, confluent parakeratosis, diminished granular layer, Munro microabscesses	Well-demarcated extensor plaques with silvery scale
Guttate psoriasis	Similar to plaque psoriasis but often less fully developed	Abrupt eruption of small papules following streptococcal infection
Pustular psoriasis	Subcorneal or intraepidermal neutrophilic pustules superimposed on psoriasiform architecture	Localized palmoplantar or generalized pustulation
Pityriasis rubra pilaris	Alternating ortho- and parakeratosis (checkerboard pattern), follicular plugging, thicker suprapapillary plates	Islands of sparing within confluent erythema
Chronic dermatophytosis	Psoriasiform hyperplasia with neutrophils in stratum corneum; PAS-D positive hyphae	Annular, expanding morphology; positive fungal culture or KOH

Seborrheic dermatitis (hyperplastic)	Milder, less regular rete elongation; follicular parakeratosis (shoulder parakeratosis)	Scalp, nasolabial fold, and central chest distribution

Anatomic and Morphologic Variants

Beyond the classic plaque, guttate, pustular, and erythrodermic forms, psoriasis presents in several site-specific morphologic variants that share the underlying psoriasiform histology while differing enough clinically to warrant separate recognition. Inverse (flexural) psoriasis involves the axillae, groin, inframammary folds, and other intertriginous sites, and, reflecting the flexural site-specific histologic variation discussed in Chapter 1, typically shows less prominent scale and a more macerated, glistening surface than classic plaque disease, though the underlying regular rete elongation and parakeratosis remain diagnostic when present. Scalp psoriasis, one of the most common and often earliest sites of involvement, can be biopsied using the transverse sectioning technique discussed in Chapter 1 when alopecia is a concurrent clinical concern, requiring the reader to apply both the psoriasiform pattern criteria developed in this chapter and the horizontal-section follicular counting principles developed in that earlier chapter simultaneously.

Palmoplantar psoriasis, whether presenting as plaque-type disease or as the pustular variant discussed above, is modified by the markedly thickened acral stratum corneum described in Chapter 1, so that parakeratosis and cornification changes must again be assessed against the correct site-specific baseline rather than the trunk-skin baseline a reader might otherwise default to, a principle first introduced in the acral psoriasis Rhythm block of Chapter 3 and directly relevant here as well. Nail psoriasis, producing the pitting, onycholysis, and subungual hyperkeratosis discussed in the clinical presentation section below, reflects psoriasiform involvement of the nail matrix and bed as described in Chapter 1's nail unit histology, and nail biopsy, though less commonly performed than skin biopsy given its technical demands, can confirm psoriasiform nail disease when the clinical picture is ambiguous.

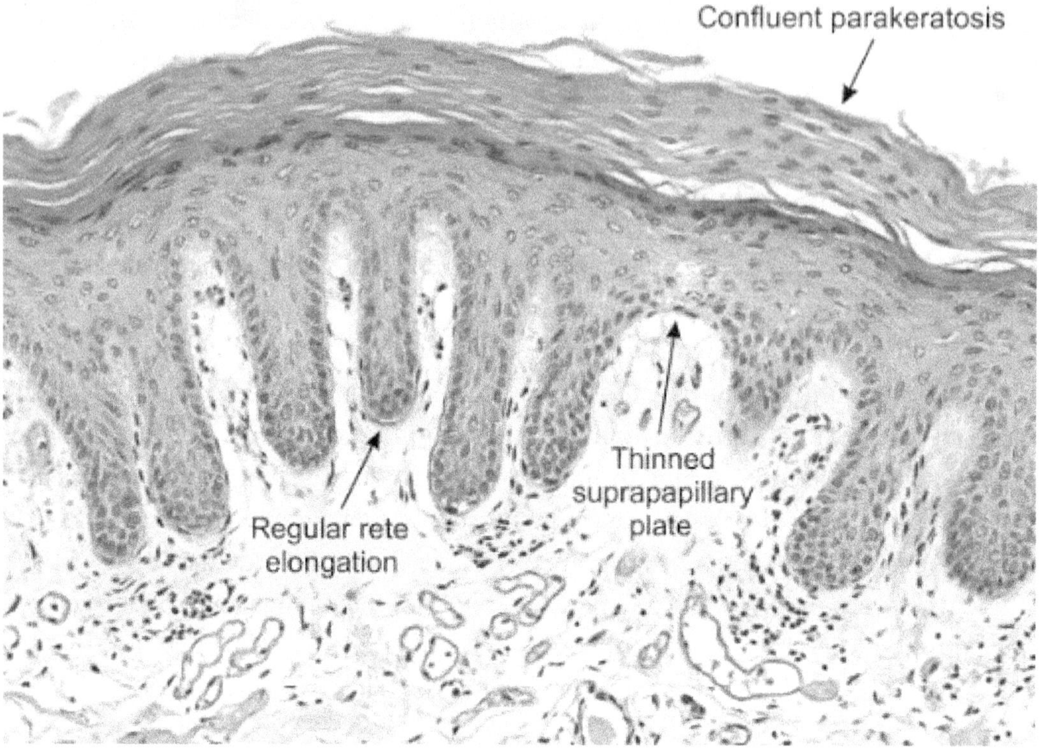

Etiology and Pathogenesis

Immunopathogenesis of Psoriasis

Psoriasis is now understood as a T cell-mediated autoimmune disease driven substantially by the interleukin-23/T helper 17 axis, in which dendritic cell-derived interleukin-23 drives differentiation and expansion of interleukin-17-producing T helper 17 cells, which in turn drive keratinocyte hyperproliferation and the recruitment of neutrophils that characterizes the pattern's histologic hallmark, the Munro microabscess, discussed further below. This mechanistic understanding, developed substantially over the past two decades, has directly informed the current therapeutic landscape, since the biologic agents that have transformed psoriasis management, including interleukin-17 and interleukin-23 inhibitors, act specifically on this pathway.

Tumor necrosis factor-alpha also plays a substantial role upstream of and alongside the interleukin-23/17 axis, contributing to the broader inflammatory milieu and explaining the efficacy of tumor necrosis factor inhibitors, an earlier generation of biologic therapy for psoriasis that remains in clinical use. The keratinocyte hyperproliferation driven by this immune cascade is dramatic in magnitude: the epidermal transit time in active psoriatic plaques is compressed to roughly three to five days, compared to the approximately four-week transit time of normal epidermis introduced in Chapter 1, a nearly tenfold acceleration that directly explains both the parakeratosis and granular layer loss that define the pattern's histology.

Genetic and Environmental Triggers

Psoriasis shows substantial heritability, with the HLA-Cw6 allele representing the most strongly and consistently replicated genetic association, particularly for early-onset, guttate-type disease, alongside numerous additional susceptibility loci identified through genome-wide association studies that converge on innate and adaptive immune pathway genes. Environmental triggers superimposed on this genetic predisposition include streptococcal infection, most classically associated with guttate psoriasis onset or flare as discussed above, physical trauma to the skin (the Koebner phenomenon, in which psoriasis develops at sites of cutaneous injury), and a range of medications recognized to trigger or exacerbate psoriasis, including lithium, beta-blockers, antimalarials, and, notably, abrupt withdrawal of systemic corticosteroids, which can precipitate a severe pustular or erythrodermic flare.

Psychological stress, alcohol use, smoking, and obesity are additionally recognized as factors that can exacerbate psoriasis severity and treatment response, reflecting the disease's substantial interaction with broader metabolic and behavioral health, an interaction developed further in the discussion of systemic associations later in this chapter. This multifactorial etiology, genetic predisposition activated by one or more environmental triggers, is a useful framework a dermatopathology report can implicitly support by noting histologic features (a background of guttate-pattern lesions, for example) that might prompt the treating clinician to specifically investigate a recent streptococcal infection or medication change.

Pathogenesis of Non-Psoriatic Psoriasiform Conditions

Pityriasis rubra pilaris, though sharing the psoriasiform architectural response, arises through a distinct pathogenesis that in a subset of cases, particularly the familial (type V) form, involves mutations in CARD14, a gene also implicated in a subset of familial psoriasis, illustrating a shared downstream inflammatory pathway despite the clinical and, as developed below, histologic distinctness of the two conditions. Sporadic pityriasis rubra pilaris is less well understood mechanistically but is similarly believed to reflect an aberrant keratinocyte differentiation and proliferation program rather than the specific interleukin-23/17-driven autoimmune process of psoriasis.

Chronic dermatophyte infection produces a psoriasiform pattern through a fundamentally different mechanism: sustained low-grade epidermal irritation and inflammatory response to fungal organisms and their metabolic byproducts within the stratum corneum drives compensatory keratinocyte hyperproliferation, a reactive rather than autoimmune process that, importantly, resolves with antifungal treatment rather than requiring the immunosuppressive or biologic therapy appropriate for true psoriasis, underscoring why the special stain exclusion discussed in the ancillary studies section of this chapter carries direct and significant treatment implications.

The Koebner Phenomenon and Its Diagnostic Relevance

The Koebner phenomenon, the development of new psoriatic lesions at sites of cutaneous trauma, whether surgical incision, sunburn, tattoo, or even a prior biopsy site, has direct relevance to specimen interpretation beyond its role as a clinical curiosity. A biopsy obtained from a site with a known preceding traumatic history in a patient with established psoriasis elsewhere may show psoriasiform change specifically attributable to this phenomenon, and recognizing this association, when the history is available, prevents misattribution of an isolated psoriasiform lesion at an unusual site (a scar, a healed laceration) to an unrelated process. The Koebner phenomenon also occurs, to varying degrees, in several of the pattern-family conditions discussed elsewhere in this book, including lichen planus and vitiligo, and its presence or absence across different diseases reflects differing degrees of dependence on local trauma-triggered inflammatory amplification as part of the underlying pathogenesis.

The therapeutic implication of the Koebner phenomenon is direct: patients with active psoriasis are counseled to minimize unnecessary cutaneous trauma, and clinicians performing procedures on psoriasis patients, including biopsies themselves, remain aware that the procedure site carries some elevated risk of subsequent koebnerization. This awareness occasionally informs biopsy site selection in clinical practice, favoring an established, representative plaque over a marginal or recently traumatized area when the clinical goal is to characterize the patient's baseline disease rather than a trauma-triggered reactive process superimposed upon it.

THE REACTION PATTERN RECOGNITION SYSTEM — The IL-23/Th17 Axis in Practice

The Pattern: Guttate Psoriasis Following Streptococcal Pharyngitis

Histologic Signature: A psoriasiform biopsy from a small, drop-like papule showing a somewhat less fully developed architecture than chronic plaque psoriasis, with prominent parakeratosis and early Munro microabscess formation but comparatively less pronounced rete elongation given the acute onset of the lesion.

The Decision: Recognize that guttate morphology and a less fully developed psoriasiform architecture together suggest recent onset, and specifically prompt inquiry into a preceding streptococcal pharyngeal infection, since this association carries both diagnostic and, in recurrent cases, therapeutic implications (tonsillectomy is occasionally considered in recurrent streptococcal-triggered guttate psoriasis refractory to standard therapy).

Trap Logic: The mimicker is pityriasis rosea, which can also present with numerous small, scaly papules and plaques. The discriminating features favoring guttate psoriasis are more confluent parakeratosis, Munro microabscesses, and a diminished granular layer, versus the more patchy parakeratosis, mild spongiosis, and extravasated erythrocytes typical of pityriasis rosea discussed in Chapter 4.

Pattern Anchor: New-onset guttate psoriasiform papules in a young patient should trigger a specific question back to the clinician: was there a sore throat in the preceding weeks. The histologic pattern alone establishes psoriasiform disease; the streptococcal link is a clinical correlation worth explicitly prompting.

Histopathologic Features and Diagnostic Criteria

Munro Microabscesses and Neutrophilic Findings

The Munro microabscess, a collection of neutrophils within the parakeratotic stratum corneum, is among the most specific histologic findings supporting a diagnosis of psoriasis, reflecting the neutrophil recruitment driven by the interleukin-17-dominated inflammatory cascade discussed above. A related but distinct finding, the spongiform pustule of Kogoj, describes neutrophil collections within the upper spinous layer of the epidermis itself rather than confined to the stratum corneum, and is more prominent in pustular psoriasis variants, where it can be extensive enough to dominate the low-power appearance of the biopsy. Neither finding is absolutely required for a psoriasis diagnosis, since early or guttate lesions may not yet have developed prominent neutrophilic collections, but their presence, when identified, substantially increases diagnostic confidence and should be specifically sought and documented when present.

Vascular and Dermal Changes

The dermal papillae in psoriasis characteristically show dilated, tortuous capillaries extending close to the thinned suprapapillary epidermal plate, a finding that correlates with the clinical Auspitz sign (pinpoint bleeding on removal of psoriatic scale) and that, together with the thinned suprapapillary plate itself, explains this classic clinical finding through direct histologic correlation. The papillary dermis typically shows a mild to moderate superficial perivascular lymphocytic infiltrate, generally less dense and less diagnostically prominent than the epidermal changes, and a notable absence of the eosinophils that frequently accompany the spongiotic pattern discussed in Chapter 4, a further discriminating feature when the psoriasiform and spongiotic patterns show some degree of histologic overlap.

Staged and Evolving Psoriasiform Histology

As with the spongiotic pattern discussed in Chapter 4, psoriasiform histology evolves with lesion duration, and recognizing the specific stage represented by a given biopsy assists both diagnostic accuracy and clinical correlation. Early or evolving psoriasis may show relatively subtle rete elongation without the fully developed regular, elongated configuration of established plaques, alongside more patchy rather than confluent parakeratosis, findings that can create diagnostic uncertainty relative to a spongiotic or nonspecific dermatitis, particularly when Munro microabscesses have not yet developed. Fully developed, established plaque psoriasis shows the complete constellation of findings developed throughout this section, while long-treated or partially resolving psoriasis, particularly following topical corticosteroid or phototherapy treatment, can show attenuated findings that no longer meet full diagnostic criteria despite ongoing clinical disease, a circumstance in which clinical history of a treated, waning lesion is essential context for interpreting an equivocal biopsy.

Histologic Features Specific to Pustular Variants

Pustular psoriasis, in both its localized palmoplantar and generalized forms, shows the psoriasiform background architecture described above with a superimposed, often extensive, neutrophilic component in the form of subcorneal or intraepidermal pustules that can be large enough to be grossly visible on the specimen and to dominate the histologic impression at low power. In generalized pustular psoriasis specifically, the pustules can be so extensive and confluent that the underlying psoriasiform architecture is less immediately apparent, and careful assessment of the surrounding, less acutely involved epidermis for the classic regular rete elongation and parakeratosis is often necessary to confirm the psoriasiform basis of the process rather than mistaking it for a primary pustular or infectious process, a distinction with direct implications given the potential severity and systemic morbidity of generalized pustular psoriasis.

Applying the Low-Power to High-Power Scanning Approach

The systematic scanning approach introduced in Chapter 1 applies directly to psoriasiform biopsies and is worth walking through explicitly given the pattern's specific diagnostic criteria. At scanning power, the reader assesses the overall silhouette for regular, evenly spaced rete ridge elongation, distinguishing this configuration from the irregular hyperplasia of a reactive or neoplastic process, and simultaneously assesses the stratum corneum for the presence and pattern of parakeratosis. At low power, the reader localizes attention to the suprapapillary plate thickness and the papillary dermal vasculature, specifically seeking the thinning and capillary dilation discussed above, while also scanning the full thickness of the stratum corneum for neutrophilic collections that would represent Munro microabscesses. Only at high power does the reader confirm specific cytologic details, including the character of the parakeratosis (confluent versus patchy, orthokeratotic admixture as in PRP), the composition of any dermal infiltrate, and, when clinically indicated, apply the special stain workup discussed later in this chapter.

This staged approach is particularly valuable for psoriasiform biopsies because, as developed throughout this chapter, the differential diagnosis includes entities (PRP, chronic dermatophytosis, mycosis fungoides) whose discriminating features are specific and easily missed if the reader moves too quickly to a presumptive diagnosis based on the low-power silhouette alone. A reader who recognizes psoriasiform architecture at scanning power but proceeds directly to a psoriasis diagnosis without systematically working through suprapapillary plate thickness, cornification pattern, and stratum corneum content at progressively higher power is skipping precisely the steps most likely to catch PRP, tinea, or an atypical lymphocytic infiltrate before the diagnosis is finalized.

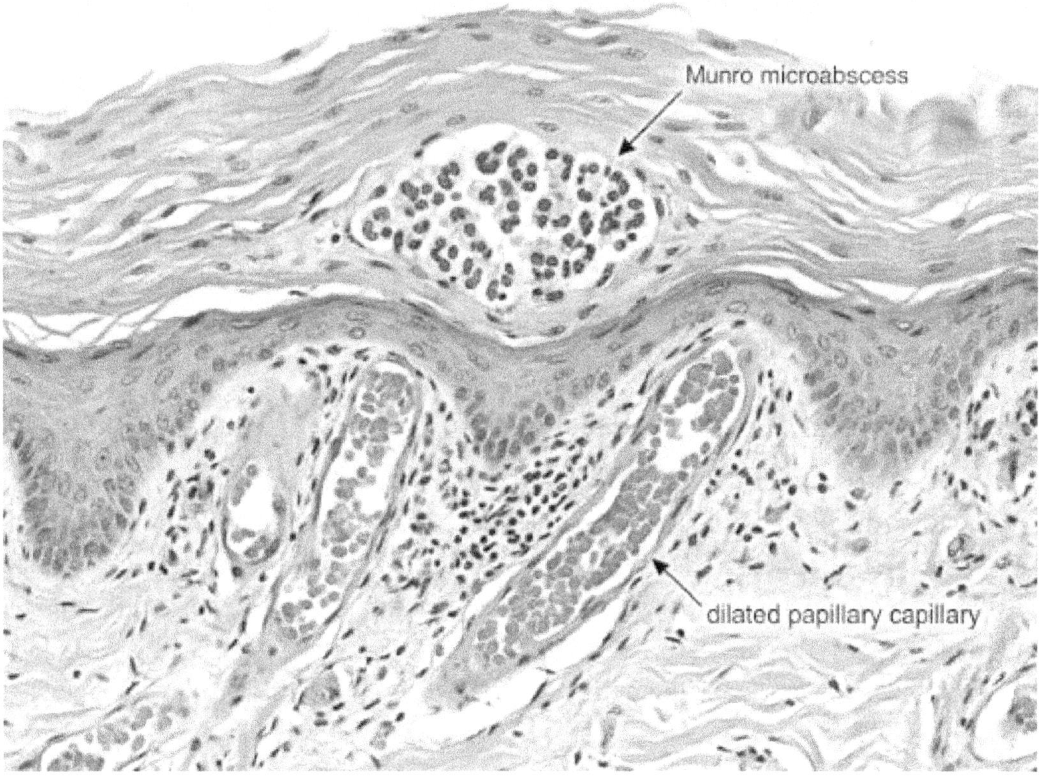

Clinical Presentation and Clinicopathologic Correlation

Clinical Morphology and Distribution

The classic clinical morphology of plaque psoriasis, well-demarcated, erythematous plaques with adherent silvery scale, favoring extensor surfaces (elbows and knees), the scalp, and the gluteal cleft, together with a chronic, relapsing course, is usually sufficiently distinctive that biopsy is reserved for atypical presentations, diagnostic uncertainty, or the exclusion of a specific mimicker such as chronic dermatophytosis or pityriasis rubra pilaris. Nail involvement, including pitting, onycholysis, and subungual hyperkeratosis, is common and, when present, supports the psoriasis diagnosis and correlates with an increased likelihood of psoriatic arthritis, discussed below, making nail examination a clinically useful piece of correlating information even when the nail itself is not the biopsied site.

Distribution carries particular discriminating weight relative to the major clinical mimickers developed in this chapter: pityriasis rubra pilaris characteristically shows a cephalocaudal progression with islands of sparing within otherwise confluent erythema, a distribution pattern that psoriasis does not typically produce, while chronic dermatophytosis typically shows an annular, centrifugally expanding morphology with a more active, scaling border and comparatively clearer center, distinct from the uniform, well-demarcated plaque morphology of psoriasis. Communicating clinical distribution details, when available, alongside the histologic findings strengthens the overall diagnostic picture presented in the final report.

Psoriatic Arthritis and Systemic Associations

Psoriatic arthritis develops in a substantial minority of psoriasis patients, typically following cutaneous disease onset by several years though occasionally preceding or co-occurring with skin involvement, and its recognition carries significant implications for systemic therapy selection, since certain biologic agents effective for cutaneous psoriasis also address the joint disease while others do not. Nail involvement, as noted above, and specific psoriasis subtypes, including scalp and inverse (flexural) psoriasis, are associated with a higher risk of psoriatic arthritis development, information that, while primarily clinical rather than histologic, is useful context for a dermatopathologist to understand given the broader clinical picture the biopsy sits within.

Beyond joint disease, psoriasis is increasingly recognized as a systemic inflammatory condition with associations extending to cardiovascular disease, metabolic syndrome, and mood disorders including depression, reflecting the broader biological consequences of chronic systemic interleukin-17 and interleukin-23-driven inflammation beyond the skin itself. While these systemic associations do not typically alter the histologic diagnosis of a given psoriasiform biopsy, awareness of them supports a more complete understanding of the disease a positive diagnosis represents and reinforces why accurate, confident psoriasis diagnosis carries value extending well beyond the immediate cutaneous finding.

Quality of Life and Psychosocial Impact

Psoriasis carries a well-documented psychosocial burden disproportionate to what its cutaneous extent alone might suggest, including elevated rates of depression, anxiety, and social withdrawal related to the visibility and chronicity of the disease, an impact that has become an increasingly explicit consideration in treatment guideline severity assessments alongside body surface area and physical symptom burden. While this psychosocial dimension does not alter the histologic diagnosis, understanding it provides useful context for why a dermatopathologist's diagnostic precision matters beyond the immediate biopsy: a confident, well-supported psoriasis diagnosis, clearly distinguished from the mimickers developed in this chapter, allows a patient to move efficiently toward effective treatment rather than experiencing the additional psychological burden of prolonged diagnostic uncertainty or a treatment course misdirected at the wrong underlying disease.

Differential Diagnosis and Histologic Mimickers

Psoriasis Versus Pityriasis Rubra Pilaris

Pityriasis rubra pilaris is among the most important and most frequently tested mimickers of psoriasis, sharing the fundamental psoriasiform architecture while showing several specific discriminating features. The alternating pattern of orthokeratosis and parakeratosis, often described as a checkerboard pattern, both horizontally across a single section and vertically within the thickness of the stratum corneum, is a characteristic and highly useful discriminator, as is follicular plugging with a shoulder of parakeratosis at the follicular ostia, a finding that reflects the clinical follicular papules characteristic of pityriasis rubra pilaris. The suprapapillary epidermal plate in pityriasis rubra pilaris is typically thicker than in psoriasis, in contrast to the thinned suprapapillary plate that is a defining feature of psoriasis, and Munro microabscesses and Kogoj spongiform pustules are characteristically absent or at most inconspicuous, in further contrast to established psoriasis.

Psoriasis Versus Chronic Dermatophytosis

As introduced above, chronic dermatophyte infection can produce a psoriasiform architecture closely resembling psoriasis, and several histologic clues should prompt specific special stain exclusion: neutrophils within the stratum corneum in a pattern that, unlike the more organized Munro microabscess, appears more diffusely scattered through a compact, often orthokeratotic (rather than purely parakeratotic) stratum corneum, and a sandwich sign as introduced in Chapter 4, in which a band of more normal-appearing stratum corneum is sandwiched between two zones of parakeratosis, reflecting episodic fungal invasion and clearance. A PAS-D stain, as discussed in Chapter 2, should be performed whenever these features are present or whenever the clinical distribution (annular, expanding, with an active border) raises tinea as a genuine consideration, since mistaking chronic dermatophytosis for psoriasis and treating with topical or systemic immunosuppressive therapy can substantially worsen the underlying fungal infection.

Psoriasis Versus Chronic Spongiotic Dermatitis and Other Mimickers

The overlap between chronic, lichenified spongiotic dermatitis and the psoriasiform pattern, extensively developed in Chapters 3 and 4, remains directly relevant here: hypergranulosis rather than granular layer loss, residual foci of spongiosis, and an eosinophil-containing infiltrate favor a chronic spongiotic process over true psoriasis. Seborrheic dermatitis, in its more chronic, hyperplastic presentations, can also show psoriasiform features, though typically milder rete elongation, a more irregular pattern, and follicular (shoulder) parakeratosis around follicular ostia rather than the confluent, diffuse parakeratosis of established psoriasis. Finally, as discussed in Chapter 4, early or patch-stage mycosis fungoides can occasionally show a psoriasiform architecture, and a treatment-refractory or atypical psoriasiform biopsy, particularly with disproportionate epidermotropism of lymphocytes relative to the degree of spongiosis or with cytologically atypical lymphocytes, should prompt consideration of this important mimicker and, when appropriate, the immunohistochemical and molecular workup discussed in Chapter 2.

A 45-year-old patient presents with a longstanding, treatment-refractory scaly plaque initially diagnosed clinically as psoriasis, and a biopsy is obtained given the poor response to standard topical therapy. Applying the three-step sequence, pattern assignment identifies a psoriasiform pattern, but differential narrowing reveals several atypical features: the parakeratosis is patchier than expected, Munro microabscesses are absent, and scattered lymphocytes within the epidermis show mild nuclear atypia with a disproportionately prominent epidermotropic distribution relative to the degree of associated spongiosis. These atypical features, considered together with the treatment-refractory clinical course, appropriately prompt immunohistochemical staining for CD3, CD4, CD8, and CD7, which in this hypothetical case shows a CD4-predominant infiltrate with aberrant loss of CD7, supporting a diagnosis of patch-stage mycosis fungoides with psoriasiform features rather than psoriasis vulgaris, a diagnosis with substantially different management implications developed fully in Chapter 18.

CAUTION: Treatment-refractory psoriasiform disease, particularly with atypical histologic features or disproportionate epidermotropism, should prompt consideration of mycosis fungoides before treatment is escalated on the assumption that the original psoriasis diagnosis was simply undertreated.

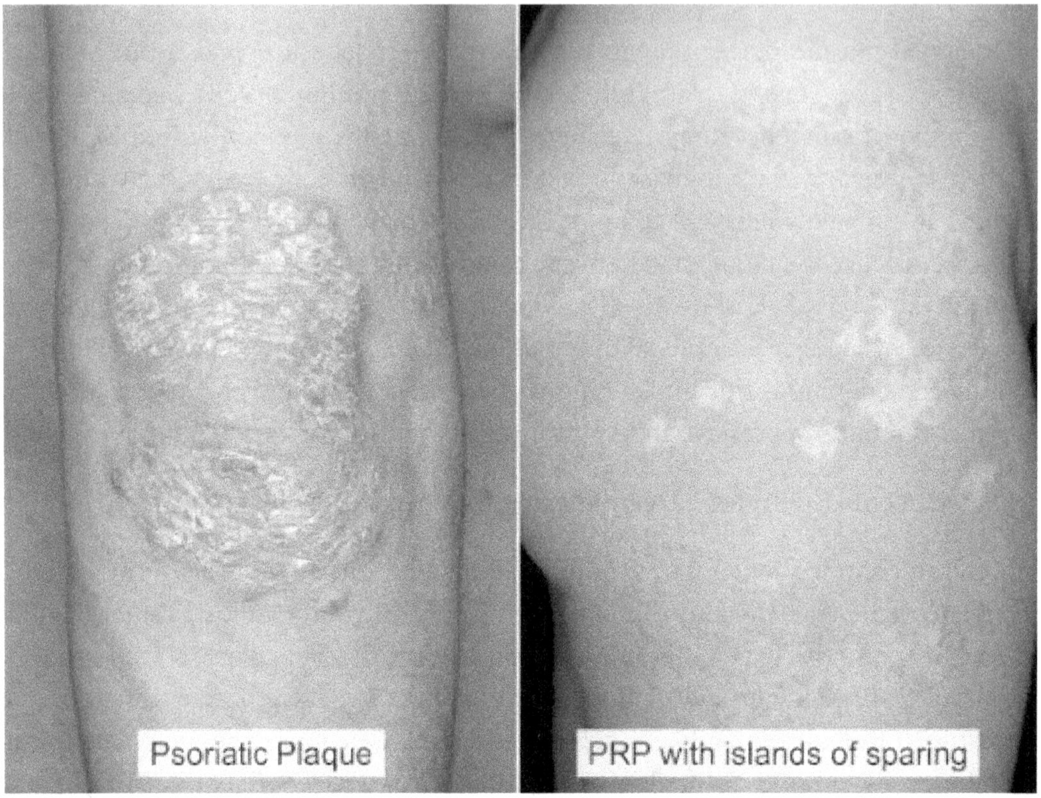

Reporting an Equivocal Psoriasiform Biopsy

Not every psoriasiform biopsy will show the complete constellation of confirmatory findings developed in this chapter, and equivocal biopsies, showing psoriasiform architecture without definitive Munro microabscesses, without a clear checkerboard pattern to suggest PRP, and with a negative PAS-D stain excluding tinea, require a reporting approach consistent with the diagnostic honesty principle established in Chapter 1. A descriptive diagnosis of psoriasiform dermatitis with a stated differential favoring psoriasis, alongside an explicit note of the specific supportive and unsupportive features observed, gives the treating clinician the most accurate and actionable picture, particularly when the clinical presentation itself is classic enough that the biopsy's primary role is confirmatory rather than diagnostically decisive on its own.

This equivocal scenario arises with some regularity in early or minimally developed lesions, in biopsies obtained from a partially treated area, and in biopsies from anatomic sites, such as flexural or acral skin, where the baseline architecture itself modifies the expected psoriasiform criteria as discussed above. Recognizing that the biopsy result exists on a spectrum of diagnostic confidence, rather than treating every psoriasiform biopsy as either definitively psoriasis or definitively something else, reflects the same nuanced, appropriately hedged reporting philosophy this book has developed since Chapter 1 and applies it specifically to the pattern most commonly encountered in routine dermatopathology sign-out volume.

Ancillary Studies

Special Stains for Excluding Infectious Mimickers

As developed extensively above, PAS-D staining is the essential ancillary study for excluding chronic dermatophytosis whenever the clinical or histologic picture raises this possibility, and should be pursued with a low threshold given the significant treatment divergence between antifungal therapy and psoriasis-directed immunosuppressive or biologic therapy. Beyond this specific and clinically important indication, special stains play a limited role in the routine diagnosis of an otherwise classic psoriasiform biopsy, consistent with the hypothesis-driven approach to ancillary testing established in Chapter 2.

Immunohistochemistry in Atypical Psoriasiform Presentations

As illustrated in the worked example above, immunohistochemistry becomes relevant when a psoriasiform biopsy shows atypical features or occurs in a treatment-refractory clinical context raising concern for mycosis fungoides, in which case the T-cell immunophenotypic panel discussed in Chapter 2, including CD3, CD4, CD8, and CD7, along with clonality studies when appropriate, is pursued. Immunohistochemistry has a more limited but occasionally useful role in confirming pityriasis rubra pilaris in ambiguous cases, where specific keratin expression patterns have been described as a research and occasionally diagnostic adjunct, though the diagnosis remains substantially clinical and histologic rather than immunohistochemistry-dependent in routine practice.

Management Implications

Connecting Diagnosis to the Psoriasis Treatment Pathway

Confirmed psoriasis diagnosis directs the treating clinician toward a treatment pathway that has been transformed over the past two decades by the biologic agents targeting the interleukin-23/17 axis discussed above, generally reserved for moderate-to-severe disease inadequately controlled by topical therapy (corticosteroids, vitamin D analogs, and topical calcineurin inhibitors), phototherapy, or, for an intermediate severity tier, conventional systemic agents such as methotrexate. The histologic confirmation of psoriasis, and specific exclusion of the mimickers developed throughout this chapter, is what allows a clinician to confidently escalate to these increasingly targeted and, in the case of biologic therapy, increasingly costly treatment tiers with appropriate confidence that the underlying diagnosis justifies that escalation.

Distinguishing Management Pathways for Look-Alike Conditions

The management divergence among the entities developed in this chapter's differential diagnosis section is substantial and underscores why accurate histologic discrimination carries direct clinical consequence beyond diagnostic precision for its own sake. Chronic dermatophytosis requires antifungal therapy and would be worsened rather than helped by psoriasis-directed immunosuppression; pityriasis rubra pilaris, while sometimes treated with agents that overlap with the psoriasis armamentarium (retinoids, methotrexate), does not reliably respond to the interleukin-17 and interleukin-23 inhibitors that have transformed psoriasis management, reflecting its distinct pathogenesis, and a diagnosis of pityriasis rubra pilaris mistaken for treatment-refractory psoriasis can lead to an unproductive and costly escalation through multiple biologic agents before the correct diagnosis is finally established. A dermatopathology report that clearly names the specific discriminating features supporting or arguing against each of these entities, rather than a generic "psoriasiform dermatitis" diagnosis, provides direct and material value to this treatment-selection process.

Severity Assessment and Its Relationship to Biopsy Findings

Psoriasis severity, and consequently treatment tier selection, is assessed clinically using measures such as body surface area involvement and composite indices including the Psoriasis Area and Severity Index, rather than through any histologic severity grading system, and a dermatopathologist should understand this division of labor to avoid overstating what a biopsy's histologic findings can contribute to severity assessment. A biopsy showing florid, fully developed psoriasiform changes with extensive Munro microabscess formation does not, by itself, indicate a more clinically severe or extensive disease burden than a biopsy showing more subtle findings, since a single biopsy samples one lesion and cannot speak to the total body surface area involved or the systemic inflammatory burden the patient experiences. The histologic report's contribution to management is diagnostic confirmation and mimicker exclusion, developed throughout this chapter, rather than severity quantification, which remains a clinical assessment performed by the treating dermatologist using validated clinical instruments.

The Dermatopathologist's Role in a Multidisciplinary Psoriasis Care Team

Psoriasis management, particularly for moderate-to-severe disease requiring systemic or biologic therapy, increasingly involves a multidisciplinary care team spanning dermatology, rheumatology when psoriatic arthritis is present, and, given the systemic associations discussed above, primary care or cardiology for cardiometabolic risk management. The dermatopathologist's contribution to this team is concentrated at specific decision points, most importantly initial diagnostic confirmation and mimicker exclusion, and secondarily at points of diagnostic uncertainty during the treatment course, such as a treatment-refractory presentation that might indicate the original diagnosis requires reconsideration, developed above in the context of mycosis fungoides. Recognizing this specific, bounded role within the larger care pathway helps calibrate what the pathology report should and should not attempt to convey, focusing its diagnostic authority on the questions histology is well positioned to answer while deferring severity assessment, treatment selection, and longitudinal monitoring to the clinical team positioned to integrate the full range of relevant information.

THE REACTION PATTERN RECOGNITION SYSTEM — The Psoriasiform Pattern Family

The Pattern: The psoriasiform reaction pattern and its major clinical subtypes and mimickers: psoriasis vulgaris and its guttate, pustular, and erythrodermic variants, pityriasis rubra pilaris, chronic dermatophytosis, and hyperplastic seborrheic dermatitis.

Histologic Signature: Regular, elongated rete ridges, thinned suprapapillary plates, confluent parakeratosis, diminished granular layer, Munro microabscesses, and dilated papillary capillaries define classic psoriasis; the checkerboard ortho-parakeratosis and follicular plugging of PRP, and PAS-D positive hyphae of tinea, are the defining discriminators for the two most important mimickers.

The Decision: Assess rete regularity, granular layer status, and the presence of Munro microabscesses to confirm psoriasis, then actively check for the specific features of PRP and chronic dermatophytosis before finalizing the diagnosis, given the substantial management divergence among these entities.

Trap Logic: PRP mimics psoriasis but shows checkerboard cornification, follicular plugging, and a thicker suprapapillary plate. Chronic dermatophytosis mimics psoriasis but shows diffusely scattered stratum corneum neutrophils, a sandwich sign, and PAS-D positive hyphae. Treatment-refractory or atypical psoriasiform disease should raise mycosis fungoides.

Pattern Anchor: Before finalizing a psoriasis diagnosis, actively look for what psoriasis should not have: checkerboard cornification (PRP), fungal hyphae (tinea), or atypical epidermotropic lymphocytes (mycosis fungoides). Each absence, confirmed rather than assumed, strengthens the diagnosis.

Summary and Key Concepts

The psoriasiform reaction pattern is defined by regular, elongated rete ridges, a thinned suprapapillary epidermal plate, and a cornification abnormality (parakeratosis with diminished granular layer) reflecting dramatically accelerated keratinocyte transit time.

Psoriasis is driven by the interleukin-23/T helper 17 immune axis, a mechanistic understanding that directly underlies the current biologic therapy landscape and explains the pattern's hallmark neutrophilic findings, Munro microabscesses and Kogoj spongiform pustules.

Pityriasis rubra pilaris and chronic dermatophytosis are the two most important histologic mimickers of psoriasis, distinguished respectively by checkerboard cornification with follicular plugging, and PAS-D positive fungal hyphae with a sandwich sign.

Clinical distribution (islands of sparing for PRP, annular expansion for tinea, extensor and scalp involvement with nail changes for psoriasis) provides essential correlating information that complements histologic findings.

Accurate discrimination among psoriasis and its mimickers carries direct management consequences, since antifungal therapy, retinoid-based treatment, and biologic immunosuppression are not interchangeable across these histologically related but etiologically distinct entities.

CHAPTER 6: THE LICHENOID AND INTERFACE REACTION PATTERN

Learning Objectives

1. Define the lichenoid and vacuolar interface reaction patterns and distinguish them by infiltrate density and distribution.
2. Describe the etiology and pathogenesis of lichen planus, lupus erythematosus, and erythema multiforme.
3. Identify the histopathologic features and diagnostic criteria that distinguish the major interface-pattern entities from one another.
4. Correlate histologic findings with clinical morphology and apply clinicopathologic correlation to an interface-pattern biopsy.
5. Construct a differential diagnosis for the interface pattern and discriminate among its major constituent diagnoses and mimickers.
6. Select appropriate ancillary studies, including direct immunofluorescence, and understand their role in interface-pattern diagnosis.

Definition and Classification

Defining the Lichenoid and Vacuolar Interface Patterns

The lichenoid and vacuolar interface patterns, introduced conceptually in Chapter 3, share a common anatomic target, the dermal-epidermal junction and basal keratinocyte layer, but are distinguished by the density and distribution of the associated lymphocytic infiltrate, a distinction with direct diagnostic consequence developed throughout this chapter. The lichenoid pattern is defined by a dense, band-like lymphocytic infiltrate that hugs the dermal-epidermal junction closely enough to substantially obscure it at low power, accompanied by basal keratinocyte vacuolar change, individual keratinocyte necrosis producing eosinophilic, anucleate Civatte bodies, and, in well-developed lesions, a sawtooth configuration of the rete ridges.

The vacuolar interface pattern shows the same fundamental basal layer injury, vacuolar change and individual keratinocyte necrosis, but with a comparatively sparse, patchy lymphocytic infiltrate that does not obscure the dermal-epidermal junction to the same degree, leaving the junction still identifiable as a discrete line at low power rather than replaced by a dense inflammatory band. This density distinction, dense and band-like versus sparse and patchy, is frequently the single most useful low-power discriminator between the lichen planus-type lichenoid pattern and the lupus erythematosus and erythema multiforme-type vacuolar interface pattern, and is explored in depth in the differential diagnosis section of this chapter.

Classification of Lichenoid Diseases

Lichen planus, the prototype of the lichenoid pattern, presents classically as violaceous, polygonal, flat-topped papules and plaques, often with fine white surface reticulation (Wickham striae), favoring the flexor wrists, ankles, and genitalia, with mucosal, nail, and scalp (lichen planopilaris) variants developed further below. Lichenoid drug eruption produces a histologically similar picture to lichen planus, distinguished by specific features developed in the differential diagnosis section, and is triggered by a wide range of medications, most classically antihypertensives, antimalarials, and nonsteroidal anti-inflammatory drugs. Lichen striatus, a distinct entity occurring predominantly in children, follows the lines of Blaschko and shows a lichenoid histology often with a more perivascular and periadnexal distribution than classic lichen planus. Lichenoid keratosis (benign lichenoid keratosis or lichen planus-like keratosis) represents a lichenoid inflammatory reaction to a preexisting benign epidermal lesion, most commonly a solar lentigo or seborrheic keratosis, and requires recognition of residual features of the underlying lesion to avoid a purely inflammatory diagnosis that misses the antecedent process.

Classification of Vacuolar Interface Diseases

Lupus erythematosus, spanning the cutaneous spectrum from acute to subacute to chronic (discoid) disease, shows a vacuolar interface pattern with several specific additional features developed below that distinguish it from other members of this category. Erythema multiforme, an acute, self-limited hypersensitivity reaction most commonly triggered by herpes simplex virus infection or, less commonly, medications, shows a vacuolar interface pattern with prominent keratinocyte necrosis that can be extensive enough to produce full-thickness epidermal necrosis in severe cases. Stevens-Johnson syndrome and toxic epidermal necrolysis represent a spectrum of severe, medication-triggered mucocutaneous reactions that share the vacuolar interface pattern and full-thickness keratinocyte necrosis of severe erythema multiforme, distinguished primarily by the extent of body surface area involvement and by a set of specific clinical and histologic severity features developed in this chapter. Graft-versus-host disease, occurring after allogeneic hematopoietic stem cell transplantation, produces a vacuolar interface pattern that can closely resemble erythema multiforme histologically, requiring clinical context (transplant history and timing) for accurate distinction.

Entity	Infiltrate Density	Key Additional Feature	Prototypical Trigger or Association
Lichen planus	Dense, band-like	Sawtooth rete, hypergranulosis, Civatte bodies	Idiopathic; hepatitis C association reported
Lichenoid drug eruption	Dense, band-like with eosinophils	Parakeratosis, deeper perivascular extension	New or changed medication
Lupus erythematosus	Sparse, patchy, superficial and deep	Basement membrane thickening, dermal	Autoimmune; photosensitivity

		mucin, periadnexal extension	
Erythema multiforme	Sparse, patchy	Prominent keratinocyte necrosis, satellite cell necrosis	Herpes simplex virus infection
Graft-versus-host disease	Sparse, patchy	Satellite cell necrosis, follicular involvement	Allogeneic stem cell transplant

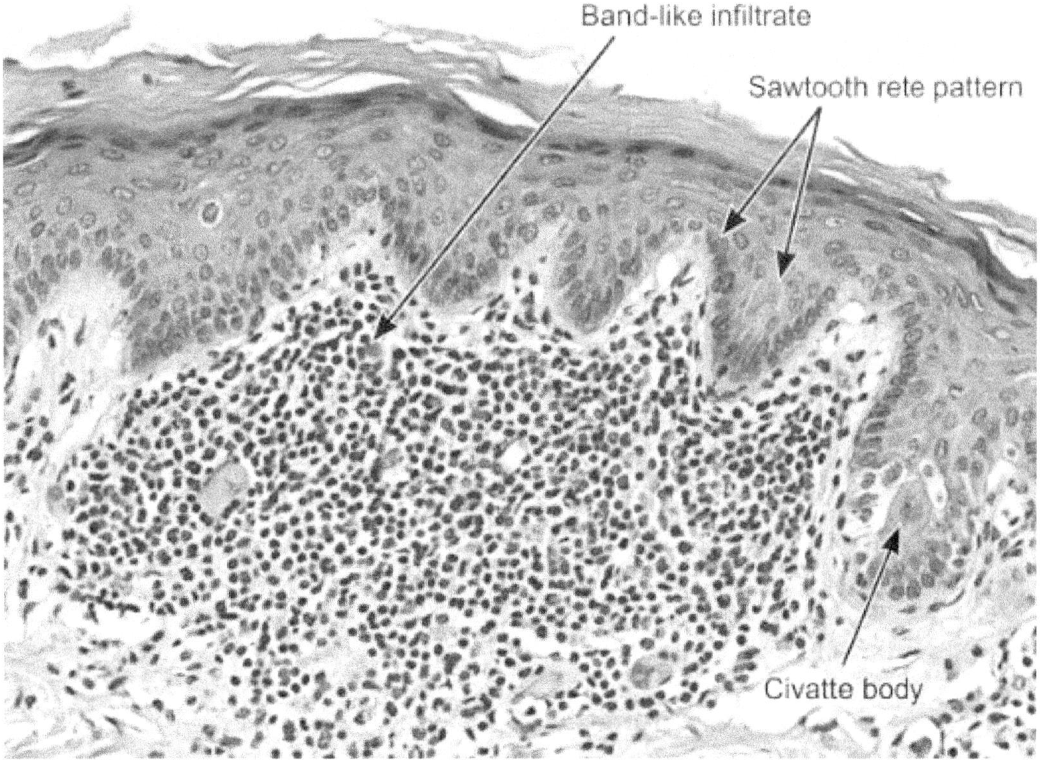

Etiology and Pathogenesis

Immunopathogenesis of Lichen Planus

Lichen planus is understood as a T cell-mediated autoimmune process in which cytotoxic CD8-positive T lymphocytes recognize an altered self-antigen on basal keratinocytes, triggering apoptotic keratinocyte death that produces the Civatte bodies characteristic of the pattern, and the dense band-like infiltrate reflects the magnitude of this cytotoxic lymphocytic response concentrated tightly at the site of antigen recognition, the basal keratinocyte layer. The specific triggering antigen remains incompletely characterized in idiopathic lichen planus, though an association with hepatitis C virus infection has been well documented in some populations, believed to reflect molecular mimicry or a related mechanism in which viral antigens or virus-altered keratinocyte proteins trigger the same cytotoxic T-cell response as the idiopathic disease.

Lichenoid drug eruption arises through a related but distinct immunologic mechanism, in which the culprit medication or its metabolite acts as a hapten or otherwise alters keratinocyte antigenicity in a way that triggers a similar cytotoxic T-cell response, typically after a longer latency period following medication initiation than is characteristic of the more rapid spongiotic and urticarial drug reactions discussed in Chapter 4, sometimes months rather than days to weeks. This longer latency, together with the specific histologic features developed in the differential diagnosis section below, assists in distinguishing lichenoid drug eruption from idiopathic lichen planus when the clinical medication history is available.

Immunopathogenesis of Lupus Erythematosus

Cutaneous lupus erythematosus reflects a complex interplay of genetic predisposition, ultraviolet light exposure, and autoantibody-mediated tissue injury, in which ultraviolet-induced keratinocyte apoptosis exposes nuclear antigens that become targets for autoantibody binding, triggering complement activation and an interferon-driven inflammatory cascade that produces the vacuolar interface pattern and, in many cases, the dermal mucin deposition characteristic of this entity, discussed further below. This ultraviolet-triggering mechanism directly explains the photosensitive distribution characteristic of cutaneous lupus and underlies the central role of photoprotection in its management.

The relationship between cutaneous and systemic lupus erythematosus varies substantially by cutaneous subtype: acute cutaneous lupus erythematosus is strongly associated with systemic disease, subacute cutaneous lupus erythematosus shows an intermediate association, often accompanied by specific autoantibodies (anti-Ro/SSA and anti-La/SSB), and chronic cutaneous (discoid) lupus erythematosus, while it can occur in the context of systemic disease, more commonly presents as a skin-limited process, though a meaningful minority of discoid lupus patients do progress to or already have systemic involvement, underscoring why appropriate clinical and serologic workup, informed by the biopsy's confirmation of the interface pattern and its specific subtype-supportive features, remains important even for apparently skin-limited presentations.

Immunopathogenesis of Erythema Multiforme and Related Severe Reactions

Erythema multiforme is understood, in its most common form, as a cytotoxic T-cell response directed against herpes simplex virus antigen-bearing keratinocytes, in which viral antigen is transported to distant, uninvolved skin sites by circulating antigen-presenting cells following an active or recent herpes simplex outbreak, explaining the characteristic distribution of erythema multiforme papules and targetoid lesions at sites remote from the primary viral infection itself. Stevens-Johnson syndrome and toxic epidermal necrolysis, by contrast, are most commonly medication-triggered, involving a cytotoxic T-cell and natural killer cell-mediated process directed against a drug-altered keratinocyte antigen, with granulysin identified as a key soluble mediator of the widespread keratinocyte apoptosis that produces the extensive epidermal necrosis characteristic of severe disease, a mechanistic distinction from the more localized, herpes-triggered process of classic erythema multiforme that helps explain the substantially greater severity and mortality risk of the Stevens-Johnson syndrome and toxic epidermal necrolysis spectrum.

Lichen Planopilaris and Follicular Lichenoid Disease

Lichen planopilaris represents the follicular expression of the same cytotoxic T-cell process that produces classic cutaneous lichen planus, targeting the follicular epithelium, particularly the isthmus and infundibulum, rather than or in addition to the interfollicular epidermis, and producing a scarring alopecia through progressive destruction and fibrous replacement of the affected follicular units, a process best appreciated using the transverse sectioning technique and follicular counting principles introduced in Chapter 1. Frontal fibrosing alopecia, considered a clinical variant of lichen planopilaris affecting the frontal and temporal hairline in a band-like distribution, shares this same underlying histologic process, and both entities show perifollicular lichenoid infiltrate concentrated at the isthmus and infundibulum with relative sparing of the deeper follicular bulb, a distribution pattern that, together with progressive loss of sebaceous glands, distinguishes early lichen planopilaris from the normal anagen follicular density discussed in the Chapter 1 Rhythm block on this exact diagnostic pitfall.

Graham-Little syndrome, an uncommon variant combining lichen planopilaris of the scalp with non-scarring alopecia of the axillary and pubic hair and a follicular, lichen planus-like eruption elsewhere on the body, illustrates the broader principle that the follicular lichenoid process can present with variable distribution and severity across different hair-bearing sites in the same patient, and recognizing the underlying shared lichenoid pathophysiology across these clinical variants, rather than treating each as an entirely separate diagnostic entity, assists in constructing an accurate and complete clinical picture when multiple sites are involved.

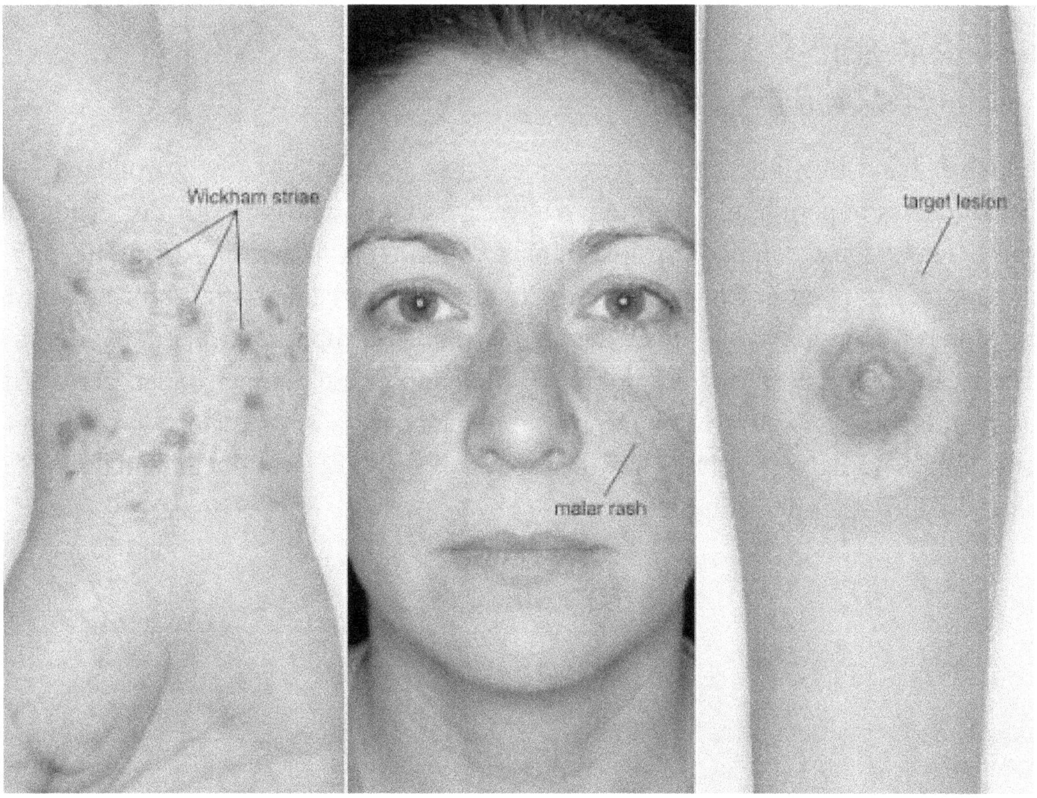

THE REACTION PATTERN RECOGNITION SYSTEM — Infiltrate Density as the Primary Discriminator

---

The Pattern: Infiltrate Density Distinguishing Lichenoid from Vacuolar Interface Disease

Histologic Signature: A dense, confluent, band-like lymphocytic infiltrate that obscures the dermal-epidermal junction (lichenoid) versus a sparse, patchy infiltrate through which the junction remains identifiable as a discrete line (vacuolar interface).

The Decision: Assess infiltrate density and junctional obscuration first, before evaluating any other feature, since this single assessment reliably sorts the great majority of interface-pattern biopsies into the lichen planus family versus the lupus erythematosus/erythema multiforme family, each with a substantially different subsequent differential diagnosis.

Trap Logic: The mimicker in each direction is the other category at an atypical stage: early or resolving lichen planus can show a less dense infiltrate than fully developed disease, and a particularly brisk lupus erythematosus flare can show a denser infiltrate than typical. When density alone is ambiguous, secondary features (sawtooth rete and hypergranulosis for lichen planus; basement membrane thickening and dermal mucin for lupus; prominent keratinocyte necrosis for erythema multiforme) resolve the distinction.

Pattern Anchor: Can you still see the dermal-epidermal junction as a distinct line at low power? If yes, think vacuolar interface (lupus, erythema multiforme). If the junction is obscured by a dense cellular band, think lichenoid (lichen planus, lichenoid drug eruption).

Histopathologic Features and Diagnostic Criteria

Diagnostic Features of Lichen Planus

Beyond the dense band-like infiltrate and sawtooth rete pattern already introduced, lichen planus characteristically shows hypergranulosis, often in a wedge-shaped configuration corresponding to the tips of the sawtooth rete ridges, compact orthokeratosis without parakeratosis, distinguishing it from the psoriasiform pattern discussed in Chapter 5, and Civatte bodies visible both within the lower epidermis and, once extruded by ongoing basal layer damage, within the superficial papillary dermis (colloid or Civatte bodies as free-lying eosinophilic globules). Melanophages, pigment-laden dermal macrophages reflecting pigment incontinence from damaged basal melanocytes, are frequently present in the papillary dermis and, in longstanding or resolving lesions, may be the most prominent remaining feature as the active lymphocytic infiltrate diminishes.

Diagnostic Features of Lupus Erythematosus

Cutaneous lupus erythematosus, beyond the sparse, patchy vacuolar interface pattern already introduced, characteristically shows basement membrane thickening, best appreciated with a PAS stain as discussed in Chapter 2, follicular plugging (keratotic material distending and plugging follicular infundibula, particularly prominent in discoid lupus), and periadnexal and perivascular extension of the lymphocytic infiltrate into the deep dermis, a depth of involvement not typically seen in lichen planus or erythema multiforme. Increased dermal mucin, assessed with Alcian blue staining when subtle, is a further characteristic finding, and the combination of interface change, basement membrane thickening, follicular plugging, and dermal mucin, when all or most are present, is highly supportive of a lupus erythematosus diagnosis over its histologic mimickers.

Diagnostic Features of Erythema Multiforme

Erythema multiforme, in addition to its sparse, patchy vacuolar interface pattern, is distinguished by prominent keratinocyte necrosis that can range from scattered individual necrotic keratinocytes (satellite cell necrosis, in which a lymphocyte is seen in close apposition to a dying keratinocyte) to, in severe cases, confluent full-thickness epidermal necrosis with subepidermal separation from the underlying dermis. Unlike lupus erythematosus, erythema multiforme characteristically lacks basement membrane thickening, follicular plugging, and significant dermal mucin, and unlike lichen planus, lacks hypergranulosis and a dense, band-like infiltrate, so that the combination of a sparse infiltrate with disproportionately prominent keratinocyte necrosis is the key discriminating combination for this entity.

Grading Severity in the Erythema Multiforme Spectrum

The extent of epidermal necrosis provides a histologic correlate to the clinical severity spectrum from erythema multiforme through Stevens-Johnson syndrome to toxic epidermal necrolysis, with more extensive, full-thickness necrosis and more prominent subepidermal separation generally corresponding to more severe clinical disease, though clinical body surface area involvement remains the primary severity determinant used for triage and management decisions rather than histologic necrosis extent alone. A frozen section assessment of epidermal necrosis extent, when clinically urgent triage decisions are needed in a patient with suspected toxic epidermal necrolysis, can provide rapid information to guide immediate management, illustrating one of the circumstances in which the frozen section technique discussed in Chapter 2, despite its general limitations for definitive diagnosis, provides genuine clinical value through speed rather than diagnostic precision.

Applying the Scanning Approach to Interface Pattern Biopsies

The low-power to high-power scanning approach introduced in Chapter 1 applies to interface-pattern biopsies with a specific emphasis on the density assessment that anchors this chapter's entire diagnostic framework. At scanning power, the reader's first and most important task is judging whether the dermal-epidermal junction remains visible as a discrete line or is obscured by a dense cellular band, a judgment that should be made deliberately before any other feature is assessed, since it determines which subsequent differential (lichenoid versus vacuolar interface) the remainder of the examination should be organized around. At low power, the reader then assesses the specific secondary features relevant to whichever branch has been selected, hypergranulosis and sawtooth architecture for the lichenoid branch, basement membrane thickening and follicular plugging for the lupus-associated vacuolar interface branch, and at high power confirms specific cytologic details including the precise character of individual keratinocyte necrosis and, when relevant, satellite cell necrosis.

This staged approach is particularly important for the interface pattern because, as developed throughout this chapter, several of its constituent diagnoses (dermatomyositis versus lupus, graft-versus-host disease versus erythema multiforme) are difficult or impossible to separate on histology alone even when every available feature has been carefully assessed, meaning that efficient, complete histologic characterization, performed once and communicated clearly, is what allows the clinical correlation this pattern so often requires to proceed efficiently rather than through repeated rounds of incomplete information exchange between pathologist and clinician.

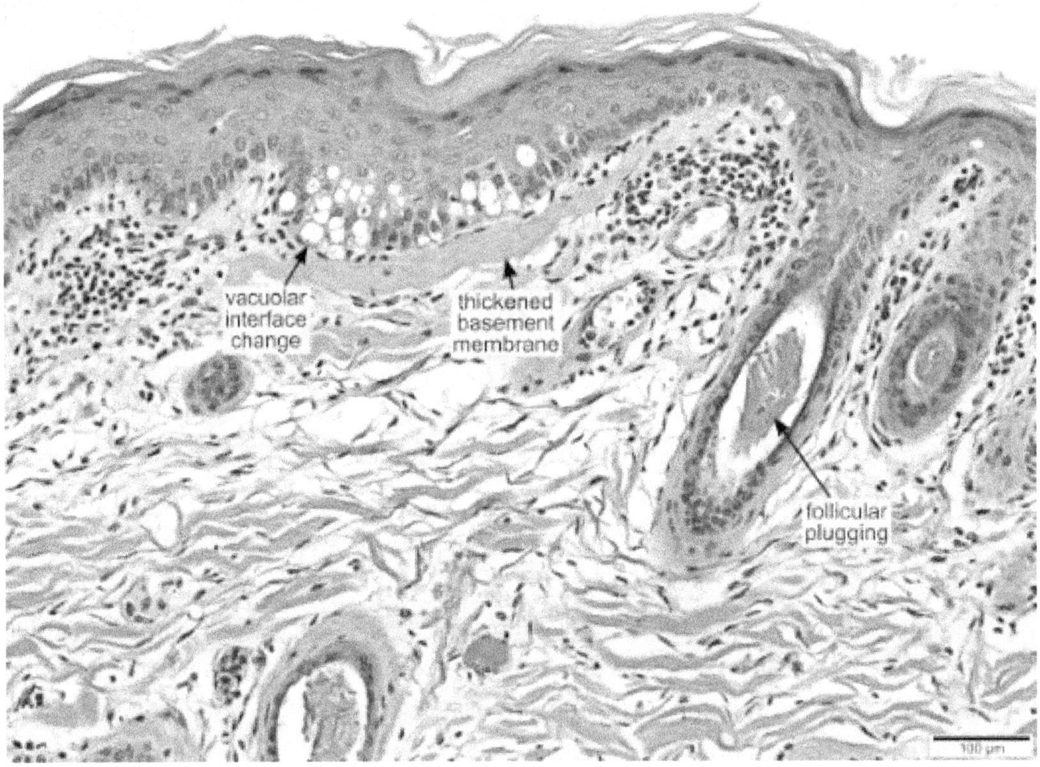

Clinical Presentation and Clinicopathologic Correlation

Lichen Planus Morphology and Variants

Classic cutaneous lichen planus presents with the violaceous, polygonal, flat-topped papules and Wickham striae described above, favoring flexural wrists and ankles, though numerous morphologic variants exist, including hypertrophic lichen planus (thick, verrucous plaques typically on the shins, which can show a somewhat different histologic emphasis with more pronounced epidermal hyperplasia), oral lichen planus (presenting as a reticulated white pattern on the buccal mucosa, erosive lichen planus, or, less commonly, a plaque-type presentation), and lichen planopilaris (a scarring alopecia in which the lichenoid infiltrate targets the follicular epithelium, discussed further in the special-site coverage of Chapter 20). Nail lichen planus produces longitudinal ridging, thinning, and, in severe cases, pterygium formation from permanent nail matrix scarring, another manifestation of the follicular and adnexal targeting capacity of this pattern's underlying immunologic process.

Lupus Erythematosus Morphology and the Cutaneous Subtypes

The three principal cutaneous lupus erythematosus subtypes show distinct clinical morphology that assists in both clinical diagnosis and biopsy interpretation. Acute cutaneous lupus erythematosus classically presents as the malar (butterfly) rash, an erythematous eruption across the cheeks and nasal bridge with characteristic sparing of the nasolabial folds, typically occurring in the context of a systemic lupus flare. Subacute cutaneous lupus erythematosus presents as annular or papulosquamous, photodistributed plaques, often on the upper trunk and extensor arms, and shows a strong association with anti-Ro/SSA antibodies as noted above. Chronic (discoid) lupus erythematosus presents as well-demarcated, scaly, atrophic plaques with follicular plugging and, in longstanding lesions, scarring and dyspigmentation, favoring the face, scalp (where it produces scarring alopecia), and ears, and showing the most pronounced basement membrane thickening and follicular plugging of the three subtypes, correlating with its typically more chronic clinical course.

Erythema Multiforme Morphology and the Target Lesion

Erythema multiforme's characteristic target (iris) lesion, a papule with three concentric zones (a dusky or necrotic center, a surrounding pale ring, and an outer erythematous ring), reflects the zonal pattern of keratinocyte necrosis and interface change described histologically above, with the necrotic center corresponding to the area of most severe epidermal injury. Mucosal involvement, when present, favors a diagnosis further along the severity spectrum toward Stevens-Johnson syndrome, and the acral and symmetric distribution of erythema multiforme, together with a history of recent or recurrent herpes labialis or genital herpes simplex infection, are the most useful clinical correlates supporting this diagnosis over lupus erythematosus, which erythema multiforme can occasionally resemble in its more subtle or early histologic presentations.

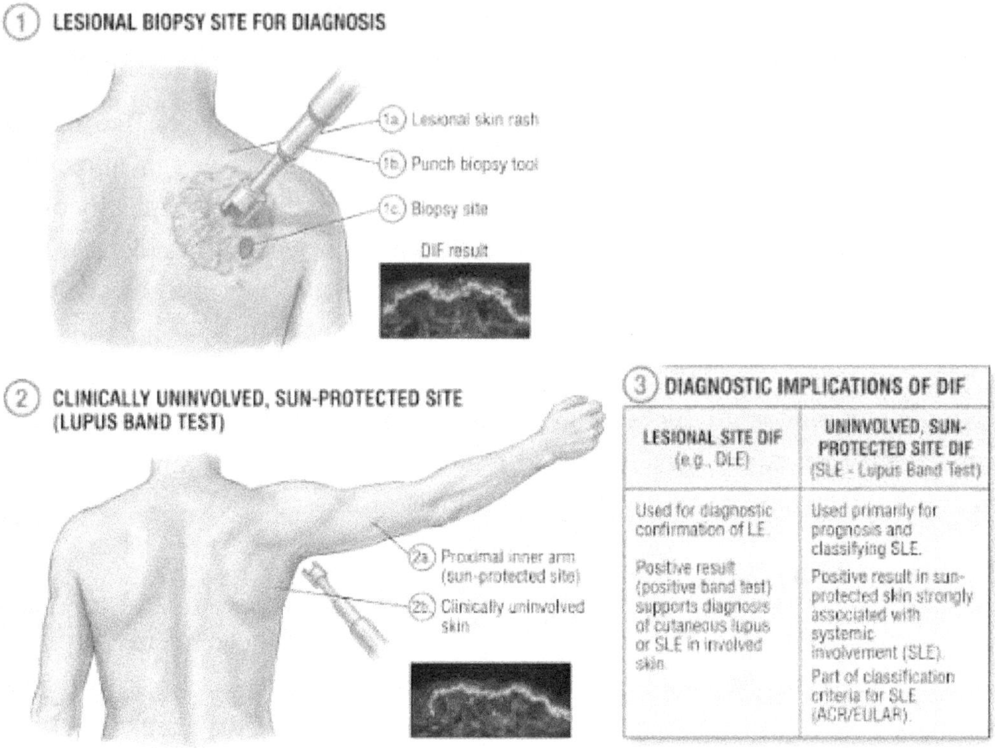

Systemic Lupus Erythematosus Classification Criteria and the Skin's Role

Cutaneous findings occupy a formal place within the classification criteria used to diagnose systemic lupus erythematosus, alongside serologic, hematologic, renal, and other organ-system criteria, and a skin biopsy confirming lupus-specific histology in a patient being evaluated for systemic disease can therefore contribute directly to meeting formal classification thresholds rather than serving only as a standalone dermatologic diagnosis. This formal role underscores why precise, criteria-aware reporting, explicitly noting whether the histologic findings meet the specific threshold typically required to support a lupus-specific interface dermatitis diagnosis (as opposed to a nonspecific interface pattern that falls short of this threshold) provides genuine value to the rheumatology or internal medicine team managing a patient's broader systemic evaluation, not only to the dermatologist managing the cutaneous disease in isolation.

This is a further illustration of a theme introduced in Chapter 1 and recurring throughout this book: a dermatopathology report frequently serves multiple clinical audiences beyond the ordering dermatologist, and awareness of how a given diagnosis feeds into broader diagnostic frameworks used by other specialties, formal lupus classification criteria in this case, staging systems for lymphoma in Chapter 18, or transplant rejection grading systems for graft-versus-host disease as discussed above, allows the report to be written with the fullest possible clinical utility in mind rather than narrowly addressing only the immediate dermatologic question.

Differential Diagnosis and Histologic Mimickers

Lichen Planus Versus Lichenoid Drug Eruption

As introduced in the Chapter 3 Rhythm block on this exact topic, lichenoid drug eruption closely mimics idiopathic lichen planus, and the discriminating features, developed in more detail here, include the presence of eosinophils within the infiltrate (uncommon in idiopathic lichen planus but frequently present in drug-triggered disease), parakeratosis (again uncommon in classic lichen planus but more frequently seen in the drug-triggered variant), and a somewhat deeper, more perivascular extension of the infiltrate beyond the tightly junctional band of idiopathic disease. A new or recently changed medication in the clinical history, particularly one from the classically implicated categories (antihypertensives, antimalarials, nonsteroidal anti-inflammatory drugs), together with these histologic features, supports the drug-induced diagnosis, and withdrawal of the culprit medication with subsequent clinical resolution provides retrospective clinical confirmation.

Lupus Erythematosus Versus Dermatomyositis

Dermatomyositis, an autoimmune connective tissue disease with prominent cutaneous involvement including the heliotrope rash and Gottron papules, shows a vacuolar interface pattern that can be histologically indistinguishable from lupus erythematosus, since both conditions share overlapping autoimmune interface pathogenesis and can show similar basement membrane thickening and dermal mucin deposition. Distinguishing between these two entities relies substantially on clinical correlation, specific distribution patterns (Gottron papules over the interphalangeal joints and periungual telangiectasia favor dermatomyositis), and, when available, specific serologic autoantibody profiles and, in dermatomyositis, evidence of associated proximal muscle weakness or elevated muscle enzymes, underscoring that this is one of the interface pattern's most challenging distinctions to resolve on histology alone.

Lichenoid Keratosis Versus Lichen Planus

Lichenoid keratosis, introduced above as a lichenoid inflammatory reaction to a preexisting benign epidermal lesion, requires the reader to specifically search the periphery of the biopsy, or, when the lesion has been extensively obscured by inflammation, to correlate with the clinical description of a solitary, often previously stable pigmented lesion that has recently become inflamed, since the diagnostic distinction from classic lichen planus rests on identifying residual features of the antecedent lesion (retained basal hyperpigmentation and elongated, club-shaped rete ridges suggestive of an underlying solar lentigo, or the characteristic squamous eddies and horn cysts of a partially obscured seborrheic keratosis) rather than on any difference in the lichenoid infiltrate itself, which can appear essentially identical to idiopathic lichen planus. Clinically, lichenoid keratosis typically presents as a solitary lesion, often on sun-exposed skin of the trunk or extremities, in contrast to the more numerous, symmetric distribution typical of classic lichen planus, and this solitary presentation should itself prompt the reader to specifically search for an antecedent lesion before finalizing a diagnosis of lichen planus in this clinical context.

Vacuolar Interface Pattern Versus Graft-Versus-Host Disease

As introduced above, acute graft-versus-host disease produces a vacuolar interface pattern with satellite cell necrosis closely resembling erythema multiforme, and the histologic distinction between these entities relies almost entirely on clinical context, since the histologic findings alone are frequently indistinguishable. A history of recent allogeneic hematopoietic stem cell transplantation, with the biopsy timing relative to transplant date informing the grading of acute graft-versus-host disease severity used by transplant clinicians, is essential information that should be explicitly requested if not provided on the original requisition, since the diagnosis and its associated grading carry direct and urgent implications for immunosuppressive management in this specific and clinically vulnerable patient population.

A 34-year-old patient three weeks post-allogeneic stem cell transplant presents with a new, diffuse maculopapular eruption, and a punch biopsy is submitted with a differential of graft-versus-host disease versus a drug eruption. Pattern assignment identifies a sparse, patchy vacuolar interface pattern with scattered individual keratinocyte necrosis and associated satellite cell necrosis, findings compatible with either leading diagnosis. Differential narrowing notes the absence of significant eosinophils, which would favor a drug eruption, and the presence of follicular involvement with individual keratinocyte necrosis within the outer root sheath, a finding more specifically associated with graft-versus-host disease than with a typical drug eruption. Diagnosis integrates these findings with the compelling clinical context, timing three weeks post-transplant is within the classic window for acute graft-versus-host disease onset, to support a descriptive diagnosis of vacuolar interface dermatitis with satellite cell necrosis and follicular involvement, favoring graft-versus-host disease, communicated promptly to the transplant team given the urgency of this clinical scenario.

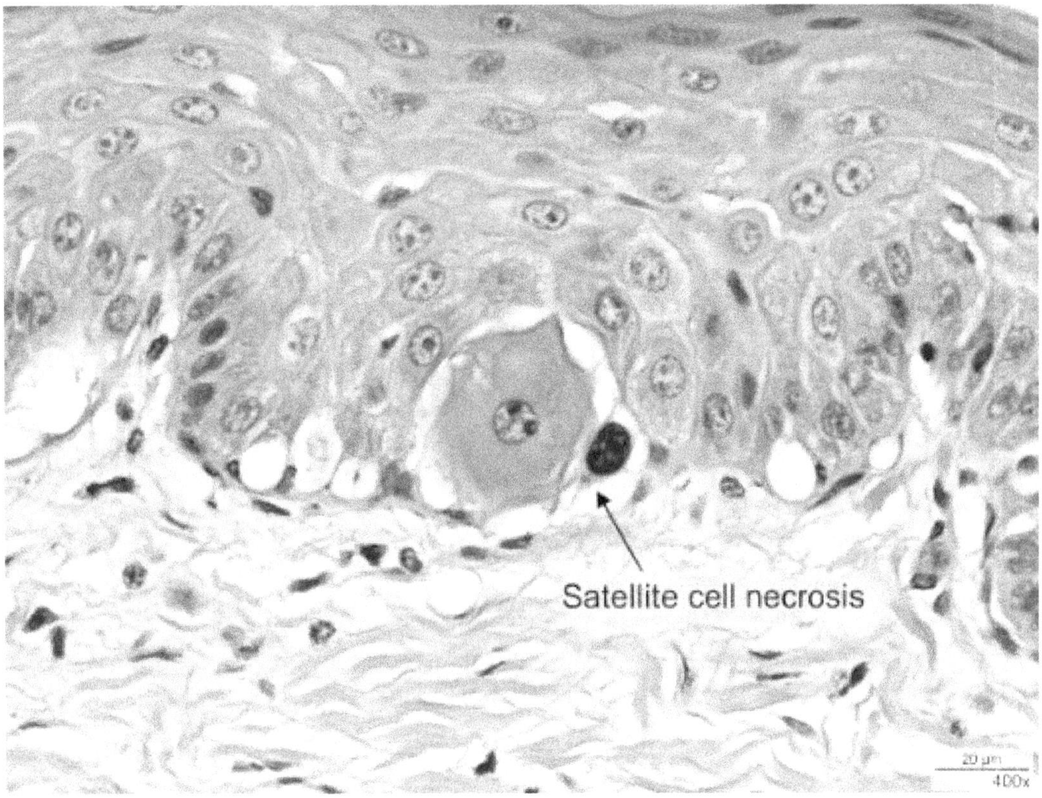

Reporting Ambiguous Interface Pattern Biopsies

As underscored throughout this chapter, several of the interface pattern's constituent diagnoses resist confident histologic separation even after careful, systematic examination, and this chapter's reporting philosophy follows directly from the diagnostic honesty principle established in Chapter 1: a descriptive diagnosis of vacuolar interface dermatitis, with a stated differential naming the specific entities under consideration and the clinical or ancillary information that would help resolve them, serves the treating clinician better than a falsely confident single diagnosis reached by arbitrarily favoring one possibility over comparably supported alternatives. This is especially true for the lupus erythematosus versus dermatomyositis distinction and the erythema multiforme versus graft-versus-host disease distinction developed above, where clinical context frequently carries more diagnostic weight than any single histologic feature.

The specific content of this differential-diagnosis communication matters as much as the decision to include one at all. A report that states "vacuolar interface dermatitis, differential includes lupus erythematosus and dermatomyositis, recommend correlation with autoantibody serologies and assessment for proximal muscle weakness" gives the clinician a concrete, actionable next step, whereas a report that lists the same two diagnoses without indicating what specific clinical information would help distinguish between them provides comparatively little additional value beyond the differential itself. This principle, that a stated differential should be paired with the specific correlating information that would resolve it, recurs throughout this book and is especially load-bearing within the interface pattern family given how frequently histology alone reaches its limit here.

Ancillary Studies

Direct Immunofluorescence in Lupus Erythematosus

Direct immunofluorescence, discussed extensively in Chapter 2, plays a specific and valuable role in lupus erythematosus diagnosis through the lupus band test, in which granular deposition of immunoglobulins (typically IgG, IgM) and complement (C3) is identified in a band-like pattern along the dermal-epidermal junction. This finding is most diagnostically useful when identified in lesional skin, supporting the lupus erythematosus diagnosis, but carries additional significance when identified in clinically uninvolved, sun-protected skin (a positive lupus band test at a non-lesional site), a finding associated with a higher likelihood of systemic disease and renal involvement, making this a circumstance in which the dermatopathologist's ancillary study directly informs systemic disease risk stratification beyond the immediate cutaneous diagnosis.

Special Stains and Immunohistochemistry in the Interface Pattern

PAS staining, as noted above, assists in confirming basement membrane thickening in lupus erythematosus when this feature is subtle on routine hematoxylin and eosin sections, and Alcian blue or colloidal iron staining, discussed in Chapter 2, confirms increased dermal mucin when this finding is similarly subtle. Immunohistochemistry plays a limited role in routine lichenoid and vacuolar interface diagnosis, though it becomes relevant in specific circumstances: CD123 immunohistochemistry, highlighting plasmacytoid dendritic cells, has been used as a research and occasionally diagnostic adjunct in distinguishing lupus erythematosus, which shows increased plasmacytoid dendritic cell infiltration reflecting the interferon-driven pathogenesis discussed above, from its histologic mimickers, though this remains a specialized rather than routine ancillary study in most practice settings.

KEY POINT: When the clinical scenario involves graft-versus-host disease or a severe drug reaction (Stevens-Johnson syndrome/toxic epidermal necrolysis spectrum), rapid communication of findings to the treating team, given the urgency of these clinical scenarios, is as important as the specific ancillary studies pursued.

Management Implications

Treatment Divergence Across the Interface Pattern Family

The entities within the lichenoid and vacuolar interface pattern family require substantially different management approaches, underscoring the clinical importance of the discriminations developed throughout this chapter. Lichen planus is typically managed with topical or, for extensive disease, systemic corticosteroids and other immunomodulatory agents, while lichenoid drug eruption management centers on identifying and discontinuing the culprit medication. Lupus erythematosus management spans topical and systemic immunomodulatory therapy calibrated to disease subtype and systemic involvement, with the biopsy's confirmation of lupus-specific features and, when performed, a positive lupus band test in non-lesional skin directly informing the intensity of systemic workup pursued. Erythema multiforme is typically self-limited and managed supportively, with antiviral prophylaxis considered for recurrent, herpes-triggered disease, while Stevens-Johnson syndrome and toxic epidermal necrolysis represent medical emergencies requiring immediate culprit medication withdrawal and, often, burn-unit-level supportive care given the extensive epidermal loss these severe reactions produce.

Urgency and Communication in Severe Presentations

Given the potential severity of Stevens-Johnson syndrome, toxic epidermal necrolysis, and acute graft-versus-host disease, the dermatopathologist's role in these specific presentations extends beyond accurate diagnosis to include appropriately urgent communication of findings, since delayed recognition of extensive epidermal necrosis or of graft-versus-host disease can meaningfully affect patient outcomes through delayed initiation of appropriate, time-sensitive management. Direct verbal or expedited written communication with the treating clinical team, rather than routine report turnaround, is warranted whenever biopsy findings support one of these severe or urgent diagnoses, reflecting a broader principle that the pathology report's value depends not only on diagnostic accuracy but on the timeliness with which that accuracy reaches the clinicians positioned to act on it.

Long-Term Monitoring Considerations for Chronic Interface-Pattern Disease

Beyond the acute and urgent scenarios discussed above, several entities within this pattern family require longitudinal monitoring that the initial biopsy diagnosis sets in motion. Discoid lupus erythematosus, given the meaningful minority of patients who develop or already have systemic disease at diagnosis, typically prompts baseline and periodic monitoring for systemic lupus erythematosus features, including relevant serologic testing and clinical assessment for renal, hematologic, and other systemic organ involvement, a monitoring pathway the biopsy's confirmed diagnosis directly initiates. Lichen planopilaris and frontal fibrosing alopecia, given their progressive and scarring nature, are typically monitored for disease activity and treatment response using standardized scalp assessment tools, with the goal of halting further follicular destruction, since already-lost follicular units, replaced by fibrous tissue, do not regenerate, making early diagnosis and treatment initiation particularly consequential for long-term hair preservation.

Erosive oral lichen planus and, in a small subset of cases, other chronic lichen planus variants carry a recognized, if modest, risk of malignant transformation to squamous cell carcinoma, particularly in longstanding erosive oral disease, and this risk informs a recommendation for periodic clinical surveillance of chronically affected mucosal sites, a consideration the dermatopathology report can appropriately note when erosive oral lichen planus is the diagnosis rendered, ensuring the treating clinician incorporates this surveillance into the patient's long-term care plan rather than treating the diagnosis as requiring only symptomatic management.

The Pattern: The lichenoid pattern (lichen planus, lichenoid drug eruption, lichen striatus) and the vacuolar interface pattern (lupus erythematosus, erythema multiforme, graft-versus-host disease), distinguished by infiltrate density.

Histologic Signature: Dense, band-like infiltrate obscuring the junction with sawtooth rete and hypergranulosis defines the lichenoid pattern; sparse, patchy infiltrate with the junction still visible, plus basement membrane thickening and dermal mucin (lupus) or prominent keratinocyte necrosis (erythema multiforme, graft-versus-host disease), defines the vacuolar interface pattern.

The Decision: Assess infiltrate density and junctional obscuration first to sort into the lichenoid or vacuolar interface family, then apply the specific secondary features and clinical context needed to resolve the diagnosis within that family.

Trap Logic: Lichenoid drug eruption mimics lichen planus (eosinophils, parakeratosis discriminate). Dermatomyositis mimics lupus erythematosus (clinical distribution and serology discriminate). Graft-versus-host disease mimics erythema multiforme (transplant history and follicular involvement discriminate).

Pattern Anchor: Junctional obscuration sorts lichenoid from vacuolar interface; within each family, the specific mimickers are resolved more by clinical context (medication history, transplant timing, distribution) than by histology alone, more so than in almost any other reaction pattern in this book.

Summary and Key Concepts

The lichenoid and vacuolar interface patterns share basal keratinocyte injury as their common target but are distinguished by infiltrate density: dense and band-like (lichenoid) versus sparse and patchy (vacuolar interface).

Lichen planus, the lichenoid prototype, shows sawtooth rete, hypergranulosis, and Civatte bodies; its histologic mimicker, lichenoid drug eruption, is distinguished by eosinophils, parakeratosis, and medication history.

Lupus erythematosus, erythema multiforme, and graft-versus-host disease share the vacuolar interface pattern; basement membrane thickening and dermal mucin favor lupus, while prominent keratinocyte necrosis favors erythema multiforme and graft-versus-host disease, which are frequently distinguished from one another primarily by clinical context.

Direct immunofluorescence, particularly the lupus band test, provides diagnostically and prognostically significant information in lupus erythematosus, including risk stratification for systemic disease when positive in non-lesional skin.

Stevens-Johnson syndrome, toxic epidermal necrolysis, and acute graft-versus-host disease are medical emergencies within this pattern family, requiring urgent, direct communication of biopsy findings to the treating clinical team.

CHAPTER 7: VESICULOBULLOUS AND VESICULOPUSTULAR DERMATOSES

Learning Objectives

1. Classify vesiculobullous disease by level and mechanism of epidermal or subepidermal split.
2. Describe the etiology and immunopathogenesis of the pemphigus and pemphigoid groups and related immunobullous diseases.
3. Identify the histopathologic features and direct immunofluorescence findings that distinguish the major immunobullous diseases from one another.
4. Correlate histologic and immunofluorescence findings with clinical presentation across the vesiculobullous disease spectrum.
5. Construct a differential diagnosis for a blistering biopsy and discriminate immunobullous disease from its major mimickers.
6. Apply direct and indirect immunofluorescence, and understand special population considerations, in the vesiculobullous workup.

Definition and Classification by Level of Split

The Level of Split as the Primary Organizing Axis

The vesiculobullous pattern, introduced in Chapter 3, is organized primarily not by a single defining histologic feature, as most of the other reaction patterns in this book are, but by the specific level and mechanism at which epidermal or subepidermal separation occurs, since this level correlates closely with the underlying disease mechanism and with the specific direct immunofluorescence pattern discussed in Chapter 2 that ultimately confirms the diagnosis. Intraepidermal splits occur within the epidermis itself and are further subdivided by mechanism into acantholytic splits, resulting from loss of keratinocyte cohesion through desmosomal disruption, and spongiotic splits, resulting from fluid-driven separation as developed in Chapter 4. Subepidermal splits occur at or just below the dermal-epidermal junction and are further subdivided by the specific target antigen within the basement membrane zone complex that the causative autoantibody or genetic defect disrupts.

This organizational framework directly parallels the compartmental logic introduced in Chapter 1 and applied throughout this book: just as identifying the anatomic compartment involved is the essential first step for the other reaction patterns, identifying the level of split is the essential first step for the vesiculobullous pattern, and every subsequent diagnostic step, from special histologic feature assessment through direct immunofluorescence interpretation, is organized around refining the diagnosis within the level of split already established at low power.

The Acantholytic (Pemphigus) Group

The pemphigus group comprises autoimmune blistering diseases in which autoantibodies target desmosomal cadherins, disrupting keratinocyte-to-keratinocyte adhesion and producing an acantholytic, intraepidermal split. Pemphigus vulgaris, the most common and clinically significant member of this group, targets desmoglein 3 predominantly, with a subset of patients also showing anti-desmoglein 1 antibodies, and produces a suprabasal split, since desmoglein 3 expression is most concentrated in the lower epidermis. Pemphigus foliaceus targets desmoglein 1 predominantly, which is more concentrated in the superficial epidermis, producing a more superficial, subcorneal split that manifests clinically as superficial erosions and scale-crust rather than the deeper, more fragile bullae of pemphigus vulgaris. Paraneoplastic pemphigus, introduced in Chapter 2, targets a broader range of antigens including desmoplakins and other plakin family proteins in addition to desmogleins, producing a combined histologic and immunofluorescence picture reflecting this broader antigenic target.

The Subepidermal (Pemphigoid) Group and Related Diseases

The pemphigoid group and related subepidermal blistering diseases are organized by the specific basement membrane zone component targeted, discussed in detail in the etiology section below, and by the resulting position of the split relative to the lamina lucida, information directly assessed using the salt-split skin technique introduced in Chapter 2. Bullous pemphigoid, the most common subepidermal immunobullous disease, targets BP180 (also known as type XVII collagen) and BP230, hemidesmosomal components, producing a split within the lamina lucida that localizes to the epidermal (roof) side on salt-split skin. Epidermolysis bullosa acquisita and anti-p200 pemphigoid target structures below the lamina lucida (type VII collagen and laminin gamma-1, respectively), producing a split that localizes to the dermal (floor) side. Dermatitis herpetiformis and linear IgA disease, while also producing subepidermal separation, are distinguished by their specific granular versus linear IgA-predominant immunofluorescence patterns, discussed in the ancillary studies section below.

Level and Mechanism	Representative Disease	Target Antigen	Key Distinguishing Feature
Intraepidermal, suprabasal, acantholytic	Pemphigus vulgaris	Desmoglein 3 (± desmoglein 1)	Deep, fragile bullae, mucosal involvement common
Intraepidermal, subcorneal, acantholytic	Pemphigus foliaceus	Desmoglein 1	Superficial erosions and scale-crust, mucosa spared
Subepidermal, lamina lucida, epidermal-side on salt-split	Bullous pemphigoid	BP180, BP230	Tense bullae over urticarial plaques, elderly patients

Subepidermal, sub-lamina densa, dermal-side on salt-split	Epidermolysis bullosa acquisita	Type VII collagen	Trauma-induced bullae, scarring, milia formation
Subepidermal, papillary tip, granular IgA	Dermatitis herpetiformis	Tissue transglutaminase (epidermal)	Intensely pruritic grouped vesicles, celiac disease association

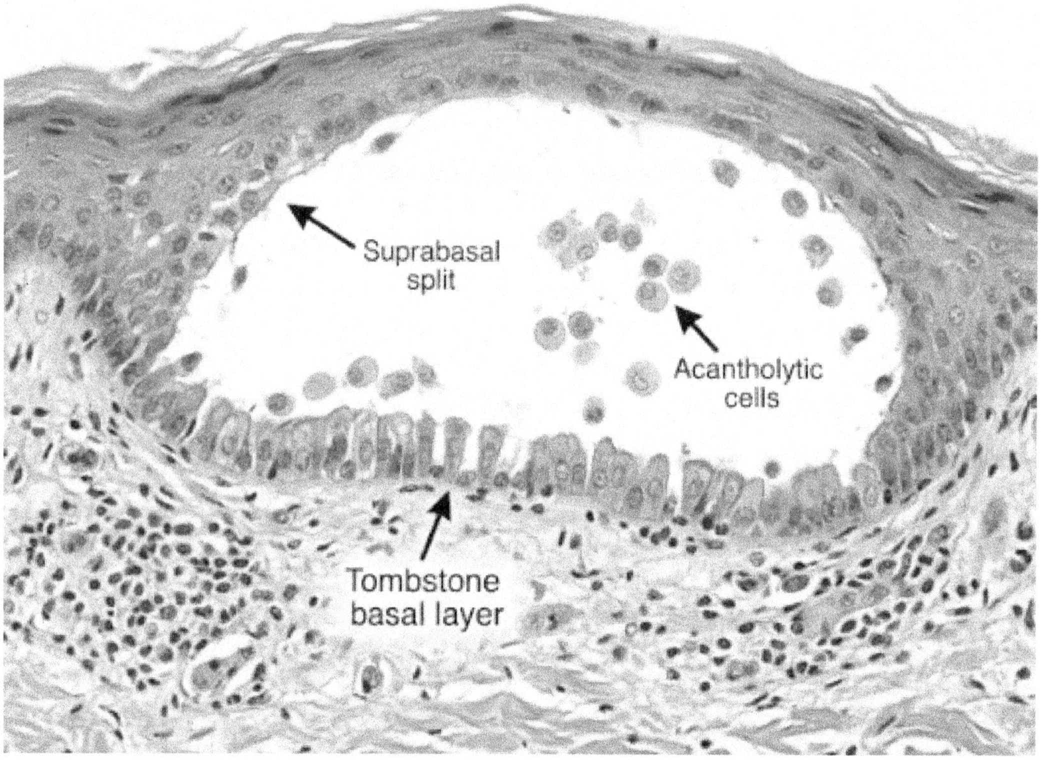

Etiology and Immunologic Mechanisms

Autoantibody-Mediated Desmosomal Disruption in Pemphigus

In the pemphigus group, circulating IgG autoantibodies bind directly to the extracellular domains of desmoglein 1 and desmoglein 3, disrupting the calcium-dependent adhesive function of these desmosomal cadherins through a combination of direct steric hindrance of cadherin binding and antibody-triggered intracellular signaling that leads to desmosome internalization and cytoskeletal reorganization, together producing the loss of keratinocyte cohesion that defines acantholysis. The relative distribution of desmoglein 1 (concentrated superficially) and desmoglein 3 (concentrated in the lower epidermis and more highly expressed in mucosal epithelium) explains both the differing level of split between pemphigus vulgaris and pemphigus foliaceus and the differing clinical distribution of mucosal involvement between these two entities, with pemphigus vulgaris showing prominent mucosal disease reflecting the mucosa's high desmoglein 3 expression relative to desmoglein 1.

Autoantibody-Mediated Basement Membrane Disruption in Pemphigoid

In bullous pemphigoid, IgG autoantibodies target the extracellular domain of BP180 and, less consistently, the intracellular BP230, triggering complement activation and recruitment of eosinophils and neutrophils that release proteolytic enzymes damaging the hemidesmosomal-lamina lucida complex, producing the subepidermal split characteristic of this disease. This complement- and eosinophil-driven mechanism explains the frequently prominent eosinophilic infiltrate seen histologically in bullous pemphigoid, discussed further below, and explains the eosinophilic spongiosis presentation of early, pre-bullous disease introduced in Chapter 4, in which the same underlying autoantibody and inflammatory process is present but has not yet produced frank subepidermal separation.

Genetic and Nutritional Mechanisms in Related Blistering Disease

Dermatitis herpetiformis, while immunologically mediated, differs mechanistically from the pemphigus and pemphigoid groups in being driven by IgA autoantibodies against tissue transglutaminase, generated as part of the immune response to gluten in genetically susceptible individuals with celiac disease, with the autoantibodies cross-reacting with epidermal transglutaminase deposited at the dermal papillary tips, producing the granular IgA deposition pattern and the neutrophil-rich papillary tip microabscesses discussed in the histopathologic features section below. This gluten-driven mechanism directly explains the disease's strong association with celiac disease and its response to a gluten-free diet, a management approach fundamentally different from the immunosuppressive therapy that anchors treatment of the pemphigus and pemphigoid groups.

Hereditary epidermolysis bullosa, distinct from the autoimmune acquired form discussed above, results from genetic mutations affecting structural proteins of the basement membrane zone or, in the simplex form, basal keratin filaments themselves, producing mechanically fragile skin that blisters with minor trauma from birth or early infancy, a fundamentally different mechanism (structural protein deficiency rather than autoantibody-mediated destruction) that nonetheless produces histologic and, in some subtypes, electron microscopic findings requiring specific expertise to characterize accurately, a specialized area of dermatopathology practice this chapter introduces but does not develop exhaustively given its relative rarity relative to the acquired immunobullous diseases that form the chapter's primary focus.

Biopsy Strategy Revisited for Suspected Immunobullous Disease

The two-specimen biopsy strategy introduced in Chapter 1, a lesional biopsy for routine histology and a perilesional biopsy for direct immunofluorescence, deserves specific reinforcement in this chapter given how central it is to accurate diagnosis across the entire vesiculobullous pattern family. The lesional biopsy should, whenever possible, capture an early, small, intact blister together with a margin of adjacent unblistered skin, since this margin preserves the transition zone where the specific level and mechanism of split is often most clearly appreciated, whereas a biopsy consisting entirely of already-separated blister roof and floor, without this transitional edge, can be considerably more difficult to interpret confidently. The perilesional biopsy for direct immunofluorescence should be taken from clinically normal-appearing skin immediately adjacent to, but not within, an active lesion, typically within a few millimeters, since skin too far from active disease may show a falsely negative or attenuated immunofluorescence pattern, while lesional skin itself, as discussed in Chapter 2, frequently shows degraded or nonspecific immunoreactant deposition.

For dermatitis herpetiformis specifically, given the intense pruritus and consequent excoriation discussed in the clinical presentation section below, biopsy site selection requires particular care, and clinicians are specifically counseled to select a subtle, minimally excoriated papule or the skin immediately adjacent to one, rather than a heavily excoriated area, for both the lesional and perilesional specimens, since excoriation can destroy or obscure both the characteristic papillary tip neutrophilic infiltrate on routine histology and the granular IgA deposition on direct immunofluorescence, potentially producing a falsely negative or uninterpretable result despite genuine underlying disease.

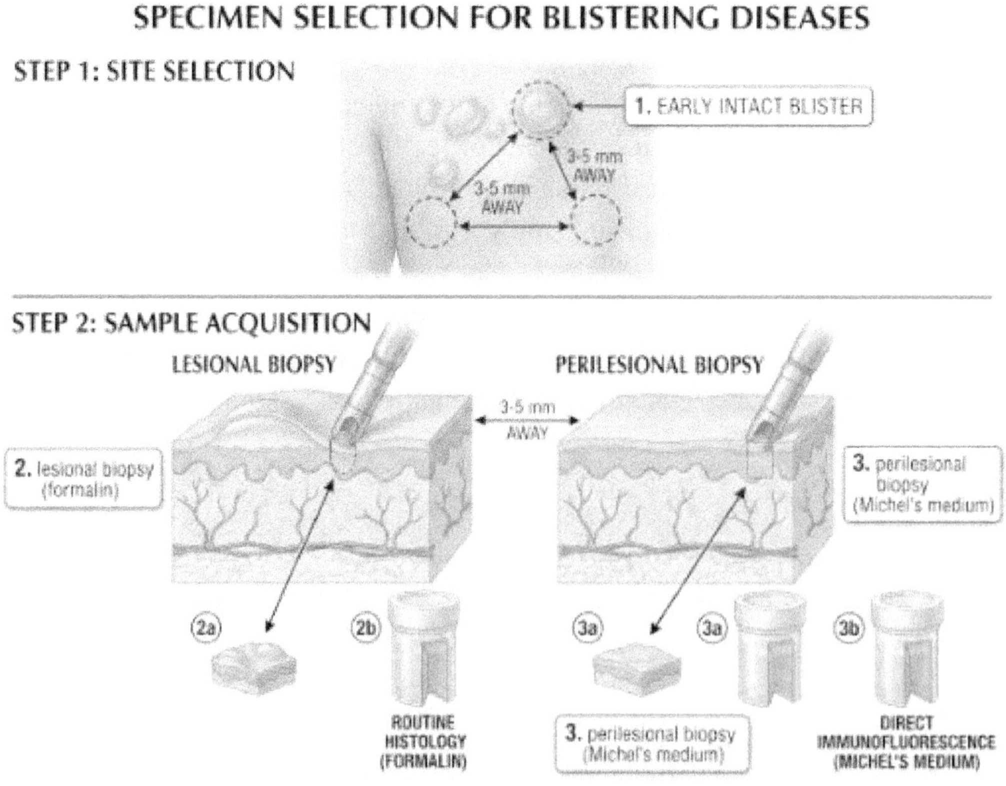

THE REACTION PATTERN RECOGNITION SYSTEM — Level of Split as the Organizing Principle

---

The Pattern: Level of Split Determines the Entire Subsequent Differential Diagnosis

Histologic Signature: An intraepidermal split with acantholytic cells and a tombstone basal layer pattern (pemphigus group) versus a subepidermal split with an intact, non-acantholytic epidermis forming the blister roof (pemphigoid group and related subepidermal diseases).

The Decision: Determine the level of split first, before assessing any other feature, since this single determination sorts the biopsy into one of two fundamentally different disease families with different target antigens, different direct immunofluorescence patterns, and different management pathways.

Trap Logic: The mimicker in each direction is a technical artifact: crush or freezing artifact, discussed in Chapter 2, can produce intraepidermal clefting that mimics true acantholysis, while an old, degenerating subepidermal blister can show secondary changes that obscure the clean subepidermal plane. The discriminating step is examining the edge of the blister, where the split first begins, rather than the most degenerated central portion of an older lesion.

Pattern Anchor: Before naming a specific immunobullous disease, answer one question: is the roof of this blister the full epidermis (subepidermal split) or only its outer portion (intraepidermal split)? Every subsequent step in this chapter follows from that answer.

Histopathologic Features and Diagnostic Criteria

Diagnostic Features of the Pemphigus Group

Beyond the level of split already established, the pemphigus group shows characteristic acantholytic cytology: rounded, retracted keratinocytes with condensed, hyperchromatic nuclei and a peripheral rim of eosinophilic cytoplasm (a corn-flake or fried-egg appearance), free-floating individually or in small clusters within the blister cavity. Pemphigus vulgaris characteristically shows a tombstone pattern along the floor of the blister, in which the residual basal keratinocytes remain attached to the underlying basement membrane despite loss of attachment to the overlying, now-separated spinous layer, resembling a row of tombstones. The inflammatory infiltrate in pemphigus is typically modest, predominantly lymphocytic with variable eosinophils, in contrast to the frequently more robust eosinophilic infiltrate of bullous pemphigoid discussed below.

Diagnostic Features of the Pemphigoid Group

Bullous pemphigoid shows a subepidermal split with an intact, non-acantholytic epidermal roof, and a blister cavity and underlying papillary dermis frequently rich in eosinophils, often with eosinophils lining up along the dermal-epidermal junction even before frank blister formation (the eosinophilic spongiosis discussed in Chapter 4). This eosinophil-rich infiltrate is one of the most useful features distinguishing bullous pemphigoid from other subepidermal blistering diseases, though it is not entirely specific, since other subepidermal diseases can show some degree of eosinophilic infiltrate, making the direct immunofluorescence and, when needed, salt-split skin studies discussed below the ultimate arbiters of specific subepidermal disease diagnosis.

Diagnostic Features of Dermatitis Herpetiformis

Dermatitis herpetiformis characteristically shows neutrophilic microabscesses concentrated at the tips of the dermal papillae, a distinctive finding that, when well developed, can progress to confluent subepidermal separation as the papillary tip neutrophilic infiltrate damages the overlying dermal-epidermal junction. This papillary tip neutrophilic pattern, together with the granular IgA deposition at the same location discussed in the ancillary studies section, is highly characteristic and, when clearly present, substantially narrows the differential before immunofluorescence confirmation, though early or subtle lesions may show only scattered neutrophils that require careful, deliberate search of multiple dermal papillae to appreciate fully.

Evaluating Blister Age and Secondary Changes

As with the other reaction patterns discussed in this book, blister age affects the histologic picture in ways a reader should account for during interpretation. An early, fresh blister shows the cleanest and most diagnostically informative architecture, while an older, degenerating blister can show reepithelialization from the blister edge, secondary infection with a superimposed neutrophilic infiltrate, and progressive loss of the specific acantholytic or subepidermal architecture as the roof and floor of the blister undergo further degenerative change. Biopsy technique, discussed in Chapter 1, directly affects the diagnostic yield here: a biopsy taken from the edge of an early, intact blister, capturing both blistered and adjacent unblistered epidermis in continuity, provides substantially more diagnostic information than a biopsy taken from the center of an older, more degenerated lesion.

Applying the Scanning Approach to Vesiculobullous Biopsies

The systematic low-power to high-power scanning approach, applied throughout this book, is organized for the vesiculobullous pattern specifically around the level-of-split determination introduced at the start of this chapter. At scanning power, the reader identifies the presence of a blister cavity and assesses, at the blister edge where the transition from intact to separated epidermis is clearest, whether the roof of the blister comprises the full epidermal thickness (subepidermal split) or only its outer portion, leaving residual basal keratinocytes on the floor (intraepidermal split). At low power, the reader characterizes the composition of the inflammatory infiltrate within and beneath the blister cavity, specifically noting the relative proportion of eosinophils, neutrophils, and lymphocytes, since this composition, as developed throughout this chapter, carries substantial discriminating weight among the specific diseases within each level-of-split category. At high power, the reader confirms specific cytologic detail, particularly the character of any acantholytic cells present, before finalizing an impression and, in nearly every case, recommending or confirming that direct immunofluorescence has been or will be performed.

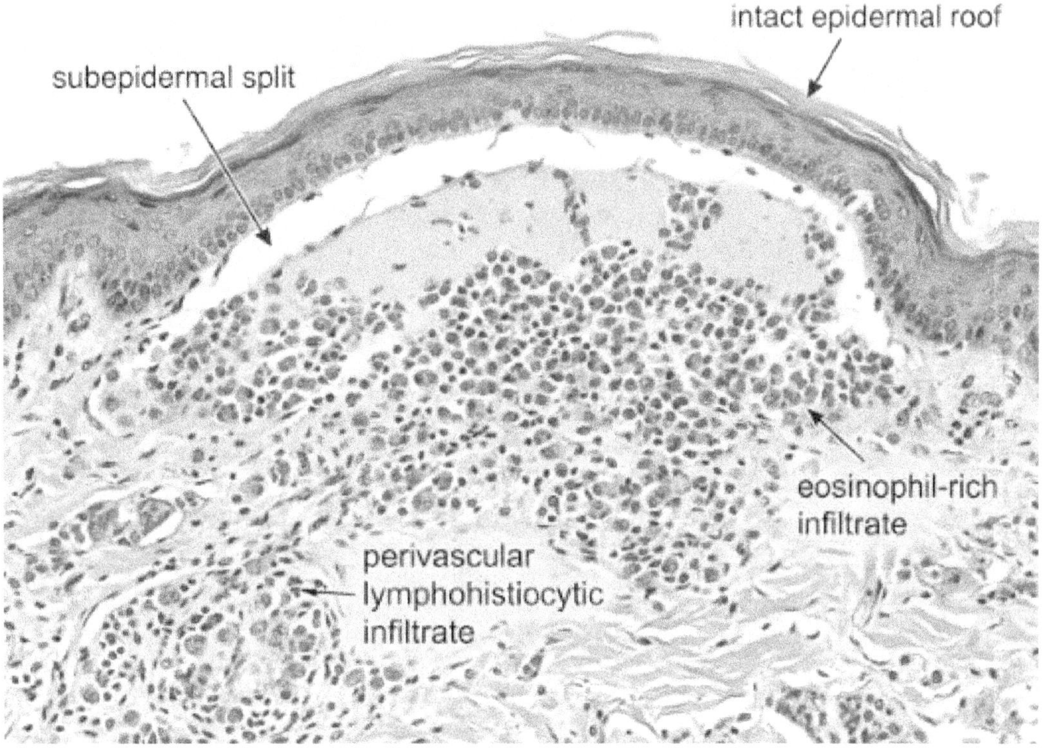

Clinical Presentation and Clinicopathologic Correlation

Clinical Morphology Across the Immunobullous Spectrum

Pemphigus vulgaris presents with flaccid, easily ruptured bullae that frequently leave behind painful erosions rather than intact blisters by the time of clinical presentation, reflecting the superficial location and mechanical fragility of the acantholytic split, together with a positive Nikolsky sign (extension of a blister or erosion with lateral pressure on adjacent clinically normal-appearing skin), and prominent, often the presenting, mucosal (oral) involvement. Bullous pemphigoid, by contrast, presents with tense, intact bullae that do not extend with lateral pressure, reflecting the more mechanically robust, full-thickness epidermal roof of the subepidermal split, frequently arising over an urticarial or eczematous background and predominantly affecting elderly patients, a demographic and morphologic pattern that should specifically raise this diagnosis, as emphasized in the Chapter 4 discussion of eosinophilic spongiosis.

Dermatitis Herpetiformis and Its Systemic Association

Dermatitis herpetiformis presents with intensely pruritic, grouped (herpetiform) vesicles and papules symmetrically distributed on extensor surfaces, particularly the elbows, knees, and buttocks, and given the intense pruritus, intact vesicles are frequently excoriated before biopsy, making biopsy site selection, favoring a fresh, minimally excoriated lesion or, ideally, perilesional skin for both routine histology and direct immunofluorescence, particularly important for this specific disease. The strong association with celiac disease, present in the great majority of dermatitis herpetiformis patients even when gastrointestinal symptoms are absent or subclinical, means that a confirmed diagnosis should prompt evaluation for celiac disease, including tissue transglutaminase serology and, when appropriate, gastroenterology referral, extending the clinical significance of this cutaneous diagnosis well beyond the skin itself.

CLINICAL PEARL: Nikolsky sign positivity (pemphigus) versus tense, non-extending bullae (pemphigoid) is a clinical bedside finding that correlates directly with the level of split established histologically, illustrating how mechanical fragility at the bedside reflects the specific plane of tissue separation at the microscope.

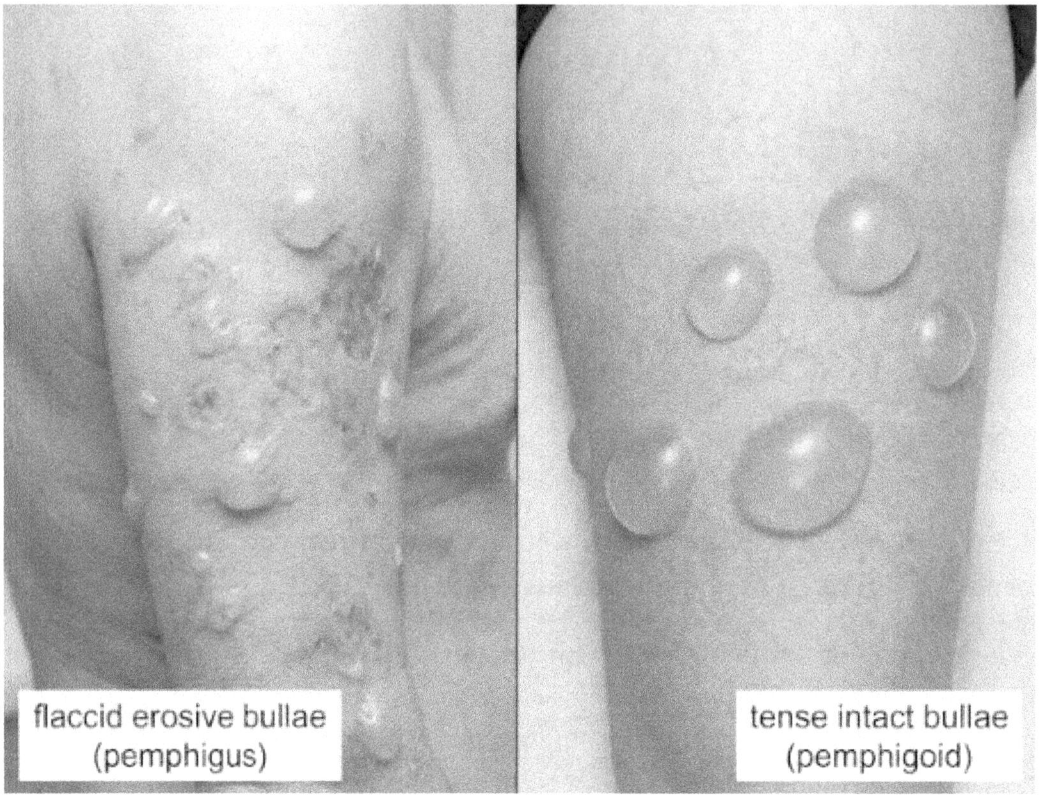

Special Populations: Neonatal, Pediatric, and Pregnancy-Associated Blistering Disease

Several vesiculobullous diseases show specific age- or pregnancy-related presentations that warrant separate mention. Neonatal pemphigus, resulting from transplacental passage of maternal pemphigus autoantibodies, produces transient blistering in the newborn of a mother with active pemphigus, typically resolving spontaneously over several weeks as maternal antibody is cleared from the neonatal circulation, a self-limited course that distinguishes it from the persistent, treatment-requiring disease seen in affected adults. Chronic bullous disease of childhood, the pediatric counterpart to linear IgA disease, shows the same linear junctional IgA deposition pattern discussed in the ancillary studies section but with a distinct clinical morphology often described as a "cluster of jewels" or "string of pearls" pattern, in which new blisters characteristically arise at the periphery of resolving older lesions.

Pemphigoid gestationis, a pregnancy-associated subepidermal immunobullous disease immunologically related to bullous pemphigoid and sharing the same BP180 target antigen, typically presents in the second or third trimester with intensely pruritic urticarial plaques progressing to tense bullae, characteristically beginning periumbilically before generalizing, and carries a recognized, if modest, association with fetal growth restriction and preterm delivery, making accurate diagnosis important for appropriate maternal-fetal monitoring beyond the immediate dermatologic management. Distinguishing pemphigoid gestationis from the more common and generally more benign polymorphic eruption of pregnancy, which does not show the linear BP180-targeted immunofluorescence pattern, relies on the same direct immunofluorescence approach developed throughout this chapter, underscoring its diagnostic centrality even in this specific and clinically distinct population.

Differential Diagnosis and Histologic Mimickers

Distinguishing Within the Pemphigus Group

Pemphigus vulgaris and pemphigus foliaceus, while sharing the fundamental acantholytic mechanism, are distinguished primarily by the level of split, suprabasal for pemphigus vulgaris and subcorneal for pemphigus foliaceus, a distinction usually apparent on routine histology but confirmed definitively by direct immunofluorescence, which shows intercellular IgG deposition throughout the epidermis in both entities but with a staining intensity gradient (stronger in the lower epidermis for pemphigus vulgaris, stronger in the upper epidermis for pemphigus foliaceus) that can assist in subtyping when the histologic level of split is ambiguous. Paraneoplastic pemphigus, as discussed in Chapter 2, should be specifically considered when a pemphigus-like presentation occurs in a patient with a known or suspected malignancy, particularly lymphoproliferative disease, given its distinct combined immunofluorescence pattern and its association with a specific, often severe and treatment-resistant, clinical course.

Distinguishing Within the Subepidermal Blistering Diseases

As discussed in Chapter 2, distinguishing among the subepidermal blistering diseases, bullous pemphigoid, epidermolysis bullosa acquisita, anti-p200 pemphigoid, and linear IgA disease, relies substantially on the specific direct immunofluorescence pattern and, when needed, salt-split skin localization, since these entities can appear similar on routine histology alone, particularly when the eosinophil-rich infiltrate that helps favor bullous pemphigoid is not prominently developed. Bullae arising specifically at sites of trauma, with subsequent scarring and milia formation, favor epidermolysis bullosa acquisita over bullous pemphigoid, reflecting the deeper, sub-lamina densa target antigen and the resulting more fragile dermal-epidermal attachment that trauma more readily disrupts, a clinical clue that complements but does not replace the definitive immunofluorescence-based distinction.

Bullous Arthropod Bite Reaction and Other Mimickers

A bullous arthropod bite reaction can produce a subepidermal or, less commonly, intraepidermal split with a prominent eosinophilic infiltrate that superficially resembles bullous pemphigoid, and is distinguished by the characteristic wedge-shaped, perivascular and interstitial dermal infiltrate extending deeper than typical bullous pemphigoid, often with a central punctum or other evidence of the causative bite, together with negative direct immunofluorescence, which excludes a genuine autoimmune process. Bullous impetigo, a superficial staphylococcal infection producing an intraepidermal, subcorneal split through the action of exfoliative toxins that specifically cleave desmoglein 1, can mimic pemphigus foliaceus both clinically and, to some degree, histologically, and is distinguished by the presence of neutrophils and, when sought, gram-positive cocci within the blister cavity, together with negative direct immunofluorescence and, when needed, bacterial culture confirmation.

Friction Blisters, Bullous Fixed Drug Eruption, and Other Uncommon Mimickers

Friction blisters, resulting from mechanical shear force at sites of repeated friction (commonly the feet in the context of new or ill-fitting footwear), produce an intraepidermal split at a characteristic level, within the mid to upper stratum spinosum, that is distinguished from the pemphigus group by the absence of true acantholysis (keratinocytes at the blister margin remain cohesive rather than showing the rounded, retracted morphology of acantholytic cells) and by a paucity of associated inflammation, reflecting the purely mechanical rather than immunologic mechanism of injury. Bullous fixed drug eruption, a distinctive variant of fixed drug eruption in which a well-demarcated, dusky plaque recurs at the same anatomic site with each exposure to the culprit medication, shows a vacuolar interface pattern with prominent keratinocyte necrosis, closely related to the erythema multiforme spectrum discussed in Chapter 6, that can progress to full subepidermal bullous separation in severe cases, and is distinguished from true immunobullous disease by negative direct immunofluorescence together with the characteristic recurrent, fixed anatomic distribution elicited on clinical history.

Bullous lupus erythematosus, an uncommon but distinct presentation in which lupus erythematosus produces subepidermal blistering through autoantibodies against type VII collagen, the same target antigen implicated in epidermolysis bullosa acquisita discussed above, illustrates a further point of overlap within the subepidermal blistering diseases: histologically and immunofluorescence-wise, bullous lupus erythematosus and epidermolysis bullosa acquisita can be difficult to distinguish, since both show a dermal-side pattern on salt-split skin, and the distinction ultimately rests on the broader clinical and serologic context of systemic lupus erythematosus (positive antinuclear antibody and other lupus-specific serologies, other systemic lupus manifestations) rather than on the immunobullous findings in isolation.

A 6-year-old child presents with rapidly spreading superficial blisters and honey-colored crusting on the face, and a biopsy is obtained given diagnostic uncertainty between bullous impetigo and a pediatric immunobullous disease. Pattern assignment identifies an intraepidermal, subcorneal split with acantholytic keratinocytes, a picture that, on histology alone, overlaps substantially with pemphigus foliaceus. Differential narrowing notes numerous neutrophils within the blister cavity and adjacent stratum corneum, a finding atypical for pemphigus foliaceus, which typically shows a comparatively sparse infiltrate. Diagnosis integrates these findings with the clinical presentation (rapid onset, honey-colored crust, pediatric age, a presentation highly atypical for pemphigus foliaceus, which is rare in children) and a negative direct immunofluorescence result to confirm bullous impetigo rather than an immunobullous disease, allowing prompt initiation of appropriate antibiotic therapy rather than unnecessary immunosuppression.

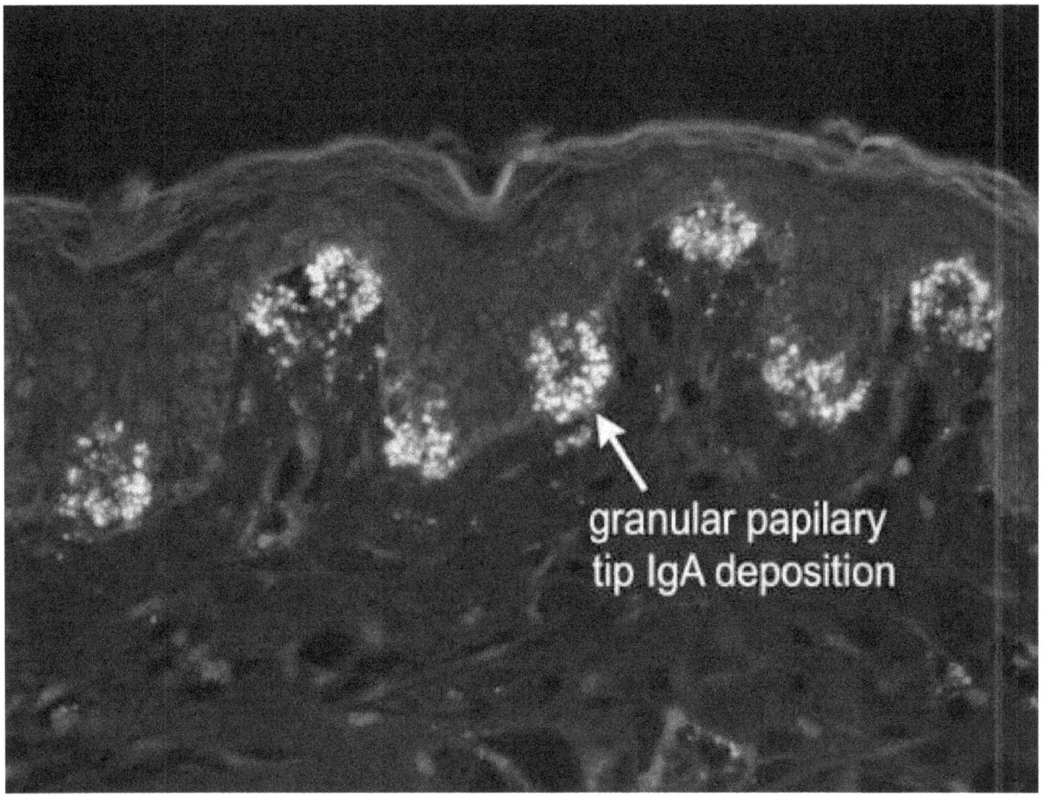

Ancillary Studies

Direct Immunofluorescence as the Diagnostic Standard

As established in Chapter 2, direct immunofluorescence of a perilesional biopsy is the diagnostic standard for definitively distinguishing among the immunobullous diseases discussed in this chapter, since it directly visualizes the specific immunoreactant and its precise location, information that routine histology alone frequently cannot provide with full confidence. Intercellular epidermal IgG deposition confirms the pemphigus group; linear junctional IgG and C3 deposition confirms the pemphigoid group, with salt-split skin localization (epidermal versus dermal side) further distinguishing bullous pemphigoid from epidermolysis bullosa acquisita and anti-p200 pemphigoid; and granular papillary tip IgA deposition confirms dermatitis herpetiformis, while linear junctional IgA deposition confirms linear IgA disease.

Indirect Immunofluorescence and Antigen-Specific Serology

As discussed in Chapter 2, indirect immunofluorescence and antigen-specific enzyme-linked immunosorbent assays provide complementary information, quantifying circulating autoantibody titers that assist in monitoring disease activity and treatment response over time, particularly valuable in the pemphigus group, where titer correlates reasonably well with clinical disease activity. Anti-desmoglein 1 and anti-desmoglein 3 enzyme-linked immunosorbent assays specifically help distinguish pemphigus vulgaris from pemphigus foliaceus and can identify the specific antibody profile (desmoglein 3 alone, desmoglein 1 alone, or both) that correlates with the specific clinical phenotype (mucosal-dominant, cutaneous-dominant, or mucocutaneous) a given patient presents with.

KEY POINT: A biopsy for routine histology alone, without an accompanying perilesional specimen for direct immunofluorescence, is frequently insufficient to definitively diagnose a suspected immunobullous disease. This two-specimen requirement, introduced in Chapter 1, is nowhere more consequential than in this chapter's disease group.

Management Implications

Treatment Pathways Across the Immunobullous Spectrum

Pemphigus vulgaris and pemphigus foliaceus, given their potential severity and, historically, substantial mortality before the advent of modern immunosuppressive therapy, are typically managed with systemic corticosteroids and, increasingly as first-line therapy in more severe or refractory disease, rituximab, a B-cell-depleting monoclonal antibody that has transformed pemphigus management by directly targeting the autoantibody-producing B-cell population. Bullous pemphigoid, generally a less immediately severe disease than pemphigus though still carrying meaningful morbidity and mortality risk particularly in elderly, comorbid patients, is managed with topical or systemic corticosteroids, with doxycycline and other steroid-sparing agents used increasingly given concerns about long-term corticosteroid toxicity in the older population bullous pemphigoid typically affects. Dermatitis herpetiformis is managed primarily with a strict gluten-free diet, addressing the underlying celiac-driven mechanism directly, with dapsone used for more rapid symptomatic control while the dietary intervention takes effect over a period of months.

The Report's Role in Directing Urgent and Long-Term Management

Given the potential severity of extensive pemphigus and the specific, targeted nature of modern immunobullous therapy, accurate and prompt diagnosis, including both routine histology and direct immunofluorescence results communicated together as an integrated diagnostic package rather than as separate, disconnected reports, directly enables the treating clinician to select the correct therapy without delay. A report that clearly states the level of split, the specific direct immunofluorescence pattern, and the resulting specific diagnosis, along with salt-split skin results when performed, gives the clinician everything needed to proceed confidently to disease-specific therapy, whereas an incomplete or ambiguous report risks delayed or empirically broad treatment that may be less effective or carry greater side-effect burden than a precisely targeted approach.

Monitoring Disease Activity Over the Treatment Course

Beyond initial diagnosis, several of the ancillary studies discussed in this chapter carry a longitudinal monitoring role that extends the dermatopathologist's contribution well past the moment of initial diagnosis. Indirect immunofluorescence titers and antigen-specific enzyme-linked immunosorbent assay values in the pemphigus group, as discussed above, are frequently followed serially to guide immunosuppressive therapy tapering, with a rising titer sometimes preceding clinical relapse and prompting earlier treatment adjustment than would occur if clinical assessment alone were relied upon. A repeat skin biopsy is occasionally obtained during the treatment course when a patient's clinical picture becomes ambiguous, for example when new blistering develops in a patient already being treated for a known immunobullous disease, since this scenario raises several possibilities, inadequately controlled original disease, a superimposed new process such as infection, or, uncommonly, evolution of the immunobullous disease itself to involve a different or additional target antigen, each of which the repeat biopsy and immunofluorescence can help distinguish.

Multidisciplinary Coordination in Severe Immunobullous Disease

Severe or extensive pemphigus, particularly when complicated by significant mucosal involvement affecting oral intake or ocular involvement threatening vision, frequently requires multidisciplinary management extending beyond dermatology to include otolaryngology, ophthalmology, and, for extensive cutaneous involvement with significant barrier disruption, wound care or burn specialists managing fluid balance and infection risk in a manner analogous to the severe cutaneous drug reaction spectrum discussed in Chapter 6. The dermatopathologist's diagnostic confirmation, and the specific subtyping developed throughout this chapter, is frequently the pivotal piece of information that activates this broader multidisciplinary response, underscoring why the urgency and clarity of communication discussed throughout this book carries particular weight for the immunobullous diseases covered in this chapter.

THE REACTION PATTERN RECOGNITION SYSTEM — The Vesiculobullous Pattern Family

The Pattern: The vesiculobullous pattern organized by level and mechanism of split: intraepidermal acantholytic (pemphigus group), subepidermal (pemphigoid group, epidermolysis bullosa acquisita, dermatitis herpetiformis, linear IgA disease).

Histologic Signature: Acantholytic keratinocytes with a tombstone basal pattern define the pemphigus group; an intact, non-acantholytic epidermal roof with a frequently eosinophil-rich infiltrate defines bullous pemphigoid; neutrophilic papillary tip microabscesses define dermatitis herpetiformis.

The Decision: Determine the level of split first, then confirm the specific disease within that level using direct immunofluorescence, the definitive diagnostic standard for this entire pattern family.

Trap Logic: Bullous arthropod bite reaction and bullous impetigo can mimic pemphigoid and pemphigus respectively on routine histology; both are resolved by direct immunofluorescence (negative in both mimickers) together with specific supporting clinical and histologic clues (wedge-shaped deep infiltrate for bite reaction; neutrophils and clinical context for impetigo).

Pattern Anchor: A vesiculobullous biopsy is incomplete without a paired perilesional specimen for direct immunofluorescence; routine histology establishes the level of split, but immunofluorescence establishes the specific diagnosis in nearly every case in this chapter.

Summary and Key Concepts

The vesiculobullous pattern is organized primarily by the level and mechanism of epidermal or subepidermal split, which correlates closely with the specific target antigen and direct immunofluorescence pattern of each constituent disease.

The pemphigus group (intraepidermal, acantholytic) targets desmogleins 1 and 3; the pemphigoid group and related subepidermal diseases target basement membrane zone components including BP180, BP230, and type VII collagen.

Dermatitis herpetiformis, driven by IgA autoantibodies against tissue transglutaminase in the context of celiac disease, shows a distinctive papillary tip neutrophilic and granular IgA pattern and is managed primarily through dietary gluten elimination.

Bullous arthropod bite reaction and bullous impetigo are important non-immunobullous mimickers, both distinguished from true immunobullous disease by negative direct immunofluorescence together with specific supporting clinical and histologic features.

Direct immunofluorescence of a perilesional biopsy, paired with routine histology of a lesional biopsy, is the diagnostic standard for this pattern family, and accurate, prompt, integrated reporting of both directly enables correct and timely treatment selection.

CHAPTER 8: THE GRANULOMATOUS REACTION PATTERN

Learning Objectives

1. Define the granulomatous reaction pattern and classify it by granuloma architecture and by infectious versus non-infectious etiology.
2. Describe the immunologic mechanisms underlying well-formed and poorly formed granulomatous inflammation.
3. Identify the histopathologic features and diagnostic criteria that distinguish the major granulomatous dermatoses from one another.
4. Correlate histologic findings with clinical presentation across the granulomatous disease spectrum.
5. Construct a differential diagnosis for the granulomatous pattern and discriminate infectious from non-infectious causes.
6. Select appropriate special stains and ancillary studies for a granulomatous biopsy, including in immunocompromised patients.

Definition and Classification

Defining the Granulomatous Pattern

The granulomatous reaction pattern, introduced in Chapter 3, is defined by aggregates of activated histiocytes, macrophages that have undergone morphologic transformation in response to sustained antigenic or particulate stimulation, often accompanied by multinucleated giant cells formed through histiocyte fusion. This pattern represents the immune system's strategy for containing material it cannot readily degrade or eliminate through simpler phagocytic mechanisms, whether that material is a persistent infectious organism, an indigestible foreign substance, or, in the non-infectious granulomatous dermatoses, a poorly understood endogenous trigger, and the resulting histiocytic aggregate functions to wall off and contain this material even when it cannot fully eliminate it.

The pattern is subdivided along two independent axes that together organize the remainder of this chapter: architecture (well-formed versus poorly formed granulomas) and etiology (infectious versus non-infectious), with the intersection of these two axes producing the specific differential diagnosis appropriate to any given granulomatous biopsy. This two-axis classification mirrors the compartmental and mechanistic organizing principles used throughout this book, and mastering it provides a systematic framework for a pattern that, more than most others in this book, spans an unusually wide etiologic range, from indolent infection to autoimmune disease to inert foreign material.

Well-Formed Versus Poorly Formed Granulomas

Well-formed (compact, epithelioid) granulomas show discrete, sharply demarcated aggregates of epithelioid histiocytes, often with a peripheral rim of lymphocytes, and are the architectural hallmark of infectious granulomatous disease (mycobacterial and deep fungal infection) and sarcoidosis, reflecting an organized, robust cell-mediated immune response capable of forming tight, well-circumscribed structures around the inciting antigen. Poorly formed (interstitial) granulomas, by contrast, show histiocytes dispersed individually or in small, loose clusters between collagen bundles without forming discrete, compact aggregates, and are the architectural hallmark of granuloma annulare and the related palisaded and interstitial granulomatous dermatitis spectrum, reflecting a different, less tightly organized immune response whose specific trigger, in most cases, remains incompletely understood.

Infectious Versus Non-Infectious Etiology

Infectious granulomatous disease encompasses mycobacterial infection (tuberculosis and non-tuberculous mycobacteria, including Mycobacterium marinum and Mycobacterium leprae), deep fungal infection (histoplasmosis, blastomycosis, coccidioidomycosis, sporotrichosis, and others, varying substantially by geographic exposure), and, less commonly encountered in routine dermatopathology practice, certain parasitic and other infectious causes. Non-infectious granulomatous disease encompasses sarcoidosis, foreign body reactions, and the granuloma annulare/interstitial granulomatous dermatitis spectrum, each with distinct architectural and associated features developed throughout this chapter, together with rarer entities such as necrobiosis lipoidica and rheumatoid nodule that share overlapping palisaded granulomatous architecture with granuloma annulare but carry distinct clinical associations.

Grading and Reporting Granulomatous Inflammation

A useful reporting discipline for granulomatous biopsies is to state the architecture observed, well-formed or poorly formed, together with the presence or absence of necrosis, a suppurative component, identifiable foreign material, and the results of any special stains performed, rather than committing prematurely to a single specific diagnosis when several remain plausible. This descriptive approach, consistent with the diagnostic honesty principle emphasized throughout this book, communicates precisely what has and has not been excluded, allowing the treating clinician to weigh the remaining possibilities against clinical context, exposure history, and systemic evaluation rather than receiving a diagnostic label that implies more certainty than the histology alone can support. Grading granulomatous inflammation by extent, focal, patchy, or diffuse, additionally provides useful information for monitoring treatment response in established diagnoses such as sarcoidosis, where serial biopsies are occasionally obtained to assess disease activity.

Entity	Granuloma Architecture	Etiology	Key Distinguishing Feature
Tuberculosis / non-tuberculous mycobacteria	Well-formed, often with caseous necrosis (TB)	Infectious	Acid-fast bacilli on Fite/Ziehl-Neelsen stain
Deep fungal infection	Well-formed, often mixed suppurative-granulomatous	Infectious	Fungal organisms on GMS/PAS-D stain
Sarcoidosis	Well-formed, "naked" (sparse peripheral lymphocytes)	Non-infectious (autoimmune/idiopathic)	Diagnosis of exclusion; negative special stains
Foreign body reaction	Well-formed to poorly formed around foreign material	Non-infectious (exogenous material)	Polarizable or visible foreign material
Granuloma annulare	Poorly formed, interstitial, palisaded around mucin	Non-infectious (idiopathic)	Increased interstitial mucin on Alcian blue stain
Necrobiosis lipoidica	Layered granulomas around necrobiotic collagen	Non-infectious (diabetes-associated)	Tiered, horizontal layering; minimal mucin
Leprosy (tuberculoid to lepromatous spectrum)	Well-formed with nerve involvement to poorly formed/foamy	Infectious	Acid-fast bacilli burden inversely tracks granuloma organization

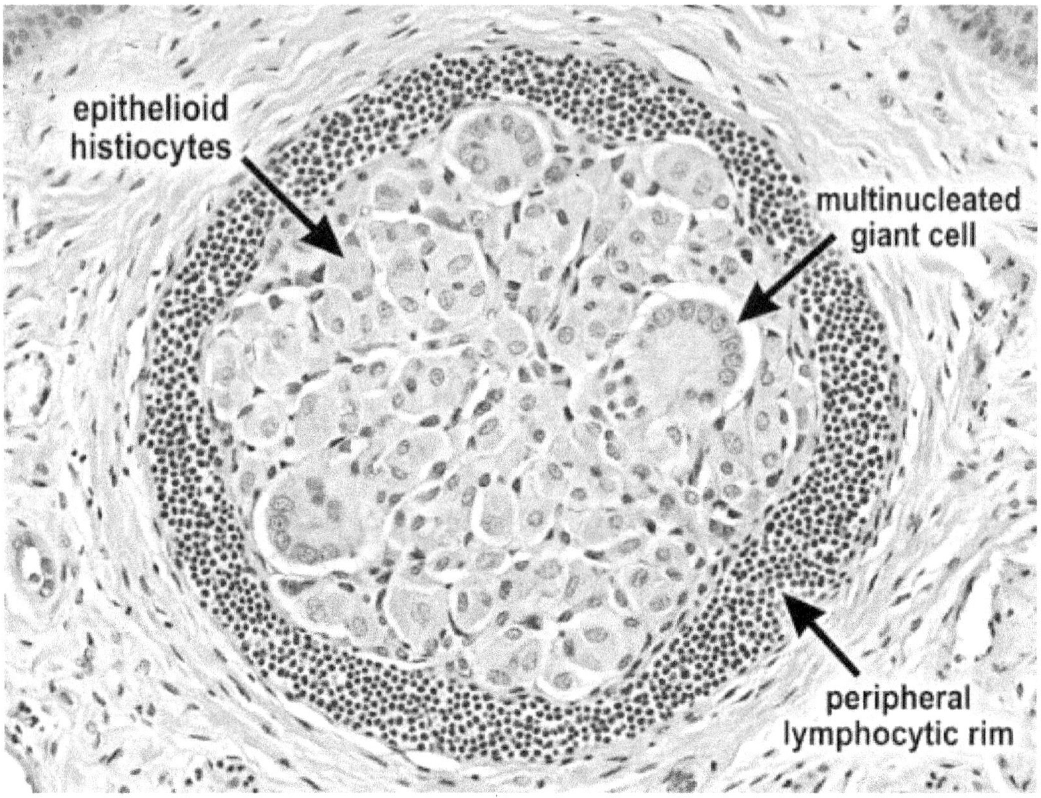

Etiology and Infectious Versus Non-Infectious Causes

Mechanisms of Mycobacterial and Deep Fungal Granuloma Formation

Mycobacterial and deep fungal organisms share a biological property that directly explains the granulomatous response they provoke: both resist straightforward elimination by neutrophils and simple macrophage phagocytosis, surviving within the phagosome through various evasion mechanisms, which triggers a sustained cell-mediated immune response involving antigen presentation to T lymphocytes, interferon-gamma-driven macrophage activation, and the eventual organization of activated macrophages into the compact, well-formed granulomas discussed above, an architecture that reflects the immune system's attempt to physically contain organisms it cannot fully eliminate. Caseous necrosis, characteristic of tuberculosis though not invariably present, reflects a more destructive element of this contained immune response, in which the center of the granuloma undergoes a distinctive form of necrosis producing an amorphous, granular, eosinophilic material that, unlike most other forms of tissue necrosis, retains its overall tissue architecture at low power despite the loss of cellular detail.

Mechanisms of Sarcoidosis

Sarcoidosis is understood as a multisystem granulomatous disease of incompletely characterized etiology, believed to reflect an exaggerated cell-mediated immune response to one or more unidentified antigens in a genetically susceptible individual, producing well-formed granulomas notable for their comparatively sparse peripheral lymphocytic rim relative to infectious granulomas, sometimes described as "naked" granulomas for this reason. Cutaneous sarcoidosis can occur as an isolated skin-limited finding or as one manifestation of systemic disease, most classically also involving the lungs, lymph nodes, and eyes, and given that sarcoidosis remains substantially a diagnosis of exclusion, established only after infectious and foreign body causes of well-formed granulomatous inflammation have been actively excluded through the special stains and, when clinically indicated, polarization discussed in the ancillary studies section below.

Mechanisms of Foreign Body Granulomatous Reactions

Foreign body granulomatous reactions arise when the immune system encounters exogenous material it cannot enzymatically degrade or otherwise eliminate, ranging from suture material and cosmetic filler substances to splinters, tattoo pigment, and a range of other implanted or embedded materials, triggering histiocyte and multinucleated giant cell recruitment that surrounds and attempts to isolate the foreign material from surrounding tissue. The specific granuloma architecture in foreign body reactions varies with the nature of the foreign material itself, ranging from tight, well-formed granulomas around discrete, larger foreign particles to a more diffuse, poorly formed histiocytic infiltrate around finely particulate or widely dispersed material, and the foreign material itself, when identifiable within the specimen, is frequently visible on routine hematoxylin and eosin staining or, for material that is not intrinsically pigmented or refractile under standard light, through polarization, discussed further below.

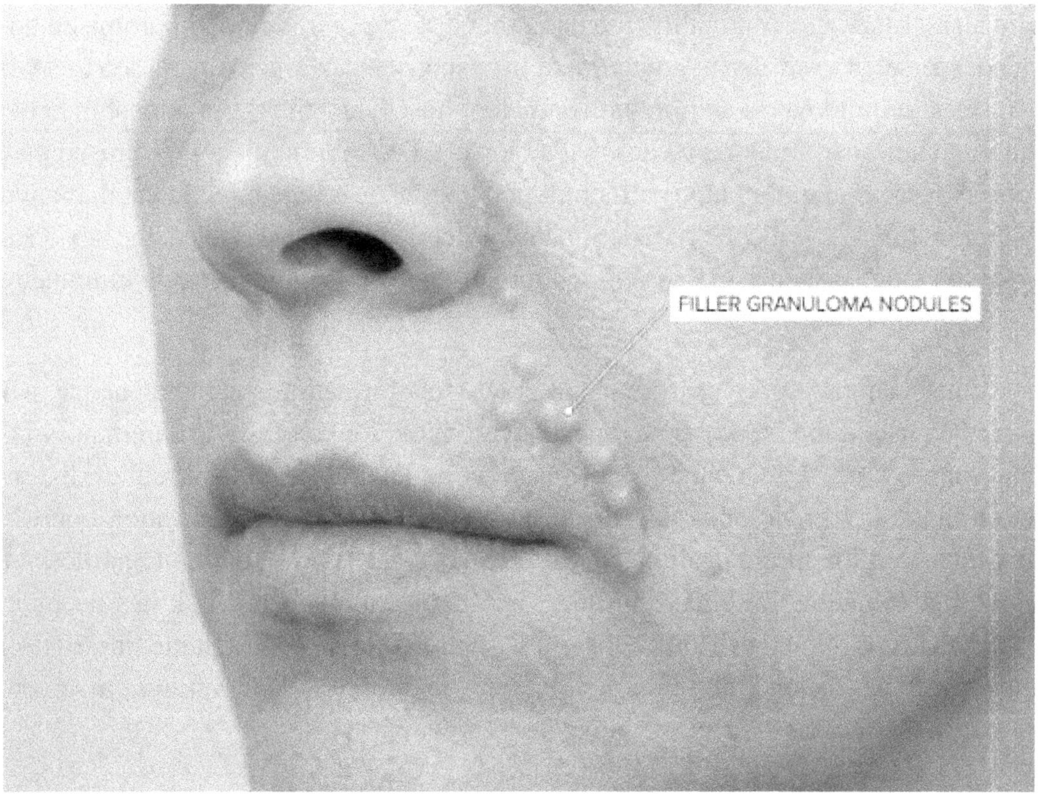

Mechanisms of Granuloma Annulare and the Interstitial Granulomatous Spectrum

Granuloma annulare's pathogenesis remains incompletely understood but is believed to involve a cell-mediated immune response, possibly triggered by minor trauma, insect bites, or other minor antigenic stimuli in a susceptible individual, that produces the poorly formed, interstitial histiocytic infiltrate discussed above, with associated dermal collagen degeneration and increased interstitial mucin deposition that together define the pattern's characteristic histology developed further below. Palisaded and interstitial granulomatous dermatitis, a related but distinct entity within this same architectural spectrum, has been associated with underlying autoimmune connective tissue disease, most notably rheumatoid arthritis, and with certain medications, illustrating that the poorly formed granulomatous pattern, like granuloma annulare itself, can arise through multiple distinct upstream triggers converging on a shared downstream histiocytic response.

Immunocompromised Hosts and Atypical Granulomatous Presentations

Immunocompromised patients, whether from HIV infection, solid organ or hematopoietic transplantation with associated immunosuppressive therapy, or biologic agents targeting tumor necrosis factor-alpha and related pathways, present a distinct diagnostic challenge because the granulomatous response itself depends on intact cell-mediated immunity, meaning that a severely immunocompromised host may show a poorly formed, sparse, or even absent granulomatous response to an organism burden that would provoke robust, well-formed granulomas in an immunocompetent host. This inverse relationship between immune competence and granuloma formation means that a biopsy from an immunocompromised patient showing minimal or poorly formed granulomatous inflammation does not exclude infection and, if anything, should heighten suspicion for an atypical or disseminated infectious process, since the absence of a well-organized granulomatous response in this setting more often reflects an inadequate immune response than an absence of organisms.

Tumor necrosis factor-alpha plays a central role in granuloma formation and maintenance, which explains why patients treated with tumor necrosis factor-alpha inhibitors for psoriasis, inflammatory bowel disease, or rheumatoid arthritis carry an elevated risk of reactivating latent tuberculosis and of disseminated deep fungal infection, and why granulomatous skin biopsies in this specific medication context warrant an especially low threshold for special staining and infectious disease consultation regardless of how sparse or atypical the granulomatous infiltrate appears. This medication-specific risk has become sufficiently well established that pre-treatment latent tuberculosis screening is now a standard requirement before initiating tumor necrosis factor-alpha inhibitor therapy in most clinical settings, a screening practice discussed further in the prevention and screening subsection below.

Leprosy and the Immunologic Spectrum of Mycobacterial Disease

Leprosy, caused by Mycobacterium leprae and the more recently characterized Mycobacterium lepromatosis, illustrates the granulomatous pattern's dependence on host immune status more clearly than perhaps any other infectious disease, presenting across a clinical and histologic spectrum that tracks directly with the strength of the host's cell-mediated immune response to the organism. Tuberculoid leprosy, occurring in hosts with a robust cell-mediated response, shows well-formed, compact granulomas with a brisk lymphocytic infiltrate often tracking along cutaneous nerves, and a correspondingly low organism burden that can make acid-fast organisms difficult to identify even with Fite staining, while lepromatous leprosy, occurring in hosts with a weak or absent cell-mediated response, shows sheets of foamy histiocytes packed with numerous acid-fast bacilli, minimal lymphocytic response, and comparatively poor granuloma organization despite the high organism burden.

This inverse relationship between granuloma organization and organism burden across the leprosy spectrum is a useful teaching illustration of the broader immunocompromised-host principle developed above, since it demonstrates within a single infectious disease that well-formed granulomas reflect a strong host response containing a low organism burden, while poorly formed or absent granulomatous organization can reflect an overwhelmed or absent host response to a high organism burden, rather than the absence of a significant infectious process. Nerve involvement, identifiable histologically as granulomatous or lymphocytic infiltration of cutaneous nerves and clinically as sensory loss in the affected skin, is a distinguishing feature of leprosy relative to other mycobacterial and granulomatous diseases discussed in this chapter and should prompt specific mention in the pathology report when identified, given its diagnostic specificity.

THE REACTION PATTERN RECOGNITION SYSTEM — Architecture as the First Diagnostic Branch Point

---

The Pattern: Well-Formed Versus Poorly Formed Granuloma Architecture as the First Diagnostic Branch Point

Histologic Signature: Discrete, compact, sharply demarcated histiocytic aggregates (well-formed) versus histiocytes dispersed individually or in small clusters between collagen bundles without forming discrete aggregates (poorly formed).

The Decision: Assess granuloma architecture first, since well-formed granulomas direct the differential toward infection and sarcoidosis, requiring special stain exclusion of organisms, while poorly formed granulomas direct the differential toward granuloma annulare and the related interstitial granulomatous dermatitis spectrum, requiring assessment of interstitial mucin instead.

Trap Logic: The mimicker in each direction is an atypical presentation: an early or resolving granuloma annulare can occasionally show more organized, semi-compact histiocytic clusters approaching a well-formed appearance, while an early or poorly developed infectious granuloma may not yet show the fully compact architecture of established disease. In an immunocompromised host, this trap is magnified, since a sparse or poorly formed granulomatous response may reflect overwhelming infection rather than a non-infectious process. When architecture alone is ambiguous, special stains (for infection) and Alcian blue (for granuloma annulare's characteristic mucin) resolve the distinction.

Pattern Anchor: Compact and discrete points toward infection or sarcoidosis and demands special stains; dispersed and interstitial points toward granuloma annulare and demands an Alcian blue stain for mucin; sparse or poorly formed in an immunocompromised host demands heightened, not lowered, suspicion for infection.

Histopathologic Features and Diagnostic Criteria

Diagnostic Features of Infectious Granulomatous Disease

Beyond the well-formed architecture already discussed, infectious granulomatous disease frequently shows necrosis, whether the caseous necrosis characteristic of tuberculosis or a suppurative component with central neutrophilic microabscess formation more characteristic of certain deep fungal infections and non-tuberculous mycobacterial infections, producing a mixed suppurative-granulomatous pattern that itself narrows the differential toward these specific etiologies over sarcoidosis, which does not typically show significant necrosis or a suppurative component. The specific organisms responsible, when identified on special stains, show characteristic morphology, discussed further in the ancillary studies section, that can suggest a specific etiologic diagnosis even before culture or molecular confirmation is available, though culture and, increasingly, molecular diagnostics remain necessary for definitive organism speciation given the morphologic overlap among related organisms on special stains alone.

Diagnostic Features of Sarcoidosis

Sarcoidal granulomas, beyond their characteristically sparse peripheral lymphocytic cuff, may contain asteroid bodies (stellate eosinophilic inclusions within giant cells) and Schaumann bodies (laminated, calcified inclusions), findings that, while suggestive, are neither sensitive nor specific for sarcoidosis and can be seen in other granulomatous processes as well, meaning their presence supports but does not independently establish the diagnosis. The absence of necrosis, of identifiable organisms on special stains, and of polarizable or otherwise identifiable foreign material together constitute the exclusionary criteria that, combined with the compact granuloma architecture and clinical correlation for systemic disease, support a sarcoidosis diagnosis, reinforcing the point made above that this remains substantially a diagnosis reached by systematic exclusion of its mimickers.

Diagnostic Features of Granuloma Annulare

Granuloma annulare shows the poorly formed, interstitial histiocytic infiltrate discussed above, palisading, when present, around zones of altered dermal collagen and increased mucin, though the palisading can be subtle or absent in the more common interstitial subtype relative to the classic palisaded subtype. Increased interstitial mucin, most confidently confirmed with Alcian blue staining as discussed in Chapter 2, is a near-universal and highly characteristic feature, appearing as pale, bluish-gray, faintly fibrillary material separating collagen bundles, and its presence, together with the poorly formed histiocytic architecture, is highly supportive of the diagnosis even when classic palisading around a central zone of altered collagen is not well developed.

Distinguishing Necrobiosis Lipoidica and Related Palisaded Entities

Necrobiosis lipoidica, strongly associated with diabetes mellitus, shows a distinctive tiered or layered pattern of granulomatous inflammation alternating with zones of necrobiotic (degenerated) collagen arranged in horizontal bands through the dermis, a "layer-cake" architecture that contrasts with the more randomly distributed interstitial pattern of granuloma annulare, together with comparatively less interstitial mucin than granuloma annulare typically shows. Rheumatoid nodule, occurring in patients with rheumatoid arthritis, shows palisaded granulomatous inflammation around a central zone of fibrinoid necrosis rather than the mucin-rich altered collagen of granuloma annulare, and typically occurs as a deeper, subcutaneous nodule rather than the more superficial dermal process typical of granuloma annulare, features that together, alongside the clinical context of established rheumatoid arthritis, distinguish this entity from its palisaded granulomatous relatives.

Elastophagocytosis and Annular Elastolytic Giant Cell Granuloma

Annular elastolytic giant cell granuloma, an uncommon entity favoring sun-damaged skin of older adults, shows histiocytes and multinucleated giant cells actively phagocytosing elastic fibers, a finding best appreciated on an elastic tissue stain showing engulfed elastic fibers within giant cell cytoplasm and a corresponding loss of elastic tissue within the affected dermis, distinguishing this entity from granuloma annulare, with which it shares clinical annular morphology but not this specific elastophagocytic mechanism. Because this entity favors chronically sun-damaged skin and shows minimal to absent interstitial mucin in contrast to granuloma annulare, correlating the biopsy site's degree of solar elastosis with the histologic findings, and obtaining an elastic tissue stain when the distinction is uncertain, resolves most cases that present overlapping clinical and low-power histologic features.

Granulomatous Rosacea and Periorificial Granulomatous Dermatitis

Granulomatous rosacea, a variant of rosacea rather than a distinct disease entity, shows well-formed to poorly formed granulomas superimposed on the background follicular and vascular changes of conventional rosacea, favoring the perioral, periocular, and centrofacial skin, and should be considered whenever a facial granulomatous biopsy is obtained, given how frequently this diagnosis is overlooked in favor of sarcoidosis or an infectious etiology when the clinical background of rosacea is not specifically communicated to the pathologist. Periorificial granulomatous dermatitis, a related pediatric-predominant entity favoring the skin around the mouth, eyes, and nose, similarly shows a granulomatous infiltrate and is thought to represent a variant within this same clinical and histologic spectrum, distinguished chiefly by patient age and the specific periorificial distribution rather than by fundamentally distinct histology.

Distinguishing granulomatous rosacea from sarcoidosis rests substantially on correlating the biopsy findings with the clinical distribution and background skin changes, since a granulomatous infiltrate confined to a background of facial erythema, telangiectasia, and follicular-centered inflammation favors granulomatous rosacea, while a similar granulomatous infiltrate without these background changes, or occurring outside the classic centrofacial distribution, favors sarcoidosis or another etiology, underscoring once again the clinicopathologic correlation this chapter has emphasized throughout. Special stains remain appropriate in either case, since granulomatous rosacea, like sarcoidosis, is ultimately a diagnosis that gains confidence from the exclusion of an infectious mimicker rather than from its own histologic features being absolutely specific.

Cutaneous Crohn Disease and Metastatic Granulomatous Involvement

Metastatic cutaneous Crohn disease, a rare manifestation of Crohn disease occurring at skin sites distant from the gastrointestinal tract and not in anatomic continuity with it, shows well-formed, non-caseating granulomas histologically indistinguishable from sarcoidosis, and should be considered in any patient with a known or suspected history of inflammatory bowel disease presenting with a granulomatous skin lesion, particularly when the lesion occurs in an intertriginous site such as the vulva, scrotum, or skin folds that is disproportionately represented in reported cases. Because the histology alone cannot reliably distinguish metastatic Crohn disease from sarcoidosis or from a granulomatous drug reaction, this diagnosis depends heavily on clinical correlation with a known or subsequently established diagnosis of Crohn disease, reinforcing this chapter's recurring theme that a well-formed, non-caseating granuloma without organisms represents a shared histologic endpoint reached by several etiologically distinct pathways rather than a single, self-evident diagnosis.

Sarcoidal Granulomas Arising Within Tattoos and Scars

Sarcoidal granulomas confined to a pre-existing tattoo or scar represent a distinct and clinically important presentation in which well-formed, naked granulomas develop in a site-specific distribution corresponding to previously deposited tattoo pigment or to a healed surgical or traumatic scar, and this presentation raises two overlapping but distinct diagnostic possibilities that the histology alone cannot always separate. The first possibility is a localized foreign body-type granulomatous reaction to the tattoo pigment or scar collagen itself, remaining confined to that site indefinitely without broader significance, and the second is that the tattoo or scar has served as a localized site of minor trauma or foreign material that has, in a susceptible individual, unmasked or triggered the first cutaneous manifestation of systemic sarcoidosis, a phenomenon sometimes discussed under the broader heading of a scar or tattoo functioning as a locus of immunologic reactivity.

Because a granulomatous reaction confined to a tattoo or scar can herald systemic sarcoidosis even when no other skin findings are present, current practice favors evaluating these patients for systemic disease, including chest imaging, in the same manner as for a cutaneous sarcoidosis diagnosis arising outside a tattoo or scar, rather than dismissing the finding as a purely local foreign body phenomenon confined to the pigment or scar tissue. Polarization remains a useful adjunct in this specific context, since tattoo pigment and certain scar-associated foreign material can themselves be polarizable, and identifying polarizable material within the granulomatous infiltrate, while not excluding a concurrent sarcoidosis diagnosis, supports at minimum a component of local foreign body reactivity contributing to the histologic picture.

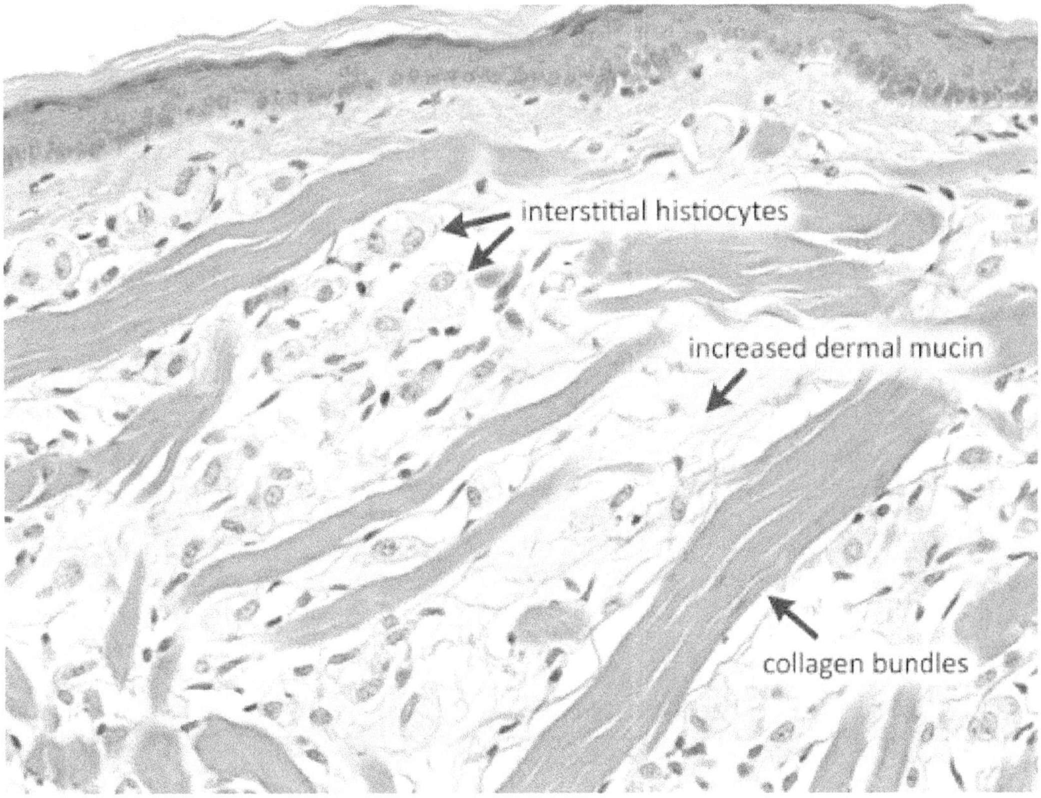

Clinical Presentation and Clinicopathologic Correlation

Clinical Morphology of Infectious Granulomatous Disease

Cutaneous tuberculosis presents in several distinct clinical forms depending on the route of inoculation and host immune status, ranging from lupus vulgaris (a chronic, slowly progressive plaque, most common in previously sensitized individuals) to tuberculous chancre (a primary inoculation lesion in a previously unsensitized individual) to miliary tuberculosis (widely disseminated lesions reflecting hematogenous spread in a severely immunocompromised host), and this clinical heterogeneity reflects varying degrees of host immune containment of the organism, itself correlating with the specific granuloma architecture and degree of necrosis observed histologically. Deep fungal infections show geographic clustering that provides important clinical context, histoplasmosis and blastomycosis in the Ohio and Mississippi River valleys, coccidioidomycosis in the southwestern United States, so that a patient's travel and residence history is essential correlating information for a granulomatous biopsy in which a deep fungal etiology is being considered.

Clinical Morphology of Sarcoidosis and Granuloma Annulare

Cutaneous sarcoidosis shows variable clinical morphology, including red-brown papules and plaques, subcutaneous nodules, and, in a distinctive variant, lupus pernio (violaceous, indurated plaques favoring the nose, cheeks, and ears), and any biopsy-confirmed cutaneous sarcoidosis diagnosis should prompt systemic evaluation, including chest imaging, given the disease's frequent, and sometimes clinically silent, systemic involvement. Granuloma annulare classically presents as annular plaques with a raised, often skin-colored to violaceous border and a clear or minimally scaly center, favoring the dorsal hands and feet, and while classic localized granuloma annulare requires no systemic workup, the generalized variant, involving numerous widespread lesions, has been associated in some studies with diabetes mellitus and, less consistently, with malignancy, associations that remain individually less robust than the necrobiosis lipoidica-diabetes association but that some clinicians consider when evaluating extensive or atypical disease.

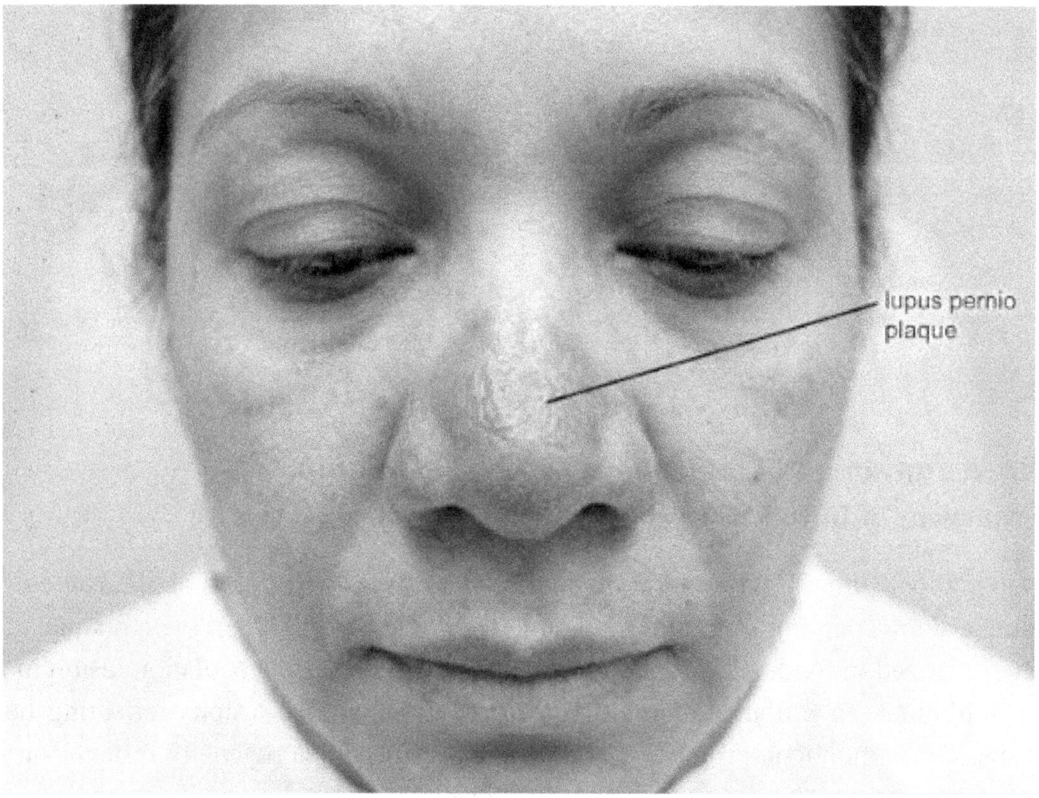

Special Populations: Pediatric and Immunosuppressed Patients

Granulomatous dermatoses in children differ in relative frequency from those in adults, with granuloma annulare representing a comparatively common pediatric presentation, often subcutaneous rather than the classic dermal annular plaque seen in adults, sometimes raising initial clinical concern for a soft tissue neoplasm before biopsy clarifies the granulomatous, non-neoplastic nature of the nodule. Blau syndrome, a rare pediatric-onset granulomatous disease resulting from mutations in the NOD2 gene, produces a triad of granulomatous dermatitis, arthritis, and uveitis, and should be considered in a child presenting with a persistent granulomatous skin eruption together with joint or ocular findings, particularly when a family history of similar findings suggests the autosomal dominant inheritance pattern this condition follows.

In solid organ and hematopoietic transplant recipients maintained on chronic immunosuppression, granulomatous skin biopsies carry a disproportionately elevated likelihood of representing infection, most often atypical mycobacterial or deep fungal disease, reflecting the same inverse relationship between immune competence and granuloma quality discussed above, and dermatopathology reports in this population should explicitly document which special stains were performed and their results, given how directly this information shapes the urgency and nature of subsequent clinical workup. Close coordination with the transplant infectious disease service, including flagging unusual or minimally organized granulomatous infiltrates for expedited communication rather than routine reporting turnaround, meaningfully improves outcomes in this specific, high-risk population.

Granuloma annulare occurring during pregnancy has been reported to occasionally flare or first present during gestation, thought to reflect the broader shift toward a distinct immunologic state during pregnancy, and while this association does not change the fundamental management approach, patients presenting with new or worsening granuloma annulare during pregnancy benefit from reassurance that this represents a recognized, benign pattern rather than an unusual or concerning finding requiring escalated workup. Hormonal contraceptive use has similarly been anecdotally associated with granuloma annulare flares in case reports, though this association is considerably less well established than the pregnancy association and should be mentioned to patients as a possible but unconfirmed contributing factor rather than a definite cause.

CLINICAL PEARL: A well-formed granulomatous biopsy without an identified organism is not, by itself, a sarcoidosis diagnosis; it is a biopsy that has excluded the infections it was tested for. Communicating this distinction, and which specific stains were performed, matters for how confidently the treating clinician can proceed.

Differential Diagnosis and Histologic Mimickers

Sarcoidosis Versus Infectious Granulomatous Disease

As emphasized throughout this chapter, distinguishing sarcoidosis from infectious granulomatous disease rests substantially on the systematic exclusion of infection through special stains, discussed in detail below, since the well-formed granuloma architecture alone cannot reliably distinguish between these etiologies, particularly for organisms present in low numbers that may not be readily identified even with appropriate staining. A granulomatous biopsy showing necrosis, a mixed suppurative component, or any organisms on special stains excludes sarcoidosis as the primary diagnosis and redirects the differential toward the specific infectious etiology suggested by organism morphology and clinical context, while a granulomatous biopsy with negative special stains, in the appropriate clinical context, supports but does not definitively prove a sarcoidosis diagnosis, given the inherent sensitivity limitations of special stains for organisms present in low burden.

Foreign Body Reaction Versus Other Well-Formed Granulomatous Processes

Foreign body reactions are distinguished from infectious and sarcoidal granulomas primarily by the identification of the foreign material itself, whether visible directly on routine hematoxylin and eosin staining (as with suture material, certain injected fillers, or larger foreign particles) or, for material that lacks intrinsic color or refractility under standard light, through polarization, which reveals birefringent material (such as certain suture types, some talc, and various other crystalline or fibrous substances) that would not otherwise be apparent. A clinical history of a preceding procedure, injection, or penetrating injury at the biopsy site is valuable correlating information, though foreign body reactions can also occur at sites without a clearly recalled inciting event, particularly for cosmetic filler material injected months to years prior, or for retained material from a remote, forgotten injury.

Granuloma Annulare Versus Necrobiosis Lipoidica and Rheumatoid Nodule

As developed in the histopathologic features section above, the tiered, layered architecture of necrobiosis lipoidica and the central fibrinoid necrosis of rheumatoid nodule distinguish these entities from granuloma annulare's more randomly distributed, mucin-rich interstitial pattern, and correlating these histologic distinctions with the relevant clinical associations, diabetes for necrobiosis lipoidica, established rheumatoid arthritis for rheumatoid nodule, strengthens diagnostic confidence in ambiguous cases. A biopsy showing overlapping or intermediate features between granuloma annulare and necrobiosis lipoidica, occasionally encountered in practice, should be reported descriptively with both possibilities named, consistent with the diagnostic honesty principle this book has emphasized since Chapter 1, particularly when the clinical distinction (a diabetic patient with an atypically annular necrobiosis lipoidica-like lesion) would benefit from this explicit acknowledgment of diagnostic uncertainty.

A 52-year-old patient with poorly controlled diabetes mellitus presents with several firm, yellow-brown, atrophic plaques with telangiectasia on the bilateral shins, and biopsy is obtained given a differential of necrobiosis lipoidica versus granuloma annulare. Pattern assignment identifies a granulomatous pattern with tiered, horizontally layered granulomas alternating with zones of necrobiotic collagen extending through the full thickness of the dermis. Differential narrowing notes minimal interstitial mucin on Alcian blue staining, arguing against granuloma annulare, and the distinctive layered architecture, strongly favoring necrobiosis lipoidica. Diagnosis integrates these findings with the clinical presentation, bilateral shin location, yellow-brown atrophic morphology with telangiectasia, and known diabetes, all classic for necrobiosis lipoidica, to confirm this diagnosis, prompting the report to note the association with diabetes control and to recommend correlation with the patient's current glycemic management, extending the biopsy's clinical value beyond the immediate dermatologic diagnosis.

A 61-year-old renal transplant recipient maintained on tacrolimus and mycophenolate presents with an enlarging, poorly demarcated, violaceous plaque on the forearm, and biopsy is obtained given clinical concern for infection versus a drug-related eruption. Pattern assignment identifies a granulomatous pattern, but one that is unusually sparse and poorly organized relative to the degree of clinical induration, with scattered, loosely aggregated histiocytes rather than discrete, well-formed granulomas. Recognizing that immunosuppression can blunt granuloma formation even in the setting of substantial organism burden, fungal and acid-fast special stains are performed despite the atypical, poorly formed appearance, and Grocott methenamine silver staining identifies scattered fungal yeast forms consistent with an atypical deep fungal infection. Diagnosis integrates the sparse granulomatous architecture, positive fungal stain, and immunosuppressed clinical context to establish a fungal infection diagnosis that would very likely have been missed had the poorly formed architecture alone been interpreted as reassuring against an infectious process, illustrating directly why immunosuppressed status escalates rather than lowers the threshold for special staining.

Interstitial Granulomatous Drug Reaction and Palisaded Neutrophilic Granulomatous Dermatitis

Interstitial granulomatous drug reaction, associated most classically with calcium channel blockers and a range of other medications, shows a poorly formed, interstitial granulomatous infiltrate that can closely mimic granuloma annulare histologically, distinguished chiefly by a temporal relationship to a new medication, a broader and more symmetric clinical distribution than typical granuloma annulare, and, in some cases, a more prominent interstitial neutrophilic component representing overlap with the related entity palisaded neutrophilic and granulomatous dermatitis. Palisaded neutrophilic and granulomatous dermatitis itself is most strongly associated with underlying autoimmune connective tissue disease, particularly systemic lupus erythematosus and rheumatoid arthritis, and shows a combination of neutrophilic and granulomatous inflammation with leukocytoclasis and collagen degeneration that places it at an overlapping intersection between this chapter's granulomatous pattern and the neutrophilic pattern discussed in Chapter 9.

Distinguishing these medication- and autoimmune disease-associated entities from idiopathic granuloma annulare depends substantially on information not always available to the pathologist at the time of initial sign-out, specifically a complete medication list and known autoimmune disease history, reinforcing the practical value of requesting this clinical information when a granulomatous biopsy shows an atypical distribution, a more symmetric or truncal pattern than classic granuloma annulare, or an unexpectedly prominent neutrophilic component alongside the granulomatous infiltrate. When this clinical information is not available and the histology is ambiguous between these overlapping entities, a descriptive diagnosis naming the differential explicitly, again consistent with this book's diagnostic honesty principle, allows the treating clinician to pursue the relevant medication history or autoimmune serologic workup rather than anchoring prematurely on granuloma annulare alone.

A 58-year-old patient with known systemic lupus erythematosus and a recently initiated calcium channel blocker presents with new, symmetric, erythematous plaques on the trunk and proximal extremities, and biopsy is obtained given a differential including granuloma annulare, interstitial granulomatous drug reaction, and a cutaneous lupus manifestation. Pattern assignment identifies a poorly formed, interstitial granulomatous infiltrate with a notable admixed neutrophilic component and scattered leukocytoclasis, a combination that does not fit cleanly with classic granuloma annulare's typically pure histiocytic, mucin-rich picture. Differential narrowing weighs the atypical truncal and symmetric distribution, the neutrophilic and leukocytoclastic component, and both a recently introduced calcium channel blocker and established systemic lupus erythematosus as plausible contributing factors, concluding that the histology is most consistent with the palisaded neutrophilic and granulomatous dermatitis-interstitial granulomatous drug reaction overlap rather than idiopathic granuloma annulare. Diagnosis is rendered descriptively, naming this differential explicitly and recommending clinical correlation with both the medication timeline and current lupus disease activity, illustrating how this overlap category is resolved through clinicopathologic correlation rather than through histology in isolation.

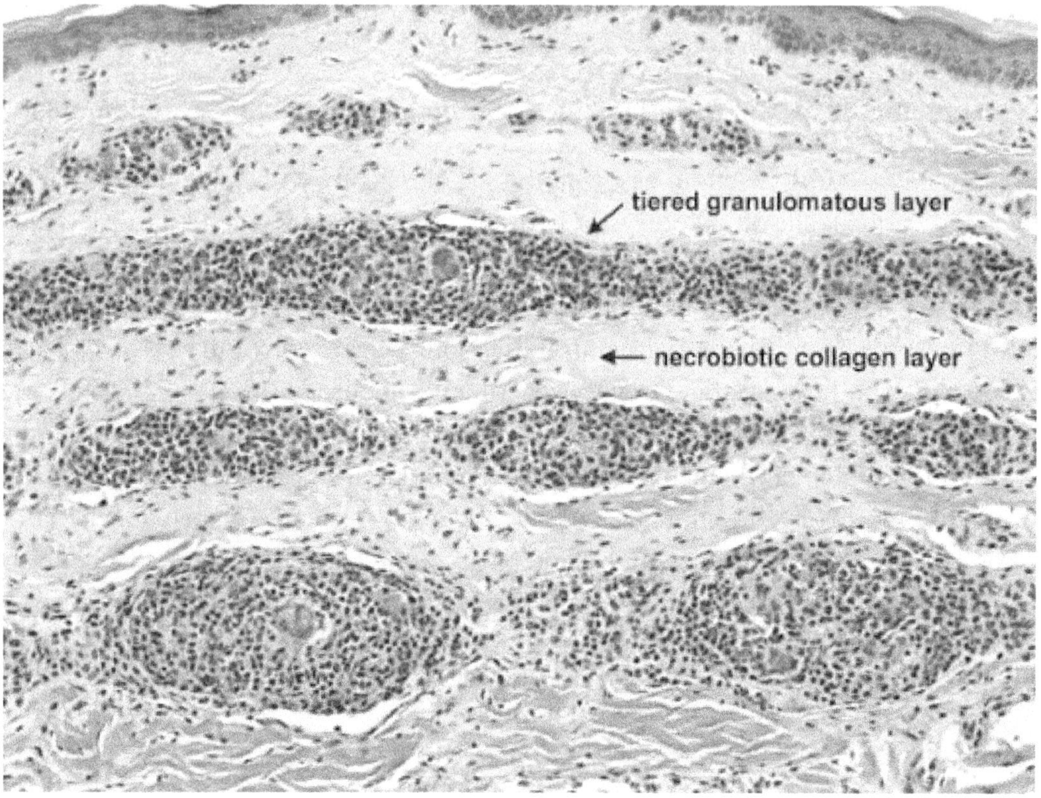

Ancillary Studies

Special Stains for Organism Identification

As developed in Chapter 2, PAS-D and Grocott methenamine silver staining identify fungal organisms, with Grocott methenamine silver generally preferred for its superior sensitivity in deep fungal infection, while Fite (modified acid-fast) staining identifies mycobacteria, preferred over standard Ziehl-Neelsen staining for its improved sensitivity for the comparatively fragile cell wall of Mycobacterium leprae specifically, though standard acid-fast staining remains appropriate and commonly used for Mycobacterium tuberculosis and most non-tuberculous mycobacteria. Given the hypothesis-driven approach to special stain selection established in Chapter 2, a well-formed granulomatous biopsy without an obvious alternative explanation (identifiable foreign material, a clear diagnosis of granuloma annulare based on architecture and mucin) should generally receive both fungal and acid-fast staining before a sarcoidosis diagnosis is entertained, given the significant treatment divergence between infection (requiring targeted antimicrobial therapy) and sarcoidosis (requiring immunosuppressive therapy that would be contraindicated in unrecognized active infection).

Polarization and Culture-Based Confirmation

Polarization of routine hematoxylin and eosin sections, performed simply by viewing the slide under polarized light, identifies birefringent foreign material that might otherwise be overlooked, and should be performed as a routine, low-cost step whenever a foreign body reaction is a genuine consideration, given its simplicity and the diagnostic information it can provide without requiring additional tissue or special stain preparation. Tissue culture, submitted at the time of initial biopsy when infectious granulomatous disease is a leading clinical consideration, provides organism speciation and, for mycobacterial infection, antimicrobial susceptibility information that special stains alone cannot supply, and this culture submission decision is generally made at the time of biopsy by the clinician rather than retrospectively by the pathologist, underscoring the value of clear communication between clinician and pathologist before, rather than only after, the biopsy is obtained whenever infectious granulomatous disease is a strong clinical consideration.

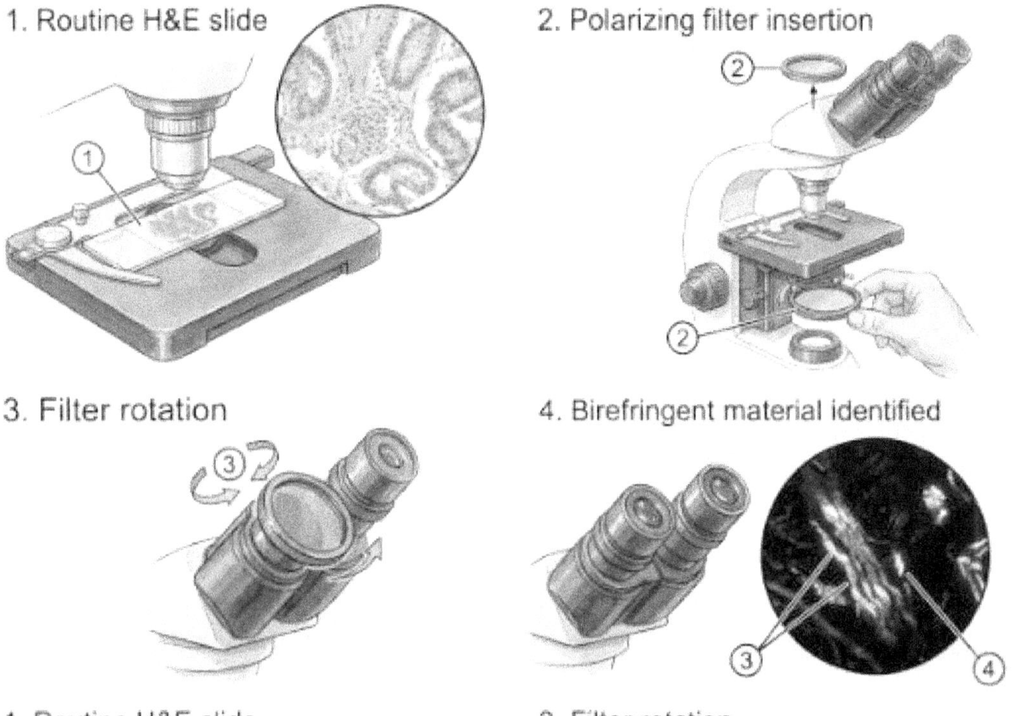

1. Routine H&E slide
2. Polarizing filter insertion
3. Filter rotation
4. Birefringent material identified

Molecular Diagnostics and PCR-Based Organism Identification

Polymerase chain reaction-based molecular testing, performed on formalin-fixed paraffin-embedded tissue or on tissue submitted fresh specifically for this purpose, offers substantially higher sensitivity than special stains for identifying mycobacterial and fungal organisms present in low burden, and can additionally provide organism speciation more rapidly than culture, which for mycobacteria in particular may require several weeks of incubation before yielding a result. Molecular testing is not a substitute for special stains and culture but a complementary tool, particularly valuable when special stains are negative despite a clinical and histologic picture that remains strongly suggestive of infection, or when rapid speciation is needed to guide urgent treatment decisions, such as in a severely immunocompromised patient with a poorly formed granulomatous infiltrate in whom empiric broad-spectrum antimicrobial therapy carries meaningful toxicity and cost.

Interpreting Negative Special Stains and When to Repeat Testing

A negative special stain result reduces but does not eliminate the probability of infection, since special stains, including molecular testing, retain imperfect sensitivity for organisms present in low burden, meaning that a granulomatous biopsy with negative fungal and acid-fast stains in a patient with a strongly suggestive clinical or exposure history should prompt consideration of repeat biopsy with additional tissue submitted for culture and molecular testing rather than immediate acceptance of a non-infectious diagnosis. This is particularly relevant in the immunocompromised populations discussed earlier in this chapter, where the combination of a genuinely low organism burden relative to disease severity and a blunted host granulomatous response can together produce a falsely reassuring initial biopsy despite clinically significant underlying infection.

CAUTION: A sarcoidosis diagnosis rendered without fungal and acid-fast special stains having been performed and reported as negative should be treated as provisional. This chapter's central diagnostic discipline, systematic exclusion before a diagnosis of exclusion is finalized, applies nowhere more directly than here.

Management Implications

Connecting Diagnosis to Treatment Pathway

The management divergence across this chapter's differential diagnosis is substantial and directly underscores the clinical stakes of accurate discrimination. Infectious granulomatous disease requires organism-specific antimicrobial therapy, often prolonged, multi-drug regimens for mycobacterial infection; sarcoidosis is managed with topical or systemic corticosteroids and other immunosuppressive agents that would be inappropriate, and potentially harmful, if applied to unrecognized infection; foreign body reactions may resolve with removal of the inciting material when feasible or may be managed expectantly when the material cannot be readily removed; and granuloma annulare, often self-limited, is managed conservatively or with topical or intralesional corticosteroids for symptomatic or cosmetically bothersome disease. This wide management divergence across a single reaction pattern is broader than in almost any other chapter of this book, reinforcing why the systematic, special-stain-supported diagnostic approach developed throughout this chapter carries such direct clinical weight.

Complications and Prognosis

Untreated or delayed-treatment infectious granulomatous disease carries the most serious potential complications discussed in this chapter, ranging from local tissue destruction and scarring to hematogenous dissemination in a severely immunocompromised host, underscoring why the diagnostic discipline developed throughout this chapter, architecture assessment followed by systematic special stain exclusion, carries such direct consequence for patient outcomes. Sarcoidosis carries a generally favorable cutaneous prognosis, though the lupus pernio variant is associated with a more chronic, treatment-resistant course and with a higher likelihood of concurrent pulmonary fibrosis, making biopsy-confirmed lupus pernio a specific indication for close pulmonary follow-up beyond the routine chest imaging recommended for cutaneous sarcoidosis generally.

Granuloma annulare, in its classic localized form, typically resolves spontaneously within one to two years even without treatment, though recurrence at the same or a new site is common, information worth conveying to patients who may otherwise pursue more aggressive treatment than the condition's natural history warrants. Necrobiosis lipoidica follows a more chronic course, with the atrophic plaques persisting indefinitely in many patients and carrying a lifetime risk of ulceration, particularly following minor trauma to the affected, atrophic skin, a risk that warrants specific patient counseling regarding trauma avoidance and prompt wound care should ulceration occur, given the impaired healing capacity of chronically diabetic, atrophic skin.

Prevention and Screening

Latent tuberculosis screening, typically with an interferon-gamma release assay or tuberculin skin testing, is now a standard requirement before initiating tumor necrosis factor-alpha inhibitor therapy and certain other biologic and immunosuppressive agents, reflecting the well-established risk of reactivation discussed earlier in this chapter, and a dermatopathology report identifying granulomatous inflammation in a patient being considered for such therapy should prompt explicit communication of this screening requirement if it has not already been addressed. Patients with a history of residence or extensive travel in a region endemic for a specific deep fungal pathogen who are being considered for biologic or other significant immunosuppressive therapy similarly warrant pre-treatment discussion of this exposure risk with the prescribing clinician, extending the same screening logic beyond tuberculosis to the geographically clustered deep fungal infections discussed throughout this chapter.

Patient Education and Counseling

Patients receiving a granuloma annulare or necrobiosis lipoidica diagnosis benefit from counseling that these are generally chronic but benign conditions, that spontaneous resolution over months to years is common for localized granuloma annulare, and that necrobiosis lipoidica, while persistent, is primarily a cosmetic and occasionally ulcerating concern rather than a marker of poorly controlled diabetes requiring treatment escalation on its own, a distinction that helps patients avoid both unwarranted anxiety and false reassurance about their underlying glycemic status. Patients receiving an infectious granulomatous disease diagnosis benefit from clear counseling regarding treatment duration, since mycobacterial and deep fungal antimicrobial regimens are often measured in months rather than weeks, and regarding the importance of treatment adherence given the consequences of undertreated infection, including antimicrobial resistance for mycobacterial disease specifically.

THE REACTION PATTERN RECOGNITION SYSTEM — The Granulomatous Pattern Family

The Pattern: The granulomatous pattern organized by architecture (well-formed versus poorly formed) and etiology (infectious versus non-infectious): mycobacterial and deep fungal infection, sarcoidosis, foreign body reaction, and the granuloma annulare/necrobiosis lipoidica/rheumatoid nodule spectrum.

Histologic Signature: Compact, discrete histiocytic aggregates with necrosis or organisms define infection; compact aggregates without necrosis or identifiable material define sarcoidosis; dispersed, interstitial histiocytes with increased mucin define granuloma annulare; tiered, layered architecture defines necrobiosis lipoidica.

The Decision: Assess architecture first (well-formed versus poorly formed), then systematically exclude infection with special stains before considering sarcoidosis, and assess interstitial mucin with Alcian blue when the poorly formed pattern is identified.

Trap Logic: Sarcoidosis is a diagnosis of exclusion mimicked by infection with low organism burden; foreign body reactions are mimicked by any well-formed granuloma unless polarization and gross/clinical correlation identify the foreign material; necrobiosis lipoidica and rheumatoid nodule mimic granuloma annulare but show distinct architecture (layered; central fibrinoid necrosis) and clinical associations (diabetes; rheumatoid arthritis); immunocompromised hosts invert the usual logic, since a sparse, poorly formed granulomatous response in this population more often signals overwhelming infection than a benign process.

Pattern Anchor: Never diagnose sarcoidosis before fungal and acid-fast special stains have been performed and reported as negative. This single discipline prevents the most consequential error this pattern family can produce: treating unrecognized infection with immunosuppression.

Summary and Key Concepts

The granulomatous reaction pattern is organized along two axes, architecture (well-formed versus poorly formed) and etiology (infectious versus non-infectious), that together determine the appropriate differential diagnosis and ancillary study workup.

Well-formed granulomas require systematic special stain exclusion of mycobacterial and fungal infection before a sarcoidosis diagnosis, itself a diagnosis of exclusion, is considered.

Poorly formed, interstitial granulomas with increased mucin define granuloma annulare, distinguished from the layered architecture of necrobiosis lipoidica, the central fibrinoid necrosis of rheumatoid nodule, and the elastophagocytosis of annular elastolytic giant cell granuloma by both histology and clinical association.

Immunocompromised patients invert the usual diagnostic logic: a sparse or poorly formed granulomatous response in this population should heighten, not lower, suspicion for infection, and warrants molecular diagnostics when special stains are negative but suspicion remains high.

Management diverges more broadly across this pattern family than in almost any other reaction pattern in this book, from antimicrobial therapy to immunosuppression to conservative management, making accurate, special-stain-supported discrimination, together with pre-treatment latent infection screening in at-risk patients, directly consequential to patient care.

CHAPTER 9: VASCULOPATHIC AND VASCULITIC REACTION PATTERNS

Learning Objectives

1. Distinguish true vasculitis from vasculopathy based on the presence or absence of vessel wall inflammation and destruction.
2. Classify cutaneous vasculitis by predominant vessel size and correlate this classification with underlying etiology.
3. Identify the histopathologic features and diagnostic criteria of leukocytoclastic vasculitis and its major mimickers.
4. Recognize the histologic patterns of thrombotic and occlusive vasculopathy and distinguish them from primary vasculitis.
5. Correlate histologic vessel findings with clinical presentation and systemic disease associations.
6. Select appropriate ancillary studies, including direct immunofluorescence, for the vasculopathic and vasculitic biopsy.

Definition and Classification

Vasculitis Versus Vasculopathy: A Foundational Distinction

The vasculopathic and vasculitic reaction pattern, introduced in Chapter 3 as one of the seven fundamental patterns organizing this book, is defined by pathology centered on the dermal or subcutaneous blood vessel wall itself, rather than by an infiltrate that happens to be perivascular in distribution, and the single most important distinction within this pattern is between true vasculitis, in which the vessel wall is directly inflamed and structurally damaged, and vasculopathy, in which the vessel is occluded or otherwise compromised without primary inflammatory destruction of the wall. This distinction carries direct clinical weight because the two processes are managed with fundamentally different strategies, immunosuppression for vasculitis and, most often, anticoagulation, correction of an underlying coagulopathy, or treatment of an occlusive etiology for vasculopathy, making the histologic discrimination between them one of the most clinically consequential distinctions a dermatopathologist renders.

True vasculitis requires histologic evidence of inflammatory cells within or destroying the vessel wall itself, evidenced by fibrinoid necrosis of the wall, endothelial cell injury, and an inflammatory infiltrate that has invaded the wall rather than merely surrounding the vessel, whereas a perivascular lymphocytic infiltrate without wall invasion or destruction, however dense, does not meet criteria for vasculitis and should not be labeled as such, a distinction developed further in the histopathologic features section below. Vasculopathy, in contrast, is defined by thrombosis, embolic occlusion, or another mechanism of luminal compromise without primary inflammatory wall destruction, though secondary inflammatory change can develop around a vasculopathic process as tissue ischemia and necrosis evolve, occasionally complicating the histologic distinction in advanced or ulcerated lesions.

Classification by Vessel Size

Cutaneous vasculitis is classified by the predominant size of vessel involved, following the same organizing logic used in the major systemic vasculitis nomenclature systems, with small vessel vasculitis affecting postcapillary venules and capillaries, medium vessel vasculitis affecting named muscular arteries typically located at the dermal-subcutaneous junction, and, less commonly encountered in isolated cutaneous disease, large vessel vasculitis affecting the aorta and its major branches. Small vessel vasculitis is by far the most common pattern encountered in dermatopathology practice, encompassing leukocytoclastic vasculitis and its many associated syndromes, while medium vessel vasculitis, though less common, carries distinct histologic features and clinical implications developed later in this chapter.

Classification of Vasculopathic Processes

Vasculopathic processes are classified by their underlying mechanism of vessel compromise: thrombotic vasculopathy, resulting from a hypercoagulable state or coagulation cascade abnormality; embolic vasculopathy, resulting from occlusion by material transported from a distant source; and calcifying vasculopathy, exemplified by calciphylaxis, resulting from vascular wall calcification and secondary luminal narrowing. Each of these mechanisms produces a broadly similar downstream histologic endpoint, luminal occlusion with resulting tissue ischemia and, in advanced cases, infarction and necrosis, meaning that the specific upstream mechanism is often inferred from a combination of subtle histologic clues and, critically, clinical and laboratory correlation rather than from occlusion morphology alone.

Entity	Vessel Size/Type	Mechanism	Key Distinguishing Feature
Leukocytoclastic vasculitis	Small vessel (postcapillary venule)	Immune complex-mediated true vasculitis	Fibrinoid necrosis, neutrophilic infiltrate with leukocytoclasis
IgA vasculitis (Henoch-Schonlein)	Small vessel	IgA immune complex-mediated	Perivascular IgA deposition on direct immunofluorescence
Polyarteritis nodosa (cutaneous)	Medium vessel (muscular artery)	Immune complex-mediated true vasculitis	Segmental necrotizing arteritis at dermal-subcutaneous junction
Thrombotic vasculopathy	Small to medium vessel	Hypercoagulability/occlusion	Fibrin/platelet thrombi without wall inflammation
Calciphylaxis	Small to medium vessel	Vascular calcification	Medial calcification with luminal narrowing, subcutaneous fat necrosis

Pigmented purpuric dermatosis	Small vessel (capillaritis)	Lymphocytic capillaritis, non-necrotizing	Extravasated erythrocytes and hemosiderin without fibrinoid necrosis
Livedoid vasculopathy	Small vessel	Thrombotic occlusion, minimal inflammation	Segmental hyalinization with fibrin thrombi, atrophie blanche scarring

Histologic Grading and Reporting Terminology

As with the granulomatous pattern discussed in the preceding chapter, a useful reporting discipline for the vasculopathic and vasculitic biopsy is to state explicitly whether the wall shows fibrinoid necrosis and true inflammatory destruction or is intact and merely occluded, together with vessel size, the presence or absence of calcification, and any ancillary study results, rather than defaulting to a single categorical label such as "vasculitis" that may not communicate the specific findings driving that interpretation. This descriptive discipline is particularly important in this pattern given how directly the wall-inflammation-versus-occlusion distinction changes management, and given that several entities in this chapter, urticarial vasculitis and early or partially treated leukocytoclastic vasculitis among them, can show comparatively subtle findings that benefit from explicit documentation of what was and was not identified.

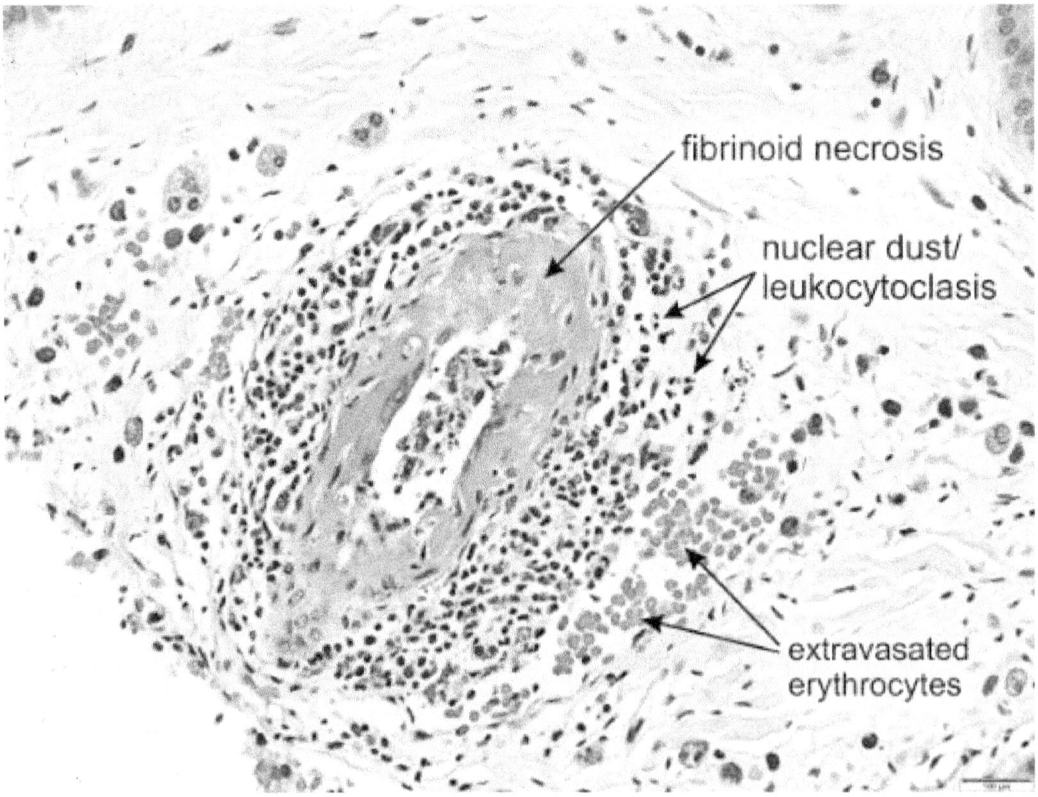

Etiology and Pathogenesis

Immune Complex-Mediated Small Vessel Vasculitis

Leukocytoclastic vasculitis is most often mediated by circulating immune complexes that deposit within postcapillary venule walls, activating the complement cascade and recruiting neutrophils whose degranulation and release of proteolytic enzymes and reactive oxygen species directly damages the vessel wall, producing the fibrinoid necrosis that defines this pattern histologically. This immune complex mechanism explains the broad and heterogeneous list of recognized triggers for leukocytoclastic vasculitis, since essentially any process capable of generating circulating immune complexes, infection, medication, autoimmune connective tissue disease, or malignancy, can precipitate this final common pathway, which is precisely why the histologic diagnosis of leukocytoclastic vasculitis functions as a starting point for etiologic investigation rather than an endpoint diagnosis in itself.

IgA vasculitis, formerly designated Henoch-Schonlein purpura, represents an immunologically distinct subset of small vessel vasculitis defined by predominant IgA deposition within affected vessel walls, identifiable on direct immunofluorescence as discussed in the ancillary studies section below, and classically associated with a preceding upper respiratory infection in children, though the disease occurs across the age spectrum and, in adults, carries a comparatively higher likelihood of renal involvement and a more protracted clinical course. The shared downstream histologic endpoint of fibrinoid necrosis and neutrophilic destruction across the immune complex-mediated vasculitides means that IgA vasculitis cannot be reliably distinguished from other leukocytoclastic vasculitis etiologies on routine hematoxylin and eosin sections alone, underscoring the diagnostic value of direct immunofluorescence in this specific clinical context.

Mechanisms of Medium Vessel Vasculitis

Cutaneous polyarteritis nodosa, like its small vessel counterparts, is understood to be immune complex-mediated, though the larger caliber of the affected muscular arteries produces a distinct histologic and clinical picture, segmental necrotizing inflammation of the arterial wall typically centered at the dermal-subcutaneous junction where named muscular arteries course, producing the deep, tender, nodular clinical lesions and the livedo pattern discussed further in the clinical presentation section below. Unlike systemic polyarteritis nodosa, cutaneous polyarteritis nodosa is generally considered a skin-limited variant without the visceral organ involvement of the systemic form, though a small subset of patients initially presenting with skin-limited disease are subsequently found to have systemic involvement, making longitudinal clinical follow-up an important component of managing this diagnosis even when the initial systemic evaluation is unremarkable.

Mechanisms of Thrombotic and Occlusive Vasculopathy

Thrombotic vasculopathy arises from a hypercoagulable state, whether inherited (protein C or S deficiency, factor V Leiden) or acquired (antiphospholipid antibody syndrome, disseminated intravascular coagulation, malignancy-associated hypercoagulability), producing intraluminal fibrin and platelet thrombi that occlude the vessel without associated inflammatory wall destruction, distinguishing this process histologically from the true vasculitides discussed above. Warfarin-induced skin necrosis, a specific and clinically important cause of thrombotic vasculopathy, results from a paradoxical transient hypercoagulable state occurring in the first several days of warfarin therapy, when protein C levels, being vitamin K-dependent and having a shorter half-life than other vitamin K-dependent clotting factors, fall more rapidly than the levels of the procoagulant factors warfarin is intended to suppress, producing a transient net procoagulant state that can precipitate extensive cutaneous thrombosis and necrosis, most classically in fatty, well-vascularized areas such as the breasts, thighs, and buttocks.

Drug-Induced and Infection-Associated Vasculitis

A substantial proportion of cutaneous leukocytoclastic vasculitis cases are attributable to a medication trigger, with antibiotics, particularly beta-lactams and sulfonamides, among the most commonly implicated culprits, alongside a specific and clinically important subset of medications, propylthiouracil, hydralazine, and minocycline prominent among them, associated with drug-induced antineutrophil cytoplasmic antibody-positive vasculitis, a distinct entity that can mimic primary systemic vasculitis serologically and clinically but generally resolves with discontinuation of the culprit medication rather than requiring the prolonged immunosuppression appropriate for primary antineutrophil cytoplasmic antibody-associated vasculitis. Establishing a clear temporal relationship between medication initiation and vasculitis onset, together with resolution following discontinuation, remains the most reliable method of confirming a drug-induced etiology, since no histologic or serologic feature definitively distinguishes drug-induced from primary vasculitis in isolation.

Infection represents the other major recognized trigger category for leukocytoclastic vasculitis, with streptococcal infection, viral hepatitis, and, less commonly in current practice, infective endocarditis among the most frequently implicated, and a thorough infectious history and, where clinically indicated, targeted infectious serologic testing should accompany the evaluation of any newly diagnosed cutaneous vasculitis case without an obvious medication trigger. Treating the underlying infection, when identified, is generally sufficient to resolve infection-triggered vasculitis without requiring immunosuppressive therapy, which would be relatively contraindicated in the setting of active, untreated infection, paralleling the same treatment-divergence logic already established for the granulomatous pattern in the preceding chapter.

Mechanisms of Calciphylaxis

Calciphylaxis, occurring predominantly in patients with end-stage renal disease, results from progressive calcification of the small and medium dermal and subcutaneous vessel walls, producing luminal narrowing and subsequent thrombosis superimposed on the calcified, structurally compromised vessel, with resulting widespread cutaneous and subcutaneous fat necrosis that carries a notably high mortality rate, driven substantially by secondary infection of the resulting necrotic, ulcerated tissue. The pathogenesis is understood to involve dysregulated calcium and phosphate metabolism in the setting of renal failure, together with additional risk factors including obesity, diabetes, and warfarin use, the last of which is thought to contribute through inhibition of a vitamin K-dependent calcification inhibitor protein, creating a mechanistic link between calciphylaxis and the warfarin-induced necrosis discussed above despite their otherwise distinct pathogenesis.

Urticarial Vasculitis

Urticarial vasculitis occupies a distinctive position at the intersection of the urticarial and vasculitic patterns, presenting clinically as urticarial wheals that, unlike ordinary urticaria, persist beyond twenty-four hours, are frequently painful or burning rather than pruritic, and resolve with residual purpura or hyperpigmentation, clinical features that should prompt biopsy to evaluate for the underlying leukocytoclastic vasculitis that defines this entity histologically. Normocomplementemic urticarial vasculitis is generally idiopathic or medication-associated and follows a comparatively benign course, while hypocomplementemic urticarial vasculitis syndrome carries a substantially higher likelihood of systemic disease, including systemic lupus erythematosus and, less commonly, an underlying paraproteinemia, and warrants a correspondingly more thorough systemic evaluation, including complement levels, once the histologic diagnosis is established.

Histologically, urticarial vasculitis shows the same fibrinoid necrosis, neutrophilic infiltrate, and leukocytoclasis that define leukocytoclastic vasculitis generally, though the intensity of these findings can be comparatively subtle relative to classic palpable purpura, since the urticarial clinical lesion does not produce the same degree of hemorrhage and tissue destruction, making careful, high-power examination of the vessel wall particularly important when this diagnosis is a clinical consideration and the initial impression at scanning power is unremarkable.

Cryoglobulinemic Vasculitis

Cryoglobulinemic vasculitis results from circulating cryoglobulins, immunoglobulins that reversibly precipitate at reduced temperature, depositing within small vessel walls and triggering the same immune complex-mediated leukocytoclastic vasculitis mechanism discussed above, with type II mixed cryoglobulinemia most strongly and classically associated with chronic hepatitis C virus infection, making hepatitis C serology a standard component of the workup for any patient with biopsy-confirmed leukocytoclastic vasculitis and a compatible risk history or unexplained purpura favoring cooler, acral skin. Type I cryoglobulinemia, associated with an underlying plasma cell dyscrasia or lymphoproliferative disorder, more typically produces a occlusive, thrombotic vasculopathy rather than true vasculitis, since the cryoglobulin in this setting precipitates directly within the vessel lumen rather than depositing as a wall-based immune complex, illustrating that the cryoglobulinemias as a group can produce either vasculitic or vasculopathic histology depending on the specific cryoglobulin subtype involved.

Livedoid Vasculopathy

Livedoid vasculopathy, despite its name, is a vasculopathic rather than a true vasculitic process, resulting from thrombotic occlusion of small dermal vessels, most often in the setting of an underlying hypercoagulable state, and producing the characteristic clinical picture of painful, recurrent ulcerations on the lower legs and ankles that heal with atrophic, porcelain-white scars historically termed atrophie blanche. Histologically, livedoid vasculopathy shows intraluminal fibrin thrombi with segmental hyalinization of the vessel wall and minimal to absent inflammatory infiltrate, distinguishing it from true vasculitis, and this distinction carries direct treatment significance, since livedoid vasculopathy responds to anticoagulant or antiplatelet therapy targeting the underlying thrombotic mechanism rather than to the immunosuppressive therapy appropriate for true vasculitis, making the histologic discrimination developed throughout this chapter directly actionable in this specific clinical presentation.

THE REACTION PATTERN RECOGNITION SYSTEM — Wall Inflammation Versus Luminal Occlusion as the First Diagnostic Branch Point

---

The Pattern: True Vasculitis Versus Vasculopathy as the First Diagnostic Branch Point

Histologic Signature: Fibrinoid necrosis and neutrophilic or lymphocytic destruction of the vessel wall itself (vasculitis) versus intraluminal thrombus or occlusive material without primary inflammatory wall destruction (vasculopathy).

The Decision: Assess the vessel wall first: is there evidence of direct inflammatory injury to the wall, or is the vessel occluded with an intact, uninflamed wall? True vasculitis directs the workup toward immune complex disease and systemic vasculitis evaluation; vasculopathy directs the workup toward hypercoagulability, embolic sources, and calciphylaxis risk factors.

Trap Logic: An advanced, ulcerated vasculopathic lesion can develop secondary inflammation around the site of infarction that mimics primary vasculitis, and a partially treated or resolving vasculitic lesion can show diminished wall inflammation alongside secondary thrombosis, blurring the distinction. Biopsying an early, untreated, non-ulcerated lesion and examining multiple vessel levels improves diagnostic accuracy in ambiguous cases.

Pattern Anchor: Fibrinoid necrosis of the wall itself means vasculitis; an occluded lumen with an otherwise unremarkable, uninflamed wall means vasculopathy. This single distinction reroutes the entire subsequent workup and treatment strategy.

Histopathologic Features and Diagnostic Criteria

Diagnostic Criteria for Leukocytoclastic Vasculitis

The histologic diagnosis of leukocytoclastic vasculitis requires fibrinoid necrosis of the postcapillary venule wall, a dense perivascular and intramural neutrophilic infiltrate, nuclear dust from neutrophil breakdown (leukocytoclasis, the finding that gives this entity its name), and extravasation of erythrocytes into the surrounding dermis, together producing the characteristic low-power appearance of a densely inflamed, hemorrhagic, and structurally disrupted small vessel. Biopsy timing meaningfully affects the histologic picture, since a lesion biopsied very early may show a predominantly lymphocytic infiltrate before the neutrophilic component becomes prominent, while a lesion biopsied late in its course may show a mixed or predominantly lymphocytic infiltrate as the neutrophilic response resolves, making biopsy of a lesion between twelve and forty-eight hours of onset optimal for capturing the classic, fully developed histologic picture.

Diagnostic Criteria for Medium Vessel Vasculitis

Cutaneous polyarteritis nodosa requires biopsy of adequately deep tissue, typically an incisional or deep punch biopsy extending into the subcutaneous fat, since the affected muscular arteries course at the dermal-subcutaneous junction and a superficial biopsy will frequently miss the diagnostic segment entirely, a practical point that should be communicated to the clinician whenever this diagnosis is a leading clinical consideration. Histologically, affected arteries show segmental fibrinoid necrosis of the wall with a mixed neutrophilic and lymphocytic infiltrate, often with concentric intimal proliferation and thrombosis in more chronic lesions, and importantly, only a segment of the vessel circumference may be involved, meaning that examining multiple tissue levels improves diagnostic yield when the diagnosis remains uncertain on initial sections.

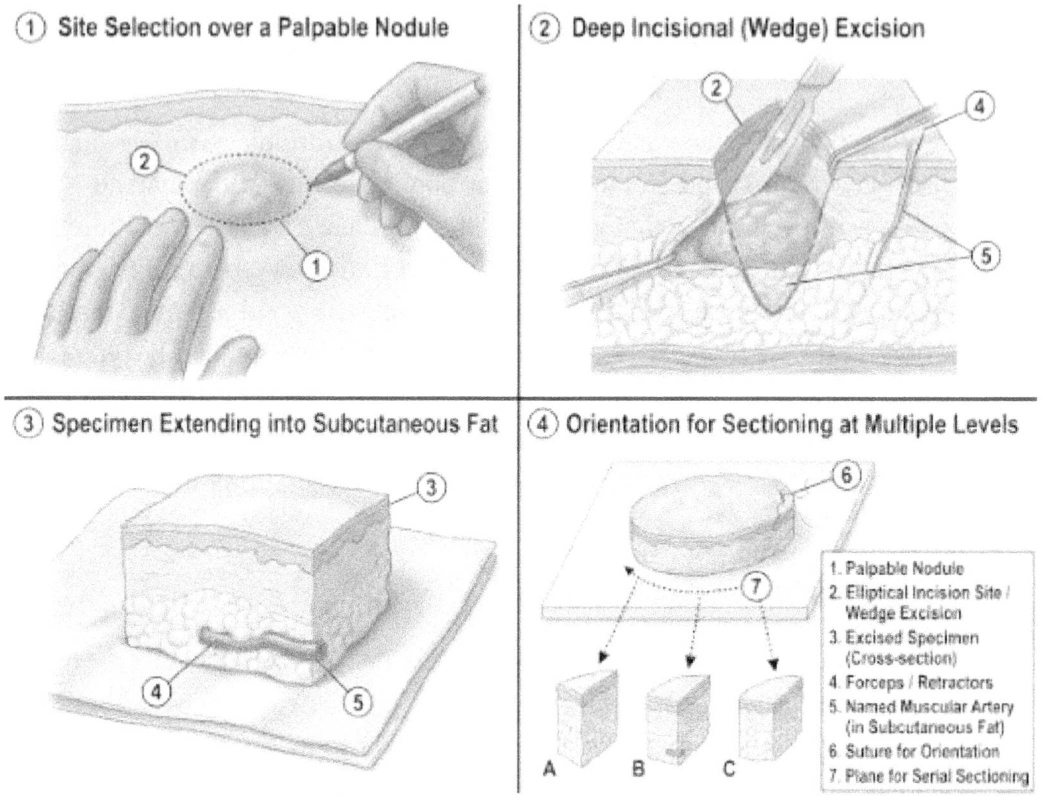

Diagnostic Criteria for Thrombotic Vasculopathy and Calciphylaxis

Thrombotic vasculopathy shows intraluminal fibrin and platelet thrombi occluding small to medium vessels without associated fibrinoid necrosis or a significant inflammatory infiltrate within the wall itself, though secondary ischemic changes in the surrounding dermis and epidermis, including epidermal necrosis in advanced lesions, may be present and should not be mistaken for primary vasculitic wall inflammation. Calciphylaxis shows the additional and diagnostically specific feature of vascular wall calcification, most readily identified within the media of small to medium subcutaneous vessels, often accompanied by extensive subcutaneous fat necrosis with characteristic basophilic calcification of the necrotic fat itself, and a von Kossa or Alizarin red special stain, discussed in the ancillary studies section, can highlight subtle calcification not immediately apparent on routine hematoxylin and eosin staining.

Diagnostic Criteria for Urticarial Vasculitis and Livedoid Vasculopathy

Urticarial vasculitis, as introduced in the etiology section above, requires the same fibrinoid necrosis and leukocytoclasis criteria applied to leukocytoclastic vasculitis generally, though examining multiple tissue levels and multiple vessels is particularly valuable in this entity given the comparatively subtle findings that can accompany its urticarial, rather than frankly purpuric, clinical presentation. Livedoid vasculopathy shows intraluminal fibrin thrombi with segmental hyalinization of the vessel wall extending into the papillary dermis, minimal to absent perivascular inflammation, and, in established or healed lesions, dermal fibrosis and epidermal atrophy corresponding to the atrophie blanche scarring described clinically, together forming a histologic picture that should prompt explicit distinction from true vasculitis in the pathology report given the differing treatment implications already discussed.

Diagnostic Criteria for Pigmented Purpuric Dermatoses

The pigmented purpuric dermatoses, a group of related entities including Schamberg disease, Majocchi purpura, and lichenoid purpuric dermatosis of Gougerot and Blum, show a lymphocytic capillaritis characterized by a superficial perivascular lymphocytic infiltrate, extravasated erythrocytes, and hemosiderin-laden macrophages, notably without the fibrinoid necrosis that defines true leukocytoclastic vasculitis, placing this group at the boundary between the vasculopathic/vasculitic pattern and the lymphocytic vasculitis-mimicker category discussed further in the differential diagnosis section. Distinguishing the specific pigmented purpuric dermatosis subtypes from one another relies substantially on clinical morphology and distribution rather than on distinct histologic features, since the underlying histology is largely shared across the group, with lichen aureus representing a localized, often unilateral variant and lichenoid purpuric dermatosis of Gougerot and Blum showing a denser, more lichenoid lymphocytic infiltrate than the other subtypes.

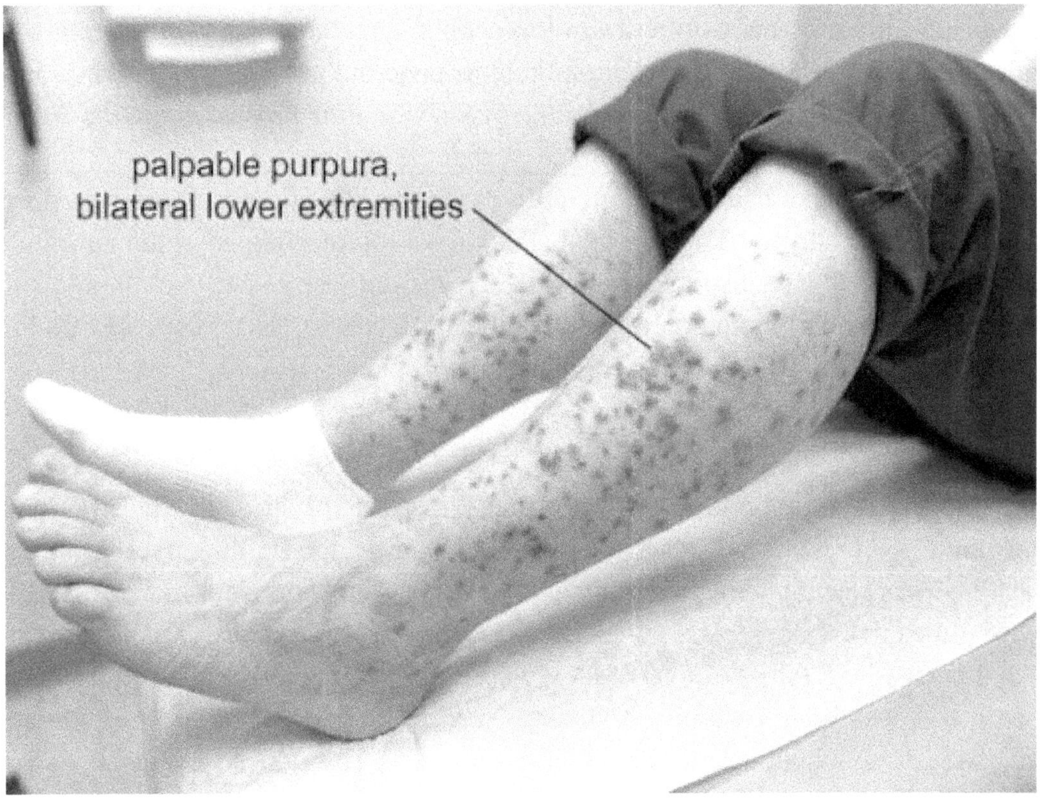

Clinical Presentation and Clinicopathologic Correlation

Clinical Morphology of Small and Medium Vessel Vasculitis

Small vessel leukocytoclastic vasculitis classically presents as palpable purpura, non-blanching, raised purpuric papules and plaques favoring dependent areas such as the bilateral lower legs, reflecting the role of hydrostatic pressure in promoting immune complex deposition within postcapillary venules in these gravitationally stressed sites, and the palpable quality of these lesions, distinguishing them from the flat, non-palpable purpura of a primary platelet or coagulation disorder, is itself a clinically useful bedside discriminator pointing toward a vasculitic rather than purely hemorrhagic process. Medium vessel cutaneous polyarteritis nodosa presents differently, with deep, tender, erythematous to violaceous subcutaneous nodules, often arranged along a livedo racemosa background pattern, a broken, irregular, net-like violaceous discoloration that reflects impaired perfusion in the watershed zones between the affected arteries, and this livedo pattern is itself a useful clinical clue distinguishing medium vessel from small vessel disease at the bedside, before biopsy confirmation.

Clinical Morphology of Vasculopathic Processes

Thrombotic vasculopathy presents with retiform (branching, angulated) purpura reflecting the geometry of the occluded vascular territory, progressing to hemorrhagic bullae and frank necrosis in more severe cases, a morphology that itself favors a vasculopathic over a vasculitic process, since the destructive vessel wall inflammation of true vasculitis less commonly produces this sharply angulated, branching pattern. Calciphylaxis presents with exquisitely painful, retiform purpuric plaques that rapidly progress to necrotic eschar, most characteristically on the proximal, fatty areas of the thighs, abdomen, and buttocks, a distribution and degree of pain disproportionate to the visible lesion size that should prompt urgent consideration of this diagnosis in an appropriate renal failure patient, given the disease's high mortality and the time-sensitive nature of the multidisciplinary management it requires.

Livedo Reticularis Versus Livedo Racemosa

Livedo reticularis, a regular, unbroken, net-like violaceous pattern typically induced or accentuated by cold exposure and resolving with warming, is a physiologic or benign finding in most patients, reflecting normal cutaneous vascular anatomy accentuated by vasospasm, and does not by itself indicate an underlying vasculitic or vasculopathic process. Livedo racemosa, by contrast, is an irregular, broken, net-like pattern that persists regardless of temperature, and reflects genuinely compromised perfusion in the vascular watershed zones between affected vessels, making it the clinically concerning counterpart to livedo reticularis and an important accompanying finding, as introduced earlier in this chapter, for cutaneous polyarteritis nodosa as well as for other occlusive and vasculitic processes, including antiphospholipid antibody syndrome, that warrant the biopsy and systemic evaluation this distinction should prompt.

Systemic Disease Associations and Special Populations

Cutaneous small vessel vasculitis warrants systematic evaluation for an underlying trigger and for systemic organ involvement, since skin findings can represent the presenting sign of a systemic small vessel vasculitis with renal, gastrointestinal, or pulmonary involvement, making urinalysis, in particular, a routine and important component of the initial workup for any patient with newly diagnosed cutaneous leukocytoclastic vasculitis regardless of how limited the cutaneous findings appear. In children, IgA vasculitis represents the most common vasculitis overall and typically follows a self-limited course, though renal involvement, when present, determines long-term prognosis and warrants closer follow-up than the cutaneous findings alone would suggest, while in elderly patients, a new vasculitis diagnosis carries a comparatively higher likelihood of an underlying malignancy or drug trigger, making a thorough medication history and age-appropriate malignancy screening more heavily weighted considerations in this population.

Special Populations: Pediatric and Elderly Vasculitis

IgA vasculitis in children typically follows a self-limited course over several weeks, with the classic tetrad of palpable purpura, arthritis, abdominal pain, and renal involvement, though not all four features need be present at initial presentation, and abdominal pain in this context warrants specific attention given the recognized association with intussusception, a complication that requires prompt clinical recognition distinct from the dermatologic workup. Long-term renal follow-up is recommended for children with IgA vasculitis even after cutaneous resolution, since renal involvement, when present, can evolve over months and determines the condition's long-term prognosis more than the cutaneous findings themselves.

In elderly patients, new-onset cutaneous vasculitis carries a meaningfully higher pretest probability of an underlying malignancy, most often a hematologic malignancy or paraproteinemia, or of a culprit medication among the frequently polypharmacy medication regimens common in this population, shifting the relative emphasis of the systemic workup toward age-appropriate malignancy screening and a systematic medication reconciliation alongside the standard evaluation applied across all age groups. Elderly patients are also disproportionately represented among calciphylaxis cases given the overlapping risk factors of renal disease, diabetes, and anticoagulant use, reinforcing the importance of maintaining calciphylaxis on the differential whenever an elderly patient with these risk factors presents with painful retiform purpura.

Pregnancy occupies a distinctive position across several entities in this chapter: the physiologic hypercoagulable state of pregnancy elevates the baseline risk of thrombotic vasculopathy and, in the peripartum period, of the rare but life-threatening entity of amniotic fluid or other embolic vasculopathy, while pre-eclampsia and the related HELLP syndrome can themselves produce a thrombotic microangiopathy with overlapping histologic features to other occlusive vasculopathies discussed in this chapter. Any pregnant or peripartum patient presenting with new retiform purpura or unexplained cutaneous necrosis warrants urgent multidisciplinary evaluation, given the range of both maternal and fetal implications spanning the differential diagnosis this presentation raises, extending well beyond the dermatologic evaluation alone.

CLINICAL PEARL: Palpable purpura on the lower legs is leukocytoclastic vasculitis until proven otherwise, but a biopsy showing fibrinoid necrosis without accompanying urinalysis and a review of medications, recent infections, and connective tissue disease symptoms leaves the workup incomplete. The biopsy establishes the pattern; it does not establish the trigger.

Differential Diagnosis and Histologic Mimickers

True Vasculitis Versus Pigmented Purpuric Dermatosis

As developed in the histopathologic features section above, the presence or absence of fibrinoid necrosis is the single most reliable discriminator between true leukocytoclastic vasculitis and a pigmented purpuric dermatosis, since both can show extravasated erythrocytes and a perivascular infiltrate, but only true vasculitis shows destructive inflammatory injury to the vessel wall itself. Clinical correlation reinforces this distinction, since pigmented purpuric dermatoses present as flat, non-palpable, golden-brown to purpuric patches reflecting their non-destructive, non-palpable capillaritis, in contrast to the palpable, raised quality of true vasculitic purpura, making the clinical morphology, when available, a useful adjunct to the histologic distinction in cases where fibrinoid necrosis is subtle or only focally present.

Vasculopathy Versus Vasculitis in the Ulcerated or Necrotic Biopsy

An ulcerated or frankly necrotic biopsy specimen presents a particular diagnostic challenge, since secondary inflammatory change surrounding an area of infarction can mimic primary vasculitic wall destruction, and the practical approach in this setting is to examine vessels at the periphery of the ulcerated or necrotic area, and ideally in adjacent, non-ulcerated tissue, where a primary vasculitic process, if present, is more likely to show clearly interpretable, uncomplicated fibrinoid necrosis rather than the secondary inflammatory change that develops around any area of tissue infarction regardless of its underlying cause. Requesting additional tissue levels and, when clinically feasible, a repeat biopsy of a less advanced, non-ulcerated lesion improves diagnostic accuracy in genuinely ambiguous cases, an approach worth explicitly recommending in the pathology report when the distinction cannot be confidently resolved on the initial specimen.

Calciphylaxis Versus Warfarin-Induced Necrosis and Other Occlusive Vasculopathies

Calciphylaxis is distinguished from warfarin-induced skin necrosis and other thrombotic vasculopathies primarily by the identification of vascular wall calcification, a feature specific to calciphylaxis among the occlusive vasculopathies discussed in this chapter, though the two entities can coexist, since warfarin use is itself a recognized risk factor for calciphylaxis as discussed in the etiology section above, occasionally producing overlapping histologic features in a single patient. The distribution of necrosis provides an additional clue, calciphylaxis favoring proximal, fatty sites (thighs, abdomen, buttocks) with extensive subcutaneous fat necrosis, while warfarin-induced necrosis, though it can occur at similar sites, is more specifically tied to the temporal relationship with warfarin initiation, typically within the first three to five days of therapy, information that should be specifically requested when this diagnosis is being considered.

A 68-year-old patient with end-stage renal disease on hemodialysis presents with exquisitely painful, retiform purpuric plaques on the bilateral thighs rapidly progressing to necrotic eschar, and biopsy is obtained given a differential of calciphylaxis versus severe vasculitis versus warfarin-induced necrosis, the patient having recently been started on warfarin for atrial fibrillation. Pattern assignment identifies extensive subcutaneous fat necrosis with small and medium vessel wall calcification, luminal narrowing, and superimposed thrombosis, without evidence of fibrinoid necrosis or an inflammatory infiltrate destroying the vessel wall itself. Differential narrowing excludes true vasculitis based on the absence of wall inflammation and distinguishes calciphylaxis from isolated warfarin necrosis based on the specific finding of vascular wall calcification, though the report notes that concurrent warfarin use likely contributed to the underlying calciphylaxis process given the mechanistic link discussed earlier in this chapter. Diagnosis of calciphylaxis is rendered, prompting urgent multidisciplinary involvement, including nephrology, wound care, and pain management, given this diagnosis's high mortality and the narrow therapeutic window for interventions such as sodium thiosulfate that can meaningfully alter the disease course when initiated early.

A 45-year-old patient with chronic hepatitis C infection presents with recurrent palpable purpura on the lower legs accompanied by acral cyanosis and joint pain that worsens in cold weather, and biopsy is obtained given a differential including cryoglobulinemic vasculitis versus another leukocytoclastic vasculitis etiology. Pattern assignment identifies small vessel fibrinoid necrosis with a neutrophilic infiltrate and leukocytoclasis, together with intraluminal eosinophilic hyaline material within several affected vessels that, on closer inspection, correlates with cryoprotein deposition. Differential narrowing correlates the cold-associated symptom pattern, the acral distribution, and the known hepatitis C infection with cryoglobulinemic vasculitis as the leading diagnosis, and the report specifically recommends properly handled cryoglobulin testing, with blood maintained at body temperature during collection, given the pre-analytic pitfalls discussed in the ancillary studies section. Diagnosis is rendered as leukocytoclastic vasculitis with a comment favoring a cryoglobulinemic etiology given the clinical and histologic correlation, prompting hepatology and rheumatology co-management addressing both the underlying hepatitis C infection and the cryoglobulinemic vasculitis it has produced.

A 6-year-old child presents with palpable purpura on the buttocks and lower legs, mild ankle arthralgia, and colicky abdominal pain one week following an upper respiratory infection, and biopsy of a purpuric papule is obtained given a differential of IgA vasculitis versus another leukocytoclastic vasculitis trigger. Pattern assignment identifies fibrinoid necrosis of postcapillary venules with a dense neutrophilic infiltrate and leukocytoclasis, confirming true small vessel vasculitis. Direct immunofluorescence performed on a concurrently obtained fresh specimen shows predominant perivascular IgA deposition, together with C3, confirming IgA vasculitis rather than another immune complex-mediated trigger. Diagnosis integrates the histologic and direct immunofluorescence findings with the classic clinical tetrad, purpura, arthralgia, abdominal pain, and the preceding upper respiratory infection, to confirm IgA vasculitis, prompting urinalysis to screen for renal involvement and specific counseling regarding the small but clinically important risk of intussusception given the abdominal pain, with a recommendation for renal function follow-up over the subsequent months given this diagnosis's occasionally delayed renal manifestations.

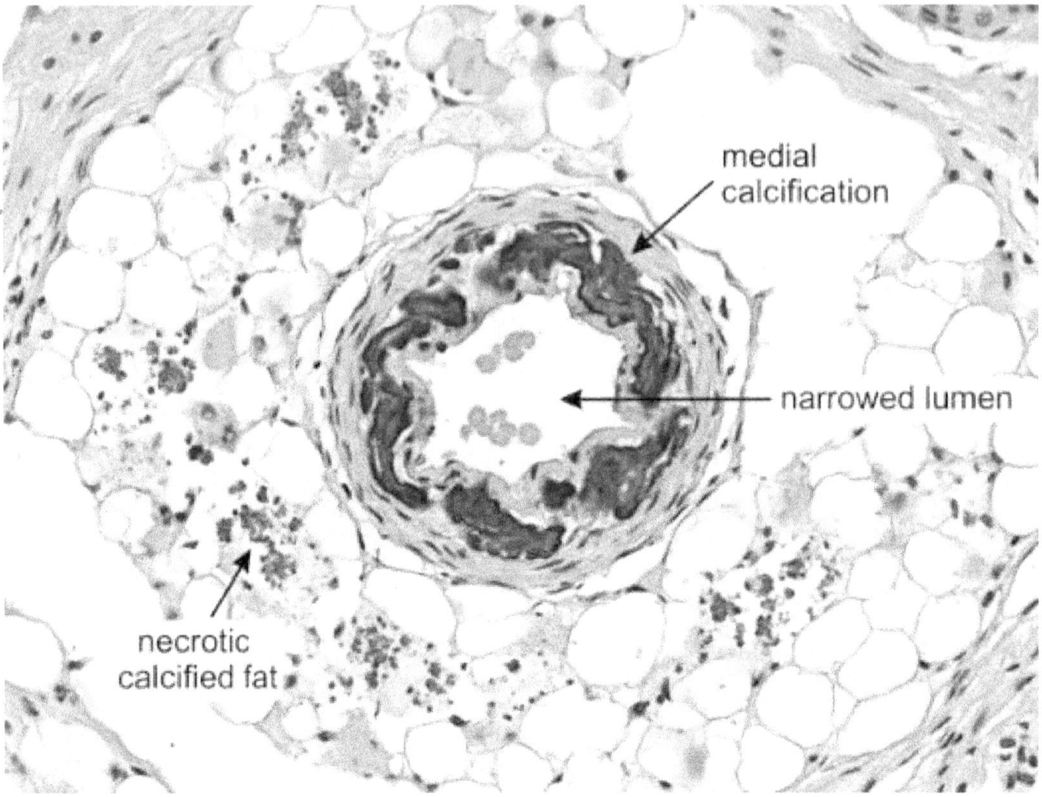

Ancillary Studies

Direct Immunofluorescence

Direct immunofluorescence, performed on a fresh or Michel's-transport-medium biopsy specimen taken from a lesion less than twenty-four to forty-eight hours old, is the single most valuable ancillary study for the vasculitic biopsy, identifying the class of immunoreactant deposited within affected vessel walls, IgA in IgA vasculitis, or a mixed pattern of IgG, IgM, and complement in other immune complex-mediated vasculitides, information that carries both diagnostic and prognostic value, particularly for distinguishing IgA vasculitis, with its associated renal risk profile, from other leukocytoclastic vasculitis etiologies. Timing is critical for this study, since older lesions show progressively diminished immunoreactant deposition as the immune complexes are cleared, meaning that a negative direct immunofluorescence result on a lesion biopsied late in its course should not be over-interpreted as excluding an immune complex-mediated process.

Special Stains for Calcification and Fibrin

A von Kossa or Alizarin red special stain highlights calcium deposition that may be subtle on routine hematoxylin and eosin staining, useful for confirming suspected but equivocal vascular wall calcification in a case where calciphylaxis is being considered, while a phosphotungstic acid-hematoxylin stain can help highlight fibrin within thrombosed vessels in ambiguous cases, though most thrombotic vasculopathy is readily identified on routine sections without requiring this additional stain. Elastic tissue staining, discussed in earlier chapters for its role in identifying elastophagocytosis and other elastic tissue abnormalities, can additionally help delineate the internal elastic lamina of a medium vessel when assessing for the segmental involvement characteristic of cutaneous polyarteritis nodosa, clarifying vessel identity and size in a biopsy where this distinction is not immediately apparent on routine staining alone.

Laboratory Correlation

Skin biopsy findings in the vasculopathic and vasculitic pattern should always be interpreted alongside the clinical timeline the treating clinician provides, since the histologic appearance of a given lesion changes meaningfully over its evolution, an early lesion showing a more purely neutrophilic, less organized infiltrate and a later or resolving lesion showing a more mixed or lymphocyte-predominant infiltrate that can be mistaken for a fundamentally different process if the lesion age is not known at the time of interpretation. Requesting lesion age and, where relevant, whether the biopsied lesion was new or represents an area of chronic, recurrent involvement is a simple but frequently underused piece of clinical information that meaningfully improves diagnostic accuracy across this entire pattern family.

Because the histologic diagnosis of leukocytoclastic vasculitis or vasculopathy functions as a starting point for etiologic investigation rather than a complete diagnosis, laboratory correlation, urinalysis, complete blood count, comprehensive metabolic panel, and, when clinically indicated, antineutrophil cytoplasmic antibody testing, cryoglobulin testing, and hypercoagulability workup, is essential for identifying the specific underlying trigger or coagulopathy responsible for the pattern identified on biopsy. The dermatopathology report itself should explicitly frame the histologic findings within this broader diagnostic context, noting that leukocytoclastic vasculitis, in particular, represents a shared histologic endpoint reached by numerous distinct etiologies rather than a single specific disease, guiding the treating clinician toward the appropriate subsequent laboratory and clinical evaluation.

Antineutrophil Cytoplasmic Antibody and Cryoglobulin Testing

Antineutrophil cytoplasmic antibody testing, though most directly relevant to the systemic small vessel vasculitides such as granulomatosis with polyangiitis and microscopic polyangiitis rather than to isolated cutaneous leukocytoclastic vasculitis, should be considered when cutaneous vasculitis is accompanied by systemic symptoms suggestive of these conditions, including sinonasal disease, pulmonary infiltrates, or renal impairment beyond isolated hematuria, since a positive result meaningfully changes both the diagnostic certainty and the intensity of systemic immunosuppressive treatment required. Cryoglobulin testing requires specific pre-analytic handling, with blood maintained at body temperature during collection and transport before allowing it to cool, since improper handling can produce a false negative result, a practical laboratory detail worth communicating to the ordering clinician whenever cryoglobulinemic vasculitis is a genuine consideration.

When antineutrophil cytoplasmic antibody testing is pursued, distinguishing the proteinase-3 and myeloperoxidase antibody subtypes, corresponding respectively to a cytoplasmic and a perinuclear immunofluorescence staining pattern on the older indirect immunofluorescence assay, carries clinical relevance beyond simple positivity, since proteinase-3 antibodies are more strongly associated with granulomatosis with polyangiitis and myeloperoxidase antibodies with microscopic polyangiitis and eosinophilic granulomatosis with polyangiitis, associations that help guide the subsequent systemic evaluation once a positive result is obtained. Drug-induced antineutrophil cytoplasmic antibody-associated vasculitis, discussed in the etiology section above, frequently shows a distinctive pattern of positivity for multiple antineutrophil cytoplasmic antibody specificities simultaneously, atypical for primary disease, an additional serologic clue that can support a drug-induced rather than primary etiology when the clinical picture is ambiguous.

CAUTION: A biopsy interpreted as "vasculitis" without explicit documentation of fibrinoid necrosis and true wall destruction may reflect a dense perivascular infiltrate that does not meet diagnostic criteria for true vasculitis. This distinction changes management from immunosuppression to an entirely different, occlusion-focused workup, and should never be assumed from a report that does not specify the wall-level findings.

Management Implications

Connecting Diagnosis to Treatment Pathway

Urticarial vasculitis is managed according to its underlying complement status and severity, ranging from antihistamines and nonsteroidal anti-inflammatory agents for mild, normocomplemententemic disease to systemic corticosteroids, dapsone, or other steroid-sparing immunosuppressive agents for hypocomplemententemic or more severe disease, again illustrating that treatment intensity across this pattern family tracks closely with the specific subtype and its systemic disease burden rather than being uniform across the broader vasculitic category.

Management across this chapter's differential diverges as sharply as in the granulomatous pattern discussed in the preceding chapter: small vessel leukocytoclastic vasculitis is managed by identifying and removing the underlying trigger, whether a medication or infection, with systemic corticosteroids or other immunosuppressive agents reserved for severe, refractory, or systemically involved disease; cutaneous polyarteritis nodosa is managed with immunosuppressive therapy tailored to disease severity, together with longitudinal monitoring for systemic progression; thrombotic vasculopathy is managed by correcting the underlying hypercoagulable state and, for warfarin-induced necrosis specifically, by discontinuing warfarin and providing vitamin K and alternative anticoagulation during the acute period; and calciphylaxis requires urgent multidisciplinary management, including sodium thiosulfate, aggressive wound care, pain control, and correction of calcium-phosphate metabolism abnormalities, given the disease's high mortality. Livedoid vasculopathy and other thrombotic vasculopathies are managed with anticoagulant or antiplatelet therapy targeted to the underlying hypercoagulable mechanism rather than with immunosuppression, a distinction this chapter has returned to repeatedly and one that bears direct practical consequence at the bedside.

Complications and Prognosis

Cutaneous polyarteritis nodosa follows a chronic, relapsing-remitting course in many patients, with periodic flares of tender nodules requiring intermittent treatment intensification, and while progression to systemic disease is uncommon once a skin-limited presentation has been established over an extended follow-up period, the small but real possibility of delayed systemic involvement justifies continued longitudinal monitoring rather than a single reassuring initial evaluation being considered definitive.

Small vessel leukocytoclastic vasculitis limited to the skin generally carries a favorable prognosis, particularly when a clear, removable trigger is identified, though chronic or recurrent disease occurs in a meaningful subset of patients and warrants ongoing evaluation for a persistent underlying cause such as an occult connective tissue disease or paraproteinemia. Calciphylaxis carries the most guarded prognosis of any entity discussed in this chapter, with mortality rates remaining substantial even with aggressive multidisciplinary treatment, driven primarily by secondary infection of necrotic tissue and by the severity of the underlying renal disease, underscoring why early recognition and urgent treatment initiation, rather than any single specific therapy, is the most important determinant of outcome in this diagnosis.

Urticarial vasculitis and livedoid vasculopathy each follow a chronic, relapsing-remitting course in a substantial proportion of patients, with hypocomplementemic urticarial vasculitis syndrome carrying the additional long-term risk of evolving systemic lupus erythematosus or another connective tissue disease over subsequent years, warranting periodic clinical reassessment even in patients whose initial systemic evaluation is unremarkable. Livedoid vasculopathy, though not immediately life-threatening in the way calciphylaxis is, carries substantial morbidity from chronic, painful, recurrent ulceration and can significantly impair quality of life and mobility over time, making early recognition of the vasculopathic rather than vasculitic mechanism, and the resulting shift toward anticoagulant or antiplatelet therapy, an important determinant of long-term functional outcome for these patients.

Prevention and Screening

For patients with recurrent leukocytoclastic vasculitis in whom a medication trigger has been identified, maintaining a clear, documented record of the culprit medication and counseling the patient to inform future prescribers helps prevent inadvertent re-exposure and recurrence, a straightforward but frequently overlooked preventive measure given how many patients see multiple prescribers over time. Patients with identified hypercoagulable states underlying thrombotic vasculopathy or livedoid vasculopathy benefit from hematology referral for consideration of long-term anticoagulation and, where relevant, family screening for an inherited thrombophilia, extending the clinical value of the dermatopathologic diagnosis beyond the immediate cutaneous findings to a broader, potentially multi-generational risk assessment.

Patient Education and Counseling

Patients diagnosed with livedoid vasculopathy or another chronic occlusive vasculopathy benefit from counseling regarding the wound care measures, compression therapy where appropriate, and trauma avoidance that support ulcer healing and prevention alongside pharmacologic management of the underlying hypercoagulable state, and from realistic expectations regarding the chronic, relapsing nature of this condition even with appropriate treatment. Patients with cryoglobulinemic or hepatitis-associated vasculitis benefit from understanding that treating the underlying viral infection, when feasible, is often central to controlling the vasculitis itself, reinforcing why hepatology and dermatology co-management, rather than dermatologic treatment in isolation, typically offers the best long-term outcome for this specific patient population.

Patients with small vessel vasculitis benefit from counseling regarding the importance of completing the recommended systemic evaluation, including urinalysis, even when cutaneous findings are limited, given the possibility of clinically silent renal involvement, and from reassurance that a clear trigger, once identified and removed, is often associated with resolution and a lower likelihood of recurrence. Patients and families facing a calciphylaxis diagnosis benefit from honest, direct communication regarding prognosis alongside emphasis on the specific, time-sensitive interventions available, allowing informed participation in the urgent multidisciplinary treatment decisions this diagnosis requires.

THE REACTION PATTERN RECOGNITION SYSTEM — The Vasculopathic and Vasculitic Pattern Family

The Pattern: The vasculopathic and vasculitic pattern organized by wall inflammation versus luminal occlusion, then by vessel size: small vessel leukocytoclastic vasculitis and IgA vasculitis, medium vessel cutaneous polyarteritis nodosa, thrombotic and calcifying vasculopathy, and pigmented purpuric dermatosis.

Histologic Signature: Fibrinoid necrosis with neutrophilic wall destruction and leukocytoclasis defines true vasculitis; intraluminal thrombus with an uninflamed wall defines thrombotic vasculopathy; medial calcification defines calciphylaxis; capillaritis without fibrinoid necrosis defines pigmented purpuric dermatosis.

The Decision: Assess the vessel wall first for evidence of true inflammatory destruction versus simple occlusion, then classify by vessel size, then correlate with direct immunofluorescence and laboratory workup to identify the specific underlying trigger or coagulopathy.

Trap Logic: Ulcerated or necrotic tissue can show secondary inflammatory change mimicking primary vasculitis; biopsy an early, non-ulcerated lesion and examine the periphery of any necrotic area. Warfarin use and calciphylaxis are mechanistically linked and can coexist, requiring specific attention to vascular wall calcification rather than assuming a single occlusive mechanism.

Pattern Anchor: Fibrinoid necrosis of the wall means vasculitis and immunosuppression; an occluded lumen with an intact wall means vasculopathy and a coagulation or calcification workup. Get the wall assessment right first, because it redirects the entire subsequent evaluation.

Summary and Key Concepts

The vasculopathic and vasculitic reaction pattern is first divided by whether the vessel wall itself shows true inflammatory destruction (vasculitis) or simple occlusion without primary wall inflammation (vasculopathy), a distinction with direct treatment implications.

Small vessel leukocytoclastic vasculitis, defined by fibrinoid necrosis, neutrophilic infiltration, and leukocytoclasis, represents a shared histologic endpoint reached by numerous distinct triggers, requiring systematic clinical and laboratory correlation rather than treatment as a single disease.

Medium vessel cutaneous polyarteritis nodosa requires deep biopsy technique to capture the affected dermal-subcutaneous junction arteries and shows segmental necrotizing arteritis that may only involve a portion of the vessel circumference.

Thrombotic vasculopathy, warfarin-induced necrosis, and calciphylaxis share an occlusive, non-inflammatory mechanism but are distinguished by vascular wall calcification (specific to calciphylaxis), distribution, and temporal relationship to medication initiation.

Direct immunofluorescence on an early, appropriately transported specimen is the single most valuable ancillary study for the vasculitic biopsy, while calciphylaxis represents a time-sensitive, high-mortality diagnosis requiring urgent multidisciplinary management.

CHAPTER 10: PANNICULITIS AND DISEASES OF SUBCUTANEOUS FAT

Learning Objectives

1. Classify panniculitis by predominant compartment of involvement: septal versus lobular.
2. Distinguish panniculitis with vasculitis from panniculitis without vasculitis and correlate this distinction with etiology.
3. Identify the histopathologic features and diagnostic criteria of erythema nodosum and the major forms of lobular panniculitis.
4. Correlate histologic findings in subcutaneous fat disease with clinical presentation and systemic associations.
5. Construct a differential diagnosis for panniculitis based on compartment, vasculitis status, and specific histologic clues.
6. Select appropriate ancillary studies, including deep biopsy technique and special stains, for the panniculitis specimen.

Definition and Classification

Defining Panniculitis and Its Compartmental Logic

Panniculitis, inflammation centered on the subcutaneous fat rather than the dermis, represents the final reaction pattern in this book's seven-pattern framework and requires a distinct diagnostic approach because the subcutaneous fat's simple lobular architecture, fat lobules separated by fibrous septa carrying the vascular supply, offers fewer histologic landmarks than the dermis, making the specific compartment of involvement, septal versus lobular, the foundational organizing axis for this entire chapter, just as architecture served this role for the granulomatous pattern and wall inflammation served this role for the vasculopathic pattern in the two preceding chapters.

Septal panniculitis, inflammation predominantly involving the fibrous septa between fat lobules with relative sparing of the lobules themselves, is exemplified by erythema nodosum, the most common panniculitis encountered in clinical practice, while lobular panniculitis, inflammation predominantly involving the fat lobules themselves, encompasses a more etiologically diverse group including infection, autoimmune connective tissue disease, pancreatic disease, alpha-1 antitrypsin deficiency, and factitial or traumatic causes, each producing distinct histologic clues developed throughout this chapter.

The Second Axis: Vasculitis Versus No Vasculitis

Historical classification schemes for panniculitis relied more heavily on clinical course and distribution than on the compartmental, mechanism-based approach this chapter emphasizes, an older nomenclature that persists in some clinical usage but has been substantially superseded as immunohistochemistry, molecular diagnostics, and a more refined understanding of specific disease mechanisms have allowed increasingly precise histologic subclassification, a theme returned to later in this chapter's discussion of Weber-Christian disease and its modern reclassification.

A second, cross-cutting classification axis asks whether the panniculitis is accompanied by vasculitis affecting vessels within the subcutaneous fat, since this distinction, much like the wall-inflammation-versus-occlusion distinction developed in the preceding chapter, carries substantial diagnostic and prognostic weight: panniculitis with vasculitis suggests entities such as erythema induratum/nodular vasculitis and cutaneous polyarteritis nodosa extending into the subcutaneous compartment, while panniculitis without vasculitis encompasses the majority of both septal and lobular panniculitis forms, including erythema nodosum itself. Applying both axes together, compartment and vasculitis status, in that order, generates a systematic four-quadrant framework that organizes the remainder of this chapter and mirrors the same architecture-first, exclusion-second diagnostic discipline established in Chapter 8.

Reporting Terminology for the Panniculitis Biopsy

Given the comparatively limited histologic vocabulary available within subcutaneous fat relative to the dermis, a panniculitis report benefits from explicitly stating the compartment involved, the presence or absence of vasculitis, the inflammatory cell composition, and any specific diagnostic clues such as fat necrosis pattern or crystal deposition, rather than defaulting to a single generic diagnosis of "panniculitis," a label that, standing alone, provides minimal actionable information to the treating clinician given how many distinct etiologies converge on this shared anatomic compartment.

Entity	Compartment	Vasculitis	Key Distinguishing Feature
Erythema nodosum	Septal	Absent	Widened septa with lymphocytes, histiocytes, and Miescher radial granulomas
Erythema induratum / nodular vasculitis	Lobular (septal extension)	Present (usually granulomatous)	Lobular granulomatous panniculitis with vasculitis, caseous necrosis
Lupus panniculitis	Lobular	Absent	Lymphocytic lobular infiltrate with hyaline fat necrosis and lymphoid follicles
Pancreatic panniculitis	Lobular	Absent	"Ghost cells" (anucleate adipocytes) with saponification

Alpha-1 antitrypsin deficiency panniculitis	Lobular	Absent	Neutrophilic infiltrate with splaying of dermal collagen bundles
Subcutaneous panniculitis-like T-cell lymphoma	Lobular	Absent	Atypical lymphocytes rimming individual adipocytes
Lipodermatosclerosis	Septal and lobular	Absent	Lipomembranous fat necrosis with background venous stasis changes
Infectious panniculitis	Lobular (variable septal)	Variable	Neutrophilic, hemorrhagic infiltrate; organisms on stain/culture

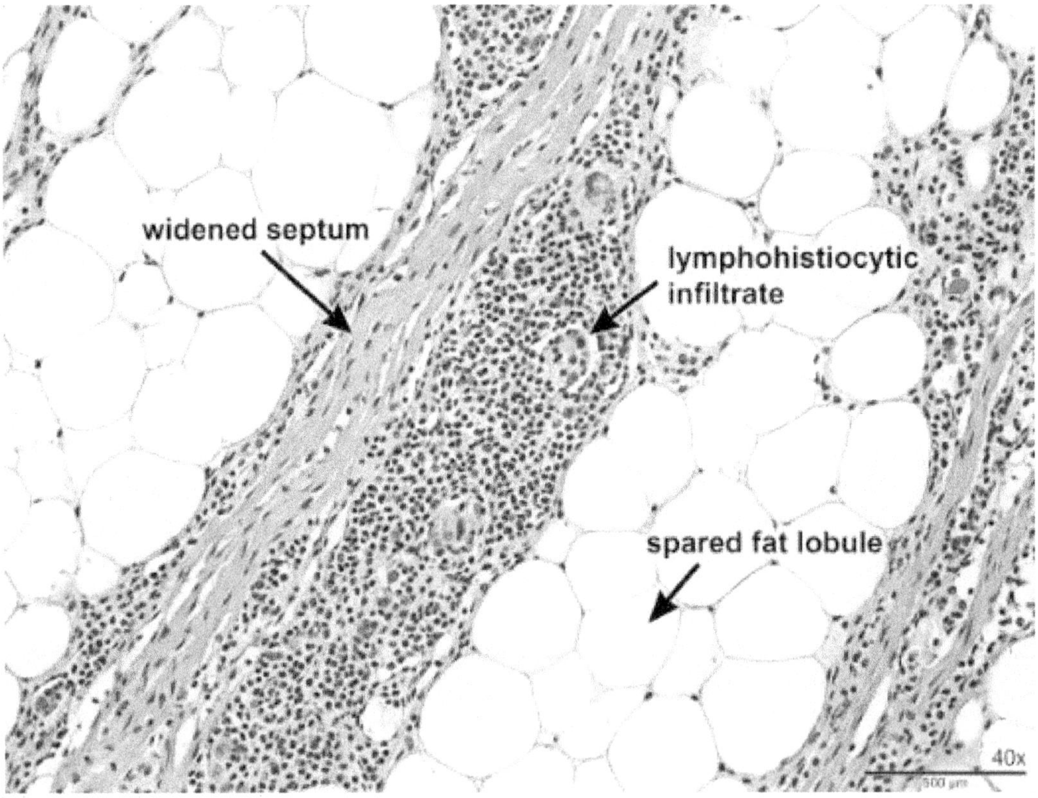

Etiology and Pathogenesis

Mechanisms of Erythema Nodosum

The seven-pattern framework this book has developed since Chapter 3 finds a particularly clear illustration in panniculitis, since the subcutaneous fat, despite its architectural simplicity relative to the dermis and epidermis, hosts a comparably wide etiologic range spanning autoimmune disease, infection, malignancy, systemic organ disease, and simple physical injury, each producing a distinguishable pattern once the compartmental and vasculitis-status framework developed in this chapter is systematically applied.

Erythema nodosum is understood as a delayed-type hypersensitivity reaction occurring in response to a wide range of antigenic triggers, streptococcal infection representing the single most common identifiable trigger, alongside other infections, medications (most notably oral contraceptives and sulfonamides), sarcoidosis, inflammatory bowel disease, and pregnancy, with a substantial proportion of cases remaining idiopathic despite thorough evaluation. This broad list of recognized triggers parallels the etiologic heterogeneity already established for leukocytoclastic vasculitis in the preceding chapter, reinforcing a theme that recurs throughout this book's later chapters: several of the reaction patterns represent a shared histologic and clinical endpoint reached through numerous distinct upstream immunologic pathways rather than a single specific disease process.

Mechanisms of Erythema Induratum and Nodular Vasculitis

Erythema induratum, when associated with an identifiable tuberculous trigger, and nodular vasculitis, the equivalent clinical and histologic entity without identifiable tuberculous association, are believed to represent a delayed-type hypersensitivity reaction to mycobacterial antigen, whether from active or remote tuberculous infection, producing a granulomatous lobular panniculitis with associated vasculitis of small and medium vessels within the subcutaneous fat, often with caseous necrosis reflecting the mycobacterial association even when organisms themselves cannot be directly demonstrated within the specimen. This entity illustrates a mechanism distinct from direct organism-mediated tissue destruction, resembling instead an immunologically mediated reaction to an antigen the host has been exposed to, whether or not viable organisms remain present at the biopsy site, a distinction with direct implications for the special stain and molecular ancillary studies discussed later in this chapter.

Mechanisms of Lupus Panniculitis

Lupus panniculitis, also termed lupus profundus, represents a subcutaneous manifestation of the autoimmune connective tissue disease spectrum discussed in Chapter 6, occurring either in isolation or in association with systemic or discoid lupus erythematosus, and is mediated by the same interface dermatitis-associated autoimmune mechanisms discussed in that chapter, extending in this presentation into the subcutaneous fat rather than remaining confined to the dermal-epidermal junction. The characteristic hyaline fat necrosis and lymphoid follicle formation discussed in the histopathologic features section below reflect a chronic, organized autoimmune inflammatory process rather than the acute hypersensitivity mechanism underlying erythema nodosum, a mechanistic distinction that correlates with lupus panniculitis's typically more indolent, chronic clinical course.

Mechanisms of Pancreatic and Alpha-1 Antitrypsin Deficiency Panniculitis

Pancreatic panniculitis results from circulating pancreatic enzymes, lipase most notably, released into the systemic circulation during acute or chronic pancreatitis or from a pancreatic neoplasm, reaching the subcutaneous fat and enzymatically hydrolyzing adipocyte triglycerides into free fatty acids that subsequently bind calcium to produce the saponification and "ghost cell" formation that define this entity's distinctive histology, discussed further below. Alpha-1 antitrypsin deficiency panniculitis results from insufficient antiprotease activity, normally provided by alpha-1 antitrypsin, allowing unchecked neutrophilic proteolytic enzyme activity to damage the subcutaneous fat and, distinctively, adjacent dermal collagen, producing the neutrophilic infiltrate with dermal collagen splaying that distinguishes this entity from most other panniculitis forms discussed in this chapter.

Mechanisms of Infectious Panniculitis

Beyond the immunologically mediated mechanisms discussed above, a further mechanistic thread connects several of this chapter's lobular panniculitis entities: each results from a discrete, identifiable biochemical or enzymatic insult to the adipocyte, circulating pancreatic lipase for pancreatic panniculitis, unchecked neutrophil proteolysis for alpha-1 antitrypsin deficiency panniculitis, cold-induced lipid crystallization for cold panniculitis, and venous hypertension-driven fibrin deposition for lipodermatosclerosis, in contrast to the more purely immune-mediated mechanisms of lupus panniculitis and subcutaneous panniculitis-like T-cell lymphoma, a mechanistic distinction that, while not always histologically obvious at first inspection, underlies much of the specific diagnostic clue-based approach this chapter has developed.

Infectious panniculitis arises from direct microbial invasion of the subcutaneous fat, most often by bacteria (including necrotizing fasciitis-associated organisms), less commonly by deep fungal or atypical mycobacterial organisms, typically in the setting of an immunocompromised host, penetrating trauma, or contiguous spread from an adjacent infected structure, and represents a distinct mechanism from the immunologically mediated panniculitis entities discussed above, in which organisms directly damage adipocytes and incite an acute, often neutrophilic and hemorrhagic inflammatory response. Recognizing infectious panniculitis promptly carries particular urgency when a necrotizing soft tissue infection is a consideration, given the rapid clinical deterioration and high mortality this specific presentation carries, making infectious panniculitis one of the few entities in this chapter where same-day communication of frozen section or preliminary findings to the surgical team can be genuinely life-saving.

Mechanisms of Lipodermatosclerosis

Lipodermatosclerosis, occurring predominantly in patients with chronic venous insufficiency, results from venous hypertension and consequent capillary damage, fibrin cuff deposition around dermal vessels, and progressive septal and lobular fibrosis, evolving from an acute, painful, erythematous phase that can clinically and even histologically mimic other forms of panniculitis to a chronic phase producing the characteristic "inverted champagne bottle" clinical deformity of the lower leg from progressive circumferential fibrosis and fat loss. Because acute lipodermatosclerosis can closely mimic infectious cellulitis or other acute panniculitis forms both clinically and histologically, correlating the biopsy findings with a background of chronic venous stasis changes, including dermal hemosiderin deposition and stasis-associated fibrosis, and with the clinical distribution over the medial ankle and lower leg, supports this diagnosis over its acute mimickers.

Weber-Christian Disease and Idiopathic Lobular Panniculitis

Erythema nodosum leprosum, a distinct entity despite its similar name, occurs as a reactional state in patients with lepromatous or borderline lepromatous leprosy, discussed in Chapter 8, and shows a neutrophilic and lobular panniculitis, sometimes with vasculitis, that is histologically and mechanistically distinct from ordinary erythema nodosum despite the overlapping name, an important distinction to draw explicitly given how easily the shared terminology can lead to diagnostic and management confusion in a patient with known or suspected leprosy presenting with new tender nodules.

Weber-Christian disease, a historical designation for idiopathic, relapsing febrile nodular panniculitis, is now understood to represent a heterogeneous group of conditions rather than a single specific entity, and a substantial proportion of cases previously classified under this label are now recognized, with the benefit of modern immunohistochemistry and molecular testing, to actually represent subcutaneous panniculitis-like T-cell lymphoma or another specific, previously unrecognized etiology, illustrating the historical evolution of this chapter's diagnostic framework and reinforcing why any panniculitis biopsy without a clear specific diagnosis after thorough histologic and ancillary evaluation warrants close clinical follow-up rather than acceptance of a purely descriptive, idiopathic label as a diagnostic endpoint. Genuinely idiopathic lobular panniculitis, once the recognized specific entities and mimickers discussed throughout this chapter have been excluded, remains a diagnosis of exclusion applied cautiously and only after this systematic process.

Cold Panniculitis and Other Physical Triggers

Cold panniculitis results from direct cold-induced adipocyte injury, occurring classically in infants and young children after prolonged exposure to a cold object or environment, reflecting the comparatively higher ratio of saturated to unsaturated fatty acids in infant subcutaneous fat, which raises its crystallization point and increases its vulnerability to cold-induced injury relative to adult subcutaneous fat, a mechanistic detail that explains this entity's strong age predilection. Popsicle panniculitis, a specific and classically described pediatric presentation resulting from prolonged contact between a cold popsicle or ice pop and the cheek, illustrates this mechanism directly and typically resolves spontaneously without specific treatment once the causative cold exposure is identified and avoided, making a directed history regarding recent cold exposure a simple but valuable component of the clinical evaluation whenever an infant presents with a firm, indurated facial or acral plaque.

THE REACTION PATTERN RECOGNITION SYSTEM — Compartment and Vasculitis Status as the First Diagnostic Branch Points

---

The Pattern: Septal Versus Lobular Compartment, Then Vasculitis Versus No Vasculitis, as the First Diagnostic Branch Points

Histologic Signature: Inflammation predominantly within the fibrous septa with relative lobular sparing (septal) versus inflammation predominantly within the fat lobules themselves (lobular); presence or absence of vasculitis affecting subcutaneous vessels within either compartment.

The Decision: Assess compartment first: septal panniculitis without vasculitis directs the differential toward erythema nodosum, while lobular panniculitis directs the differential toward a broader group requiring further subclassification by vasculitis status and specific histologic clues (necrosis pattern, cell composition, crystal or ghost cell formation).

Trap Logic: Advanced or long-standing septal panniculitis can develop secondary lobular extension that mimics primary lobular disease, and inadequately deep biopsies can fail to capture the full septal-to-lobular architecture needed for accurate compartment assignment. A deep incisional or wedge biopsy extending well into the subcutaneous fat, rather than a standard punch biopsy, is essential for reliable compartment and vasculitis assessment.

Pattern Anchor: Septum-predominant without vasculitis points toward erythema nodosum; lobule-predominant with granulomatous vasculitis points toward erythema induratum/nodular vasculitis; lobule-predominant without vasculitis requires further subclassification by cell composition and necrosis pattern. Get the compartment right first, using adequately deep tissue.

Histopathologic Features and Diagnostic Criteria

Diagnostic Features of Erythema Nodosum

Erythema nodosum shows widened, fibrotic septa infiltrated by lymphocytes, histiocytes, and, in a minority of cases, eosinophils, with the diagnostically useful Miescher radial granuloma, a small, well-defined cluster of histiocytes arranged radially around a central cleft-like space, frequently identifiable within the septa in early or evolving lesions, though this finding becomes less prominent and more difficult to identify in older, more fibrotic lesions. The fat lobules themselves remain largely uninvolved in classic erythema nodosum, with inflammation confined to the septa and only minimal, secondary extension into the immediately adjacent lobular periphery, a compartmental purity that itself supports the diagnosis when present and that becomes progressively less distinct as the lesion ages and septal fibrosis extends further into the surrounding tissue.

Diagnostic Features of Erythema Induratum and Nodular Vasculitis

Erythema induratum and nodular vasculitis show a lobular, granulomatous panniculitis with well-formed and poorly formed granulomas admixed with lymphocytes and, characteristically, vasculitis affecting small to medium vessels within the subcutaneous septa and lobules, with caseous necrosis a common though not universal accompanying feature that, when present, further supports the tuberculous or mycobacterial-antigen association discussed in the etiology section above. The combination of lobular granulomatous inflammation and vasculitis together distinguishes this entity from other lobular panniculitis forms discussed later in this chapter, none of which characteristically show this specific granulomatous vasculitis combination, making the identification of vasculitis within a granulomatous lobular panniculitis specimen a specific and diagnostically useful finding.

Diagnostic Features of Lupus Panniculitis

Lupus panniculitis shows a lymphocytic lobular panniculitis with characteristic hyaline fat necrosis, adipocytes that have lost their normal architecture and taken on a smudged, eosinophilic, hyalinized appearance, together with lymphoid follicle formation, organized aggregates of lymphocytes resembling germinal centers, a finding that, while not entirely specific to lupus panniculitis, is highly suggestive when combined with the other features of this pattern. Overlying epidermal and dermal changes of discoid or subacute cutaneous lupus erythematosus, interface dermatitis, basement membrane thickening, and increased dermal mucin as discussed in Chapter 6, may or may not be present in a given lupus panniculitis specimen, and their absence does not exclude the diagnosis, since lupus panniculitis can occur with minimal or no overlying epidermal involvement in a meaningful subset of cases.

Diagnostic Features of Pancreatic and Alpha-1 Antitrypsin Deficiency Panniculitis

Pancreatic panniculitis shows the pathognomonic finding of "ghost cells," anucleate adipocytes with thickened, shadowy cell membranes reflecting saponification of the cell contents, together with basophilic calcium deposition and a neutrophilic infiltrate, findings sufficiently distinctive that their identification should prompt immediate correlation with pancreatic function testing and imaging even when a pancreatic history has not been specifically provided to the pathologist. Alpha-1 antitrypsin deficiency panniculitis shows a lobular neutrophilic infiltrate with a distinctive pattern of splaying between individual dermal collagen bundles at the dermal-subcutaneous junction, a finding that, together with hemorrhage and fat necrosis, should prompt alpha-1 antitrypsin level testing, particularly in a patient with a personal or family history of early-onset emphysema or liver disease that might otherwise suggest this underlying deficiency.

Diagnostic Features of Lipodermatosclerosis and Infectious Panniculitis

Acute lipodermatosclerosis shows septal and lobular fibrosis, fat necrosis with lipomembranous (membranocystic) change, a distinctive arcaded, feathery membrane lining necrotic fat spaces, and, in the acute phase, hemorrhage and a mixed inflammatory infiltrate, while the chronic phase shows progressive, dense sclerosis of both septa and lobules with relatively diminished inflammation, together with the background dermal stasis changes discussed above that support this diagnosis over its histologic mimickers. Infectious panniculitis shows a predominantly neutrophilic, often hemorrhagic and necrotic infiltrate with variable vasculitis and, importantly, organisms that may or may not be identifiable on routine or special stains depending on organism burden and prior antimicrobial exposure, making tissue culture, submitted at the time of biopsy whenever infectious panniculitis is a genuine consideration, an essential complement to histologic examination given the limitations of special stains alone in this specific, urgent clinical context.

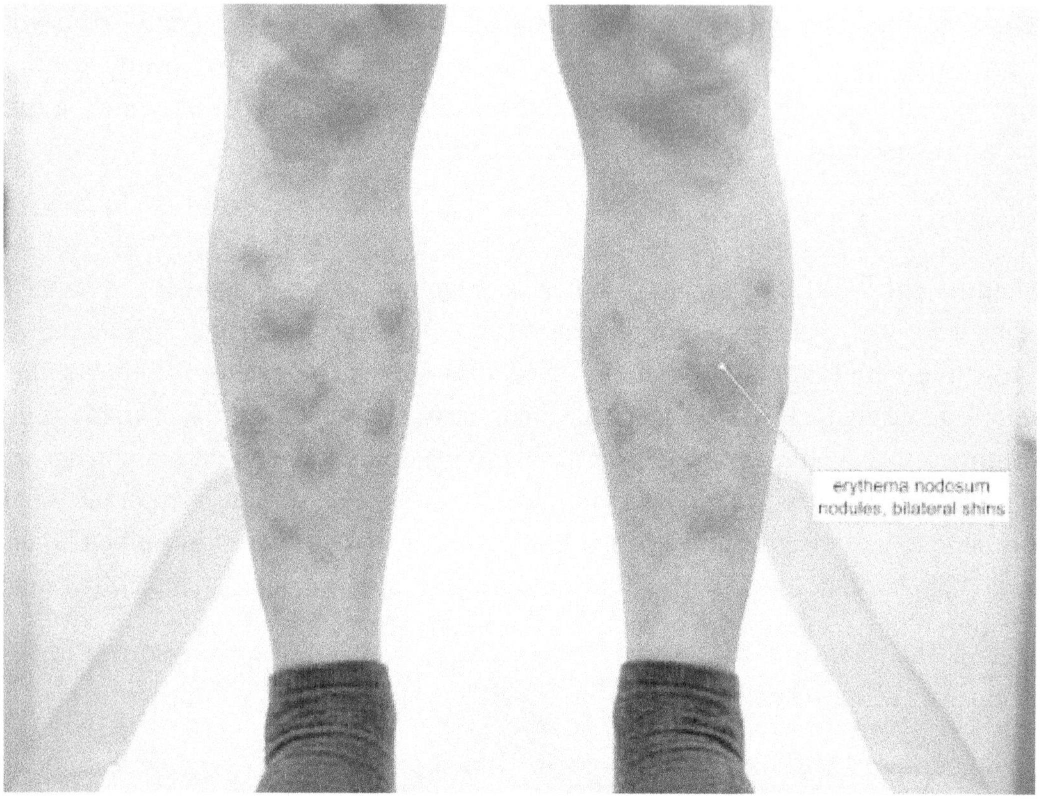

Clinical Presentation and Clinicopathologic Correlation

Clinical Morphology of Erythema Nodosum

Erythema nodosum presents as tender, erythematous to violaceous, poorly demarcated subcutaneous nodules, classically bilateral and symmetric on the anterior shins, evolving through a bruise-like color progression over one to two weeks before resolving without scarring or ulceration, a self-limited course that itself provides useful clinicopathologic correlation supporting this diagnosis over the other panniculitis entities discussed in this chapter, most of which follow a more chronic or ulcerating course. Given the broad list of recognized triggers discussed in the etiology section, the clinical evaluation of erythema nodosum should include a directed history for recent infection, new medications, and symptoms of sarcoidosis or inflammatory bowel disease, together with a chest radiograph, given the recognized association between erythema nodosum and hilar lymphadenopathy in both sarcoidosis and certain infections.

Clinical Morphology of Lobular Panniculitis Entities

Erythema induratum and nodular vasculitis present with tender, erythematous to violaceous nodules and plaques favoring the posterior calves, in contrast to the anterior shin predominance of erythema nodosum, frequently ulcerating, a clinical distinction that, together with the more chronic course typical of this entity relative to erythema nodosum, should prompt biopsy to confirm the diagnosis and evaluate for an underlying tuberculous trigger. Lupus panniculitis presents as deep, firm, occasionally tender subcutaneous nodules and plaques favoring the proximal extremities, face, and trunk, healing with a characteristic depressed, lipoatrophic scar reflecting the destructive fat necrosis discussed above, a healing pattern distinct from any other panniculitis entity in this chapter and itself a useful clinical clue.

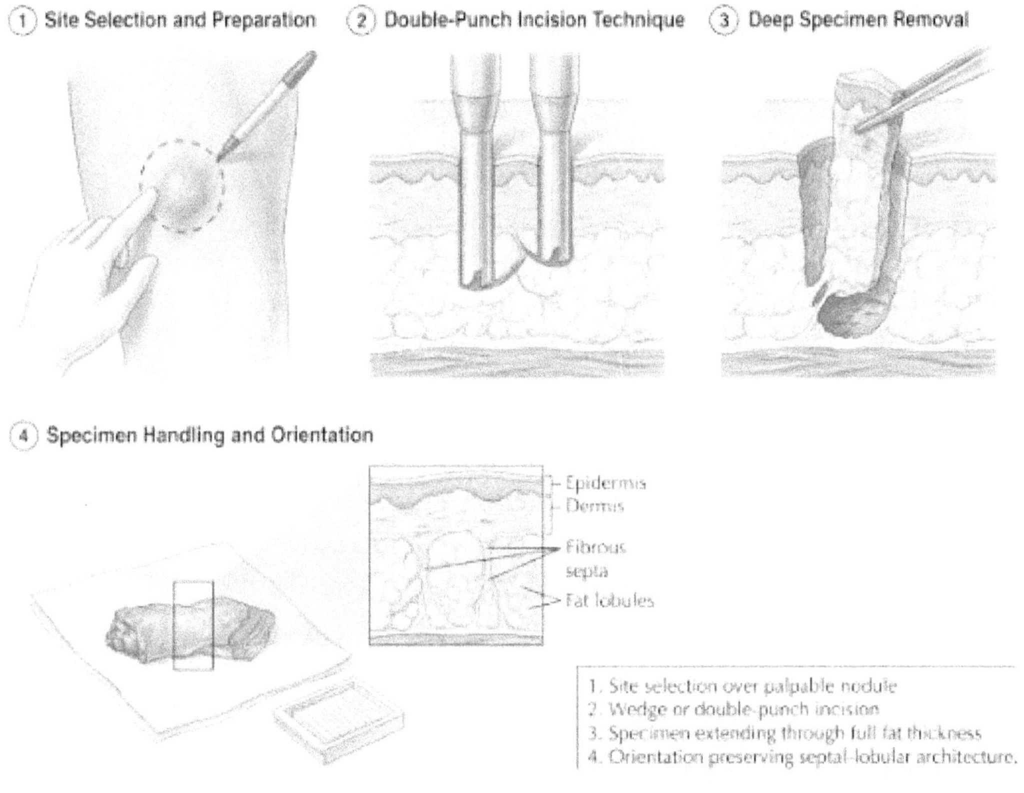

Clinical Morphology of Lipodermatosclerosis and Infectious Panniculitis

The clinicopathologic correlation this book has emphasized since Chapter 1 applies with particular force throughout this chapter, since panniculitis as a category is more heavily dependent on this correlation than perhaps any other reaction pattern discussed in this book, given the subcutaneous fat's comparatively limited independent histologic vocabulary; a pathology report that omits clinical distribution, lesion duration, and relevant systemic history when signing out a panniculitis specimen forfeits diagnostic precision that is readily available and specifically important for this pattern.

Acute lipodermatosclerosis presents with a tender, erythematous, indurated plaque over the medial lower leg or ankle in a patient with underlying chronic venous insufficiency, frequently misdiagnosed clinically as cellulitis given the overlapping erythema and tenderness, a misdiagnosis that biopsy, together with careful attention to the chronic venous stasis background, can help avoid, sparing the patient an unnecessary course of antibiotics for a condition that will not respond to antimicrobial therapy. Infectious panniculitis presents with rapidly progressive erythema, warmth, and tenderness, frequently with systemic signs of infection, fever, and, in the specific and urgent case of a necrotizing soft tissue infection, pain disproportionate to the visible clinical findings, a red flag finding that should prompt emergent surgical evaluation independent of and in parallel with any pathology workup rather than awaiting biopsy results before escalating care.

Special Populations and Systemic Correlation

Erythema nodosum in children most commonly follows streptococcal pharyngitis and carries an excellent prognosis with spontaneous resolution, while erythema nodosum arising during pregnancy is a recognized, generally benign association not requiring treatment beyond symptomatic management, illustrating that the same histologic pattern carries a substantially different clinical significance and required workup depending on the specific patient population and clinical context. Subcutaneous panniculitis-like T-cell lymphoma, introduced in the classification table above and discussed further in the differential diagnosis section, is a rare but clinically important consideration in any patient presenting with persistent, non-resolving lobular panniculitis-like lesions, particularly when accompanied by systemic symptoms such as fever, weight loss, or cytopenias suggestive of an associated hemophagocytic syndrome, a recognized and potentially life-threatening complication of this specific lymphoma.

Obesity itself is increasingly recognized as a contributing factor across several entities discussed in this chapter beyond lipodermatosclerosis specifically, both through its direct association with chronic venous insufficiency and through a distinct, poorly understood association with a more generalized, sometimes termed "lipedema-associated," subcutaneous inflammatory process in some patients, an evolving area of clinical and histologic characterization that underscores this chapter's broader theme of the subcutaneous fat functioning as a metabolically and immunologically active organ rather than an inert structural layer.

Lipodermatosclerosis occurs disproportionately in patients with obesity and long-standing venous insufficiency, populations in whom compression therapy adherence can be practically challenging, making patient-specific counseling regarding compression device selection and realistic adherence expectations an important, often underemphasized component of effective long-term management beyond the histologic diagnosis itself. Infectious panniculitis in immunocompromised patients, paralleling the discussion of immunocompromised hosts in Chapter 8, can present with a comparatively subtle or atypical inflammatory response despite significant underlying organism burden, reinforcing why tissue culture should be pursued liberally in this population even when the neutrophilic infiltrate expected in classic infectious panniculitis is not prominently displayed.

CLINICAL PEARL: Tender nodules on the anterior shins with a bruise-like color evolution and spontaneous resolution over several weeks is erythema nodosum until proven otherwise; nodules that ulcerate, persist beyond several weeks, or favor the posterior calves warrant biopsy rather than presumptive erythema nodosum management.

Differential Diagnosis and Histologic Mimickers

Erythema Nodosum Versus Erythema Induratum/Nodular Vasculitis

As developed above, the presence of a predominantly lobular, granulomatous infiltrate with vasculitis distinguishes erythema induratum/nodular vasculitis from the septal, non-vasculitic pattern of erythema nodosum, though an inadequately deep biopsy that fails to capture the full extent of subcutaneous involvement can obscure this distinction, underscoring once again the critical importance of adequate biopsy depth for any panniculitis specimen, a point this chapter shares directly with the medium vessel vasculitis discussion in the preceding chapter. When the histologic distinction remains ambiguous on available tissue, correlating with the clinical distribution, anterior shin favoring erythema nodosum and posterior calf favoring erythema induratum/nodular vasculitis, provides additional supportive information pending, where clinically warranted, repeat deeper biopsy.

Lupus Panniculitis Versus Subcutaneous Panniculitis-Like T-Cell Lymphoma

Distinguishing lupus panniculitis from subcutaneous panniculitis-like T-cell lymphoma represents one of the most clinically consequential differential diagnoses in this chapter, since both present with a lymphocytic lobular panniculitis, but subcutaneous panniculitis-like T-cell lymphoma shows atypical lymphocytes rimming individual adipocytes in a distinctive pattern sometimes described as "beads on a string," karyorrhectic debris, and cytologic atypia not present in the reactive lymphocytic infiltrate of lupus panniculitis, features that, together with immunohistochemical and molecular studies discussed in the ancillary studies section, are essential for confident distinction given the substantially different management and prognosis these two entities carry. Overlap and diagnostic difficulty between these entities is well recognized in the literature, and a subset of cases require immunohistochemistry, T-cell receptor gene rearrangement studies, and close clinical correlation, including evaluation for an associated or evolving connective tissue disease, before a confident final diagnosis can be rendered.

A 34-year-old patient with a history of discoid lupus erythematosus presents with a firm, mildly tender subcutaneous nodule on the proximal thigh that has persisted for several months, and deep biopsy is obtained given a differential of lupus panniculitis versus subcutaneous panniculitis-like T-cell lymphoma. Pattern assignment identifies a lymphocytic lobular panniculitis with hyaline fat necrosis and scattered lymphoid follicles, without adipocyte rimming by atypical lymphocytes and without significant cytologic atypia on careful high-power examination. Differential narrowing supports lupus panniculitis over lymphoma based on the absence of adipocyte rimming and atypia, further supported by immunohistochemistry showing a mixed, predominantly reactive-appearing T-cell and B-cell population without the CD8-predominant, cytotoxic T-cell phenotype characteristic of subcutaneous panniculitis-like T-cell lymphoma. Diagnosis of lupus panniculitis is rendered, correlating with the patient's known discoid lupus erythematosus, and the report recommends clinical follow-up to monitor for the characteristic lipoatrophic scarring this entity produces, together with continued dermatologic surveillance given this patient's underlying connective tissue disease.

Lipodermatosclerosis Versus Infectious Panniculitis and Erythema Nodosum

Distinguishing acute lipodermatosclerosis from infectious panniculitis or cellulitis relies substantially on the absence of organisms on special stains and culture, together with the identification of the lipomembranous fat necrosis and background chronic venous stasis changes discussed above, a distinction that carries direct and immediate treatment consequence, since lipodermatosclerosis does not respond to antimicrobial therapy and instead requires compression therapy and management of the underlying venous insufficiency. Lipodermatosclerosis can additionally be distinguished from erythema nodosum, with which it may share a lower leg location and tender, erythematous clinical appearance, by its combined septal and lobular involvement, in contrast to erythema nodosum's predominantly septal, lobule-sparing pattern, and by the lipomembranous fat necrosis specific to lipodermatosclerosis, features that together resolve this distinction in the substantial majority of cases.

A 61-year-old patient with a long history of chronic venous insufficiency and bilateral lower extremity edema presents with a new, tender, erythematous, indurated plaque over the medial right ankle, and has been treated with two courses of oral antibiotics for presumed cellulitis without improvement. Biopsy is obtained given a differential of infectious panniculitis versus lipodermatosclerosis versus erythema nodosum. Pattern assignment identifies combined septal and lobular fibrosis with lipomembranous fat necrosis and background dermal hemosiderin deposition and stasis-associated changes, without a significant neutrophilic infiltrate and without organisms identified on Grocott methenamine silver and Fite staining. Differential narrowing excludes infectious panniculitis based on the absence of organisms and the non-neutrophilic infiltrate composition, and excludes erythema nodosum based on the combined septal-lobular involvement and lipomembranous necrosis pattern, favoring lipodermatosclerosis given these findings together with the background venous stasis changes and the clinical history of chronic venous insufficiency. Diagnosis of lipodermatosclerosis is rendered, sparing the patient a third unnecessary antibiotic course, and the report recommends compression therapy and vascular surgery or phlebology referral for management of the underlying venous insufficiency driving this process.

Traumatic and Factitial Panniculitis

Cold panniculitis, introduced in the etiology section above, is distinguished from other lobular panniculitis entities primarily by the clinical history of preceding cold exposure and the affected patient's typically young age, since the histologic findings, crystallization-associated adipocyte necrosis with a mixed lymphohistiocytic infiltrate and, in some cases, needle-shaped cleft formation reflecting the crystallized lipid, are less specific in isolation than the other diagnostic clues emphasized throughout this chapter, making clinical correlation particularly important for this specific entity relative to most others discussed here.

The differential diagnosis approach developed throughout this chapter, compartment assessment first using adequately deep tissue, vasculitis assessment second, and specific histologic clue identification third, applies with equal rigor to traumatic and factitial panniculitis, since both can, in principle, produce findings overlapping with several of the more specific entities discussed above, making the correlating clinical history, preceding trauma, a procedure, or a suspected self-inflicted process, an essential component of confident diagnosis in this specific context rather than a mere supplementary detail.

Traumatic fat necrosis, resulting from blunt trauma, surgery, or injection, shows lobular fat necrosis with hemorrhage, foamy macrophages, and, in resolving lesions, cystic change and fibrosis, generally without the specific diagnostic clues, ghost cells, adipocyte rimming, dermal collagen splaying, characteristic of the more specific entities discussed above, making a clinical history of preceding trauma or a procedure at the biopsy site essential correlating information whenever this diagnosis is being considered. Factitial panniculitis, resulting from self-injected substances, ranges in histologic appearance depending on the specific material injected, occasionally showing foreign material identifiable directly or through polarization as discussed in Chapter 8, and should be considered, with appropriate clinical sensitivity, when the clinical distribution and history suggest a self-inflicted rather than spontaneous process.

A 29-year-old patient with recurrent, painful, ulcerating nodules on the bilateral posterior calves over the past several months, previously treated presumptively as erythema nodosum without improvement, undergoes deep incisional biopsy given persistent symptoms. Pattern assignment identifies a lobular, granulomatous panniculitis with admixed lymphocytes, scattered caseous necrosis, and vasculitis affecting small vessels within the fat lobules, a pattern inconsistent with the septal, non-vasculitic pattern expected in erythema nodosum. Differential narrowing favors erythema induratum over erythema nodosum given the lobular, granulomatous, vasculitic pattern and posterior calf distribution, and an interferon-gamma release assay sent following this histologic finding returns positive, supporting a mycobacterial antigen-driven mechanism even though Fite and Grocott methenamine silver stains performed on the specimen do not directly demonstrate organisms. Diagnosis of erythema induratum is rendered, correcting the prior erythema nodosum working diagnosis, and antituberculous therapy is initiated in coordination with infectious disease, illustrating directly why compartment and vasculitis assessment, rather than clinical impression alone, is essential for accurate diagnosis and appropriate treatment selection in this specific differential.

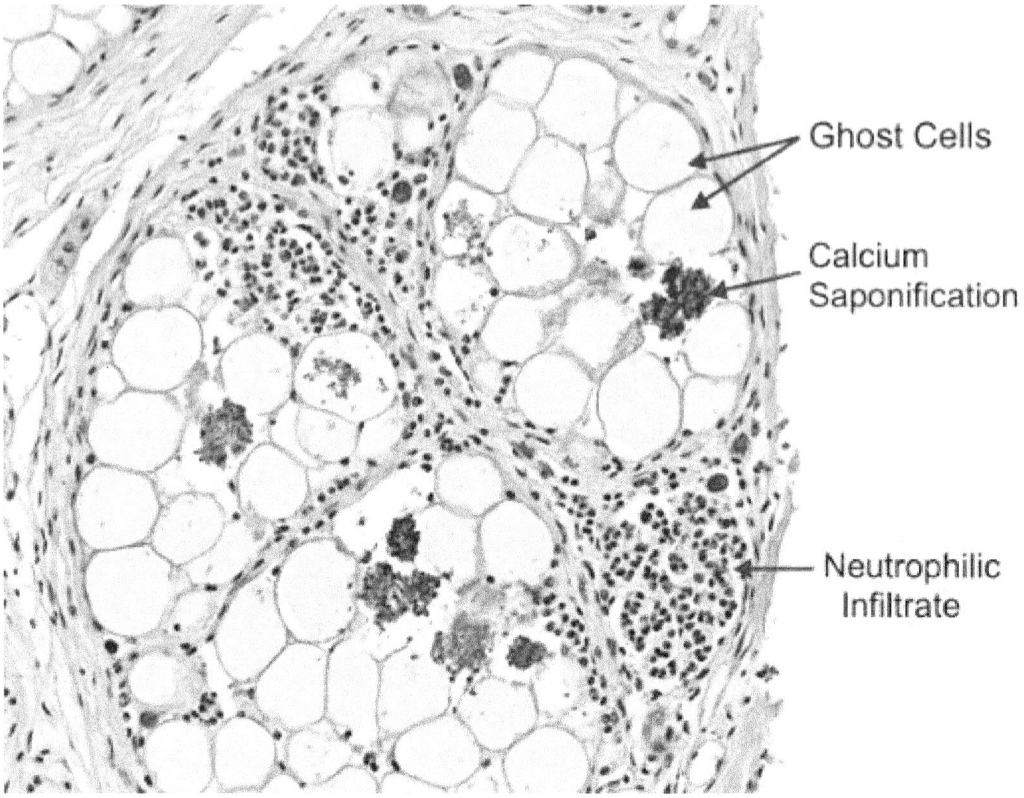

Ancillary Studies

Immunohistochemistry for Lymphoma Evaluation

When subcutaneous panniculitis-like T-cell lymphoma is a genuine consideration, an immunohistochemical panel including CD3, CD4, CD8, CD56, and cytotoxic markers such as TIA-1 and granzyme B is essential, with the characteristic phenotype showing a CD8-predominant, cytotoxic T-cell population, and CD56 positivity, when present, raising consideration of the more aggressive natural killer/T-cell lymphoma variant that requires distinction from the more indolent alpha-beta T-cell subtype of subcutaneous panniculitis-like T-cell lymphoma given the substantially different prognosis and treatment approach between these two related entities.

Molecular Studies and Special Stains

T-cell receptor gene rearrangement studies can support a diagnosis of subcutaneous panniculitis-like T-cell lymphoma by demonstrating a clonal T-cell population, though a polyclonal result does not entirely exclude the diagnosis and must be interpreted alongside the morphologic and immunohistochemical findings, given the known limitations of clonality testing sensitivity in this and other cutaneous lymphoma contexts discussed further in later chapters of this book. Fite and Grocott methenamine silver staining, discussed in Chapter 8, should be performed on any lobular granulomatous panniculitis with vasculitis to evaluate for erythema induratum/nodular vasculitis's mycobacterial association, though organisms are frequently not directly demonstrable even when the clinical and histologic picture strongly supports this diagnosis, reflecting the delayed hypersensitivity, rather than direct organism burden-driven, mechanism discussed in the etiology section above.

Laboratory Correlation

Complete blood count with differential and inflammatory markers, erythrocyte sedimentation rate and C-reactive protein, provide useful general supporting information across most entities in this chapter, elevated inflammatory markers supporting an active inflammatory or infectious process and cytopenias raising concern for the hemophagocytic syndrome discussed above in the context of subcutaneous panniculitis-like T-cell lymphoma, though none of these tests carry the specific diagnostic weight of the targeted studies discussed throughout this section.

Antinuclear antibody and extractable nuclear antigen serologic testing should accompany any diagnosis of lupus panniculitis without an already-established systemic or discoid lupus erythematosus diagnosis, given the recognized possibility that lupus panniculitis represents the initial presenting manifestation of previously undiagnosed disease, extending the biopsy's diagnostic value beyond the cutaneous finding into the broader systemic evaluation this diagnosis warrants.

This chapter closes this book's core seven-pattern framework begun in Chapter 3, and the diagnostic discipline it has reinforced, compartment or architecture first, a secondary structural axis (vasculitis status, wall inflammation, etiology) second, specific histologic clues third, and clinical and laboratory correlation throughout, is the same discipline applied across every reaction pattern this book has covered, a unifying approach the Reaction Pattern Master Atlas at the end of this book consolidates across all chapters for rapid clinical reference.

Serum lipase and amylase testing, together with pancreatic imaging when clinically indicated, should be pursued whenever ghost cells and saponification suggest pancreatic panniculitis, while alpha-1 antitrypsin level testing should be pursued whenever the distinctive collagen-splaying neutrophilic pattern of alpha-1 antitrypsin deficiency panniculitis is identified, in each case extending the biopsy's diagnostic value directly into a specific, actionable systemic evaluation. Interferon-gamma release assay or tuberculin skin testing, together with chest imaging, should accompany any diagnosis of erythema induratum/nodular vasculitis given its mycobacterial antigen association, paralleling the same latent tuberculosis evaluation logic already established for the granulomatous pattern in Chapter 8.

Frozen Section and Rapid Communication in Suspected Infectious Panniculitis

When a necrotizing soft tissue infection is a clinical consideration, intraoperative frozen section evaluation for the extent of fat and fascial necrosis, thrombosed vessels, and organisms can provide rapid information supporting the surgical team's debridement decisions, and same-day verbal communication of these preliminary findings, followed by a complete written report once permanent sections and special stains are available, represents an appropriate and clinically important deviation from routine reporting turnaround given the time-sensitive nature of this specific diagnosis. Gram stain performed on frozen or fresh tissue can provide additional rapid information regarding organism morphology, gram-positive versus gram-negative and cocci versus rods, that can meaningfully guide empiric antimicrobial selection before culture results, typically requiring one to several days, become available.

Vascular Studies and Correlation for Lipodermatosclerosis

Venous duplex ultrasonography, evaluating for venous reflux and confirming the underlying chronic venous insufficiency, provides valuable correlating information for a lipodermatosclerosis diagnosis and additionally identifies candidates for definitive venous intervention, such as endovenous ablation, that can address the underlying cause rather than only the downstream cutaneous manifestation, extending the biopsy's clinical value into the vascular treatment pathway beyond dermatologic management alone. Ankle-brachial index testing, distinguishing coexisting arterial insufficiency from purely venous disease, is a useful adjunct in patients being considered for compression therapy, since compression is relatively contraindicated in the setting of significant arterial insufficiency, making this a practically important test to obtain before initiating treatment rather than an optional addition to the workup.

CAUTION: A lymphocytic lobular panniculitis diagnosed as "lupus panniculitis" without careful high-power assessment for adipocyte rimming and cytologic atypia, and without immunohistochemistry when any uncertainty exists, risks missing subcutaneous panniculitis-like T-cell lymphoma, an error with substantially different prognostic and treatment consequences than a missed diagnosis elsewhere in this chapter.

Management Implications

Connecting Diagnosis to Treatment Pathway

Erythema nodosum is managed symptomatically, with nonsteroidal anti-inflammatory agents, rest, and leg elevation, together with identification and treatment of any underlying trigger, given this entity's generally self-limited course; erythema induratum/nodular vasculitis is managed with antituberculous therapy when an active or latent tuberculous trigger is identified, or with other anti-inflammatory or immunosuppressive approaches for idiopathic nodular vasculitis; lupus panniculitis is managed with antimalarial agents, most often hydroxychloroquine, and other systemic lupus-directed therapy; pancreatic and alpha-1 antitrypsin deficiency panniculitis are managed by treating the underlying systemic disease, pancreatic disease or enzyme replacement therapy respectively, rather than by direct treatment of the cutaneous findings; and subcutaneous panniculitis-like T-cell lymphoma is managed with immunosuppressive therapy or, for more aggressive or refractory disease, systemic chemotherapy, underscoring yet again the wide management divergence this book has repeatedly emphasized across its later chapters. Lipodermatosclerosis is managed with compression therapy, treatment of the underlying venous insufficiency, and, in select candidates, definitive venous intervention, while infectious panniculitis is managed with organism-directed antimicrobial therapy and, when a necrotizing soft tissue infection is confirmed or strongly suspected, emergent surgical debridement, a time-sensitive intervention in which delay measured in hours, rather than days, can meaningfully affect outcome.

Complications and Prognosis

Erythema nodosum carries an excellent prognosis with resolution over several weeks in the great majority of cases, though recurrence is possible if the underlying trigger persists or recurs, while erythema induratum/nodular vasculitis follows a more chronic, relapsing course with a tendency toward ulceration and scarring that can cause meaningful long-term morbidity in affected patients. Lupus panniculitis, while not immediately life-threatening, produces disfiguring lipoatrophic scarring that can be cosmetically significant, particularly on the face, making early diagnosis and treatment initiation valuable for limiting the extent of eventual fat loss, while subcutaneous panniculitis-like T-cell lymphoma carries a generally favorable prognosis for the alpha-beta phenotype but a substantially more guarded prognosis when hemophagocytic syndrome develops, a complication requiring urgent recognition and treatment given its associated mortality risk. Lipodermatosclerosis follows a chronic course punctuated by acute flares, with progressive circumferential lower leg fibrosis and fat loss occurring over years if the underlying venous insufficiency remains inadequately treated, while infectious panniculitis carries a prognosis ranging from excellent, for a localized process treated promptly, to guarded and occasionally life-threatening, for a confirmed necrotizing soft tissue infection, making the speed of diagnosis and treatment initiation the single most important determinant of outcome across this specific entity's clinical spectrum.

Pancreatic and alpha-1 antitrypsin deficiency panniculitis each carry a prognosis tied directly to the underlying systemic disease rather than to the cutaneous findings themselves, reinforcing the recurring principle developed throughout this chapter that a panniculitis biopsy functions as a window into systemic disease at least as often as it represents a primary, self-contained dermatologic diagnosis, and that the dermatopathologist's role extends meaningfully beyond the skin specimen itself whenever one of this chapter's specific diagnostic clues is identified.

Prevention and Screening

Patients with an identified predisposing factor for lipodermatosclerosis, established chronic venous insufficiency in particular, benefit from proactive compression therapy and venous insufficiency management before lipodermatosclerosis develops, an opportunity for genuine primary prevention that distinguishes this entity from most others in this chapter, where the panniculitis itself is typically the first clinical sign prompting evaluation rather than a preventable downstream complication of an already-recognized condition. Patients with recurrent erythema nodosum should undergo a systematic re-evaluation for a persistent or previously unidentified trigger, particularly inflammatory bowel disease and sarcoidosis, given that recurrent disease more strongly suggests an ongoing underlying process than the single-episode presentation typical of infection-triggered erythema nodosum.

Patient Education and Counseling

Patients with erythema nodosum benefit from reassurance regarding the condition's self-limited course and from counseling that the bruise-like color evolution they observe over several weeks is an expected part of the healing process rather than a sign of worsening disease. Patients with lupus panniculitis benefit from counseling regarding the risk of permanent lipoatrophic scarring and the value of early treatment in limiting this outcome, while patients diagnosed with subcutaneous panniculitis-like T-cell lymphoma benefit from clear communication distinguishing this entity's generally favorable prognosis from the more aggressive connotation the word "lymphoma" often carries in a patient's mind, alongside specific counseling regarding the systemic symptoms that should prompt urgent evaluation for hemophagocytic syndrome.

Patients with lipodermatosclerosis benefit from clear explanation that this condition, despite its erythematous, indurated, sometimes cellulitis-mimicking appearance, does not represent an infection and will not respond to antibiotics, information that can help patients understand why treatment focuses on compression and venous management rather than antimicrobial therapy, together with realistic counseling regarding the chronic, fluctuating course this condition typically follows even with appropriate treatment. Families of infants diagnosed with cold panniculitis benefit from simple, practical counseling regarding avoidance of prolonged direct cold contact against a child's skin, together with reassurance regarding this condition's benign, self-limited course once the causative exposure has been identified and avoided.

THE REACTION PATTERN RECOGNITION SYSTEM — The Panniculitis Pattern Family

The Pattern: The panniculitis pattern organized by compartment (septal versus lobular) and vasculitis status: erythema nodosum, erythema induratum/nodular vasculitis, lupus panniculitis, pancreatic and alpha-1 antitrypsin deficiency panniculitis, and subcutaneous panniculitis-like T-cell lymphoma.

Histologic Signature: Widened septa with sparing of lobules defines erythema nodosum; lobular granulomatous infiltrate with vasculitis defines erythema induratum/nodular vasculitis; lymphocytic lobular infiltrate with hyaline necrosis and follicles defines lupus panniculitis; ghost cells define pancreatic panniculitis; adipocyte rimming by atypical lymphocytes defines subcutaneous panniculitis-like T-cell lymphoma.

The Decision: Assess compartment first (septal versus lobular) using adequately deep tissue, then assess vasculitis status, then apply the specific histologic clues (ghost cells, collagen splaying, adipocyte rimming, lymphoid follicles) that distinguish the lobular panniculitis entities from one another.

Trap Logic: Inadequately deep biopsies obscure compartment assessment; advanced septal panniculitis can show secondary lobular extension; lupus panniculitis and subcutaneous panniculitis-like T-cell lymphoma share a lymphocytic lobular pattern and require careful assessment for adipocyte rimming and cytologic atypia, supported by immunohistochemistry, to distinguish confidently; and acute lipodermatosclerosis can mimic infectious cellulitis both clinically and, to a lesser degree, histologically.

Pattern Anchor: Deep tissue first, compartment second, vasculitis status third, specific histologic clue last. Never diagnose lupus panniculitis without explicitly excluding adipocyte rimming by atypical lymphocytes at high power, and never diagnose infectious panniculitis or lipodermatosclerosis without correlating necrosis pattern against organism stains, culture, and the venous stasis background respectively.

Summary and Key Concepts

Panniculitis is organized first by compartment, septal versus lobular, and second by the presence or absence of vasculitis, a two-axis framework that requires adequately deep tissue, incisional or wedge biopsy rather than standard punch biopsy, for reliable assessment.

Erythema nodosum, the most common panniculitis in practice, shows a septal, non-vasculitic pattern with Miescher radial granulomas and follows a self-limited course reflecting its delayed-type hypersensitivity mechanism to a broad range of triggers.

Erythema induratum/nodular vasculitis shows a lobular, granulomatous panniculitis with vasculitis and an association with mycobacterial antigen exposure, distinguishing it from the non-vasculitic lobular panniculitis entities.

Ghost cells and saponification identify pancreatic panniculitis, dermal collagen splaying identifies alpha-1 antitrypsin deficiency panniculitis, and hyaline fat necrosis with lymphoid follicles identifies lupus panniculitis, each prompting a specific, targeted systemic evaluation.

Subcutaneous panniculitis-like T-cell lymphoma must be actively excluded whenever a lymphocytic lobular panniculitis is encountered, given its histologic overlap with lupus panniculitis and its distinct management, prognosis, and hemophagocytic syndrome risk.

CHAPTER 11: CONNECTIVE TISSUE DISEASES OF THE SKIN

Learning Objectives

1. Classify the cutaneous connective tissue diseases by predominant histologic pattern: interface, sclerosing, and mucin-predominant, and by overlap syndrome presentation.
2. Distinguish the histologic subtypes of cutaneous lupus erythematosus, including neonatal and tumid variants, and correlate them closely with clinical presentation and systemic risk.
3. Identify the histopathologic features and diagnostic criteria of morphea/scleroderma, systemic sclerosis, and dermatomyositis.
4. Correlate histologic findings across the connective tissue diseases with clinical presentation, systemic organ risk, and relevant serologic and antibody associations.
5. Construct a full differential diagnosis distinguishing the connective tissue diseases from one another and from their histologic mimickers.
6. Select appropriate ancillary studies, including direct immunofluorescence, nailfold capillaroscopy, and serologic correlation, for the connective tissue disease biopsy.

Definition and Classification

The Autoimmune Connective Tissue Disease Spectrum

As this book's final individual reaction pattern chapter, this chapter also stands somewhat apart from the six pattern chapters preceding it, since the connective tissue diseases are less a single unified reaction pattern than a disease category that draws on two of this book's previously established patterns, the interface pattern from Chapter 6 and, newly introduced here, the sclerosing pattern, applying the same architecture-first, mechanism-second, clinical-correlation-third diagnostic discipline this book has used throughout to a disease group defined more by shared autoimmune etiology than by a single shared histologic starting point.

The connective tissue diseases of the skin comprise a group of autoimmune disorders, lupus erythematosus, dermatomyositis, morphea and systemic sclerosis, and the overlap syndromes among them, that share a common underlying autoimmune mechanism directed against components of the skin and, in the systemic forms, other organs, while producing histologically and clinically distinguishable patterns that this chapter organizes around three dominant histologic themes: interface dermatitis, dermal sclerosis, and, cutting across both, increased dermal mucin deposition. This chapter extends the interface dermatitis discussion introduced in Chapter 6 into its full connective tissue disease context and introduces the sclerosing pattern as a distinct entity, together completing this book's coverage of the major immune-mediated dermal reaction patterns.

Lupus erythematosus and dermatomyositis are both fundamentally interface-pattern diseases, sharing significant histologic overlap that can make their distinction challenging on histology alone, while morphea and systemic sclerosis are fundamentally sclerosing diseases, and increased dermal mucin, while not unique to this disease group, appears with sufficient frequency and diagnostic usefulness across several of these entities that its assessment forms a recurring diagnostic thread throughout this chapter, much as it did for granuloma annulare in Chapter 8.

Classification of Cutaneous Lupus Erythematosus

Cutaneous lupus erythematosus is subclassified into acute cutaneous lupus erythematosus, subacute cutaneous lupus erythematosus, and chronic cutaneous lupus erythematosus (discoid lupus erythematosus being the most common chronic subtype), a classification that correlates meaningfully with systemic disease risk, acute cutaneous lupus erythematosus carrying the highest association with systemic lupus erythematosus, and discoid lupus erythematosus, particularly when localized rather than generalized, carrying a comparatively lower though still clinically relevant systemic association. Each subtype shares the fundamental interface dermatitis pattern discussed in Chapter 6 but differs in the intensity and specific distribution of histologic findings, developed further in the histopathologic features section below.

Classification of Sclerosing Connective Tissue Disease

The term "scleroderma" is frequently used loosely in clinical practice to refer to either morphea or systemic sclerosis, and this imprecision can create genuine confusion between patients and clinicians, or even among clinicians themselves, regarding whether a given "scleroderma" diagnosis carries the systemic implications of systemic sclerosis or the more limited, skin-confined implications of morphea, making precise terminology in both clinical documentation and patient communication a small but meaningful point of practice this chapter's classification framework is intended to support.

Morphea (localized scleroderma) and systemic sclerosis share the fundamental histologic finding of progressive dermal collagen sclerosis but differ substantially in clinical distribution and systemic involvement, morphea remaining confined to the skin and subcutaneous tissue in defined plaques or bands, and systemic sclerosis involving the skin diffusely or in an acral-predominant pattern alongside internal organ fibrosis, most critically pulmonary, renal, and gastrointestinal, that determines this disease's substantially more guarded overall prognosis relative to morphea. This clinical distinction, rather than the histology itself, which is often similar or indistinguishable between the two entities on a single biopsy, is the primary basis for their diagnostic separation, underscoring the centrality of clinicopathologic correlation throughout this chapter.

Mucin as a Cross-Cutting Diagnostic Clue

Increased dermal mucin, identifiable on routine hematoxylin and eosin staining as pale, faintly basophilic, stringy interstitial material separating collagen bundles, and more confidently confirmed with Alcian blue or colloidal iron staining as discussed in Chapter 2, appears across this chapter's disease spectrum with varying intensity and diagnostic significance: prominent and diagnostically useful in dermatomyositis and tumid lupus erythematosus, present but comparatively less prominent in the other lupus erythematosus subtypes, and notably increased in the mucin-rich sclerosing mimickers, scleredema and scleromyxedema, discussed in the differential diagnosis section below. This cross-cutting relevance means that mucin assessment functions as a secondary diagnostic axis throughout this chapter, complementing but never substituting for the primary interface-versus-sclerosing distinction that organizes the chapter's overall diagnostic approach.

The specific pattern of mucin deposition, diffusely interstitial versus more focally accentuated around vessels and adnexal structures, together with its intensity relative to the degree of accompanying interface change or collagen sclerosis, provides additional discriminating information in ambiguous cases, though this chapter emphasizes, consistent with the diagnostic honesty principle established in Chapter 1, that mucin quantity alone is rarely sufficient for a specific diagnosis without integration with the other histologic, clinical, and serologic findings this chapter has developed.

Entity	Dominant Pattern	Key Histologic Feature	Systemic Association
Acute cutaneous lupus erythematosus	Interface	Subtle vacuolar change, minimal scarring	Strong (SLE)
Subacute cutaneous lupus erythematosus	Interface	Prominent vacuolar change, superficial infiltrate	Moderate; strong Ro/SSA association
Discoid lupus erythematosus	Interface	Follicular plugging, basement membrane thickening, deep perivascular/periadnexal infiltrate	Lower (localized); higher (generalized)
Dermatomyositis	Interface	Similar to lupus; increased dermal mucin, less follicular plugging	Myositis; malignancy (adult-onset)
Morphea	Sclerosing	Thickened, homogenized collagen with loss of periadnexal fat	Absent (localized to skin)

Systemic sclerosis	Sclerosing	Similar to morphea; acral distribution, nailfold capillary changes	Strong (pulmonary, renal, GI)

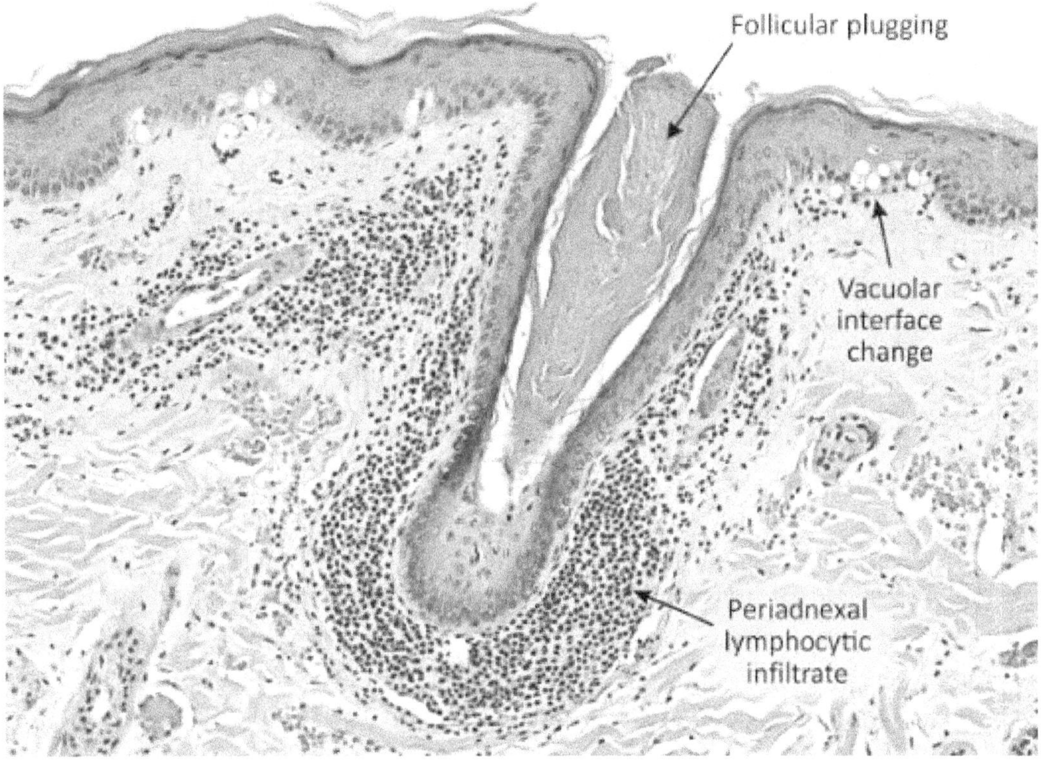

Etiology and Pathogenesis

Mechanisms of Cutaneous Lupus Erythematosus

The etiologic mechanisms across this chapter's disease spectrum, while individually distinct, together illustrate a recurring theme in autoimmune skin disease first introduced with the interface pattern in Chapter 6: an initiating injury, whether ultraviolet-induced keratinocyte apoptosis, complement-mediated microangiopathy, or microvascular endothelial injury, triggers a cascade of immune activation that ultimately produces the tissue-level histologic changes this chapter catalogs, meaning that understanding the specific upstream mechanism for each entity directly informs both the expected histologic pattern and the rationale for the targeted therapies discussed in the management implications section.

Cutaneous lupus erythematosus results from a complex interplay of genetic susceptibility, ultraviolet light exposure, and dysregulated innate and adaptive immunity, with ultraviolet exposure inducing keratinocyte apoptosis and the release of nuclear autoantigens that, in a genetically susceptible individual, trigger autoantibody production and a type I interferon-driven inflammatory cascade culminating in the cytotoxic T-cell-mediated basal keratinocyte injury that defines the interface dermatitis pattern histologically. This ultraviolet-triggered mechanism explains the pronounced photodistribution of cutaneous lupus lesions and the well-established clinical practice of counseling affected patients regarding strict photoprotection as a component of disease management, discussed further in the management implications section below.

Mechanisms of Dermatomyositis

Dermatomyositis is understood as a complement-mediated microangiopathy targeting the capillaries of skin and skeletal muscle, with complement membrane attack complex deposition on endothelial cells triggering capillary damage, tissue ischemia, and a secondary interface dermatitis pattern that closely parallels, but is mechanistically distinct from, the more directly cytotoxic T-cell-mediated interface injury of lupus erythematosus, a mechanistic distinction that helps explain the shared histologic interface pattern despite the two diseases' otherwise different systemic manifestations. Adult-onset dermatomyositis carries a well-established and clinically important association with underlying malignancy, particularly ovarian, lung, gastrointestinal, and lymphoid malignancies, occurring in a substantial minority of adult patients and typically diagnosed within the first one to two years surrounding the dermatomyositis diagnosis, making age-appropriate malignancy screening a standard and important component of the evaluation for any newly diagnosed adult dermatomyositis patient.

Mechanisms of Morphea and Systemic Sclerosis

Morphea and systemic sclerosis share a pathogenesis believed to involve initial microvascular endothelial injury, triggering a cascade of immune activation and fibroblast stimulation, ultimately producing excessive collagen deposition through mechanisms involving transforming growth factor-beta and related profibrotic signaling pathways, a mechanism that helps explain why early, active lesions in both conditions can show an inflammatory infiltrate that diminishes as the lesion progresses to the densely sclerotic, relatively acellular late-stage histology more classically associated with these diseases. Systemic sclerosis additionally involves a well-characterized vasculopathic component, including the Raynaud phenomenon that frequently precedes cutaneous involvement by months to years and the nailfold capillary changes discussed in the clinical presentation section below, distinguishing its pathogenesis from morphea's more purely localized, skin-confined process.

Genetic and Environmental Risk Factors

Genetic susceptibility across this chapter's disease spectrum involves a complex polygenic architecture, with specific human leukocyte antigen associations, complement deficiency states (particularly early complement component deficiencies conferring elevated systemic lupus erythematosus risk), and a growing list of identified susceptibility loci contributing incremental risk rather than any single deterministic genetic cause, explaining why these diseases, while showing clear familial clustering in some cases, do not follow simple Mendelian inheritance patterns. Environmental factors beyond ultraviolet light exposure, including smoking (associated with more severe and treatment-resistant cutaneous lupus erythematosus), silica and organic solvent exposure (associated with systemic sclerosis), and certain viral infections proposed as potential triggering or modifying factors, together illustrate that these autoimmune connective tissue diseases, like several other reaction pattern categories discussed throughout this book, arise from a convergence of genetic predisposition and environmental triggering rather than from either factor operating in isolation.

Neonatal Lupus Erythematosus

Neonatal lupus erythematosus results from transplacental passage of maternal anti-Ro/SSA and, less commonly, anti-La/SSB antibodies into the fetal circulation, producing transient annular or targetoid cutaneous lesions, often periorbital in distribution, that typically resolve over the first several months of life as maternal antibody is cleared from the infant's circulation, together with the substantially more clinically significant, and typically permanent, complication of congenital heart block, resulting from antibody-mediated injury to the developing fetal cardiac conduction system. Given the risk of congenital heart block, any infant with suspected neonatal lupus erythematosus warrants cardiology evaluation, and any mother found to carry anti-Ro/SSA antibodies, whether or not she carries a clinical lupus erythematosus diagnosis herself, warrants fetal cardiac monitoring during subsequent pregnancies given the recognized recurrence risk this maternal antibody status carries.

Overlap Syndromes and Mixed Connective Tissue Disease

Antisynthetase syndrome, defined by anti-Jo-1 or another anti-aminoacyl-tRNA synthetase antibody together with a characteristic clinical constellation of myositis, interstitial lung disease, arthritis, Raynaud phenomenon, and "mechanic's hands" (fissured, hyperkeratotic skin along the radial fingers), represents another well-characterized overlap presentation most closely related to dermatomyositis, illustrating that the specific antibody identified in a given patient can itself define a recognizable overlap phenotype with its own characteristic pattern of organ involvement and, for antisynthetase syndrome specifically, a comparatively higher risk of interstitial lung disease than other dermatomyositis-spectrum presentations.

A meaningful subset of patients present with overlapping clinical, serologic, and histologic features spanning more than one of this chapter's connective tissue diseases, mixed connective tissue disease, characterized by high-titer anti-U1-ribonucleoprotein antibodies together with overlapping features of lupus erythematosus, systemic sclerosis, and myositis, representing the most well-characterized example of this overlap phenomenon. Skin biopsy in overlap syndrome patients frequently shows a combination of interface and sclerosing features that does not cleanly fit a single entity discussed in this chapter, reinforcing that the diagnostic framework this chapter presents, while organizing the great majority of cases into recognizable patterns, should be applied with the same descriptive flexibility and explicit acknowledgment of overlapping findings that this book has emphasized since Chapter 1 whenever a biopsy genuinely does not fit a single category.

THE REACTION PATTERN RECOGNITION SYSTEM — Interface Versus Sclerosing as the First Diagnostic Branch Point

The Pattern: Interface Dermatitis Versus Dermal Sclerosis, With Mucin as a Cross-Cutting Secondary Axis, as the First Diagnostic Branch Point in Connective Tissue Disease

Histologic Signature: Vacuolar or lichenoid injury to the basal keratinocyte layer with an associated lymphocytic infiltrate (interface: lupus, dermatomyositis) versus thickened, homogenized dermal collagen with loss of periadnexal fat and progressive adnexal entrapment (sclerosing: morphea, systemic sclerosis), with increased dermal mucin cutting across both categories.

The Decision: Assess the epidermal-dermal junction first for interface change, then assess the dermal collagen for sclerosis; interface findings direct the differential toward lupus and dermatomyositis, requiring further distinction by infiltrate depth, distribution, and mucin, while sclerosing findings direct the differential toward morphea and systemic sclerosis, requiring clinical distribution and nailfold capillary correlation for further distinction.

Trap Logic: Long-standing discoid lupus erythematosus can develop secondary dermal sclerosis that mimics a primary sclerosing process, and early, inflammatory-stage morphea can show a lymphocytic infiltrate that is occasionally mistaken for an interface process before the underlying collagen changes are appreciated. Careful assessment of the epidermal-dermal junction specifically, rather than the overall dermal cellularity, resolves most such ambiguous cases, aided by mucin assessment as a tie-breaking secondary clue when needed.

Pattern Anchor: Vacuolar basal layer injury means interface and directs toward lupus/dermatomyositis; thickened, homogenized collagen with adnexal entrapment means sclerosing and directs toward morphea/systemic sclerosis. Assess the junction first, the collagen second, mucin third.

Histopathologic Features and Diagnostic Criteria

Diagnostic Features Distinguishing the Lupus Erythematosus Subtypes

Acute cutaneous lupus erythematosus shows comparatively subtle vacuolar interface change with a sparse superficial perivascular lymphocytic infiltrate and minimal basement membrane thickening, reflecting this subtype's typically brief, self-limited individual lesion duration relative to the chronic discoid subtype, while subacute cutaneous lupus erythematosus shows more prominent vacuolar interface change with a band-like superficial infiltrate, occasionally with a psoriasiform epidermal component, and a strong association with anti-Ro/SSA antibodies discussed in the ancillary studies section below. Discoid lupus erythematosus shows the most florid histologic changes among the three subtypes: prominent vacuolar interface change, follicular plugging with keratotic material distending dilated follicular infundibula, thickened basement membrane readily demonstrated with periodic acid-Schiff staining, and, distinctively, a deep perivascular and periadnexal lymphocytic infiltrate extending around hair follicles and eccrine structures well into the deep dermis, a depth and distribution of infiltrate not typically seen in the other two subtypes.

Diagnostic Features of Dermatomyositis

Dermatomyositis shows an interface dermatitis pattern similar to lupus erythematosus but with several distinguishing features that, while individually not entirely specific, together support this diagnosis over lupus: comparatively less follicular plugging and less deep periadnexal infiltrate than discoid lupus erythematosus, more prominent increased dermal mucin than typically seen in lupus subtypes other than lupus panniculitis discussed in Chapter 10, and, in some cases, epidermal atrophy that can be more pronounced than the epidermal changes typical of lupus erythematosus. Given this substantial histologic overlap, the distinction between dermatomyositis and lupus erythematosus frequently relies as much or more on clinical correlation, proximal muscle weakness and the characteristic cutaneous findings discussed in the clinical presentation section, and serologic testing, as on histology in isolation.

Diagnostic Features of Morphea and Systemic Sclerosis

Early, inflammatory-stage morphea and systemic sclerosis show a superficial and deep perivascular and interstitial lymphoplasmacytic infiltrate with early collagen thickening, while established, later-stage lesions show the more classically recognized findings of thickened, homogenized, eosinophilic collagen bundles with loss of the normal clear separation between individual bundles, progressive entrapment and eventual loss of eccrine glands and periadnexal fat, and a relatively diminished or absent inflammatory infiltrate, together producing a distinctive low-power appearance of dense, homogeneous, hypocellular dermis extending into the subcutaneous fat in more advanced lesions. Distinguishing morphea from systemic sclerosis is generally not possible on histology alone, since both conditions produce essentially identical dermal sclerosis, making the biopsy's role in this specific distinction limited primarily to confirming the presence of a sclerosing process, after which clinical distribution, nailfold capillaroscopy, and serologic testing determine the specific diagnosis.

Lupus Erythematosus Panniculitis and Tumid Lupus Erythematosus

Lupus erythematosus panniculitis (lupus profundus), introduced in Chapter 10, and tumid lupus erythematosus, a distinct lupus subtype showing minimal to absent interface change but prominent dermal mucin and a dense superficial and deep perivascular and periadnexal lymphocytic infiltrate without significant epidermal involvement, together illustrate that the lupus erythematosus spectrum extends beyond the three classically taught interface subtypes discussed above, and that mucin assessment, rather than interface change alone, can be the more diagnostically salient finding in specific lupus subtypes. Tumid lupus erythematosus presents clinically as succulent, edematous, erythematous plaques without significant surface scale, a morphology that, combined with its comparatively subtle or absent interface change, can lead to initial confusion with other mucin-rich or edematous dermal infiltrates, including polymorphous light eruption and, occasionally, the early inflammatory-stage sclerosing dermatoses discussed later in this chapter, before the characteristic deep periadnexal lymphocytic pattern is specifically recognized.

Special Stains for Mucin and Collagen Assessment

Alcian blue or colloidal iron staining, discussed above and in Chapter 2, confirms and highlights increased dermal mucin when this finding is subtle or its presence is diagnostically important, particularly for distinguishing tumid lupus erythematosus and dermatomyositis from their respective histologic mimickers, while a Masson trichrome stain can help delineate the specific pattern and extent of dermal collagen sclerosis in morphea and systemic sclerosis, particularly useful for assessing the depth of sclerotic extension into the subcutaneous septa in deep morphea or for distinguishing early, subtle sclerosis from a normal dermis in an equivocal case. Periodic acid-Schiff staining, as introduced earlier in this chapter, remains valuable for confirming basement membrane thickening in discoid lupus erythematosus, a finding that can be difficult to appreciate confidently on routine hematoxylin and eosin staining alone, particularly in early or subtle lesions.

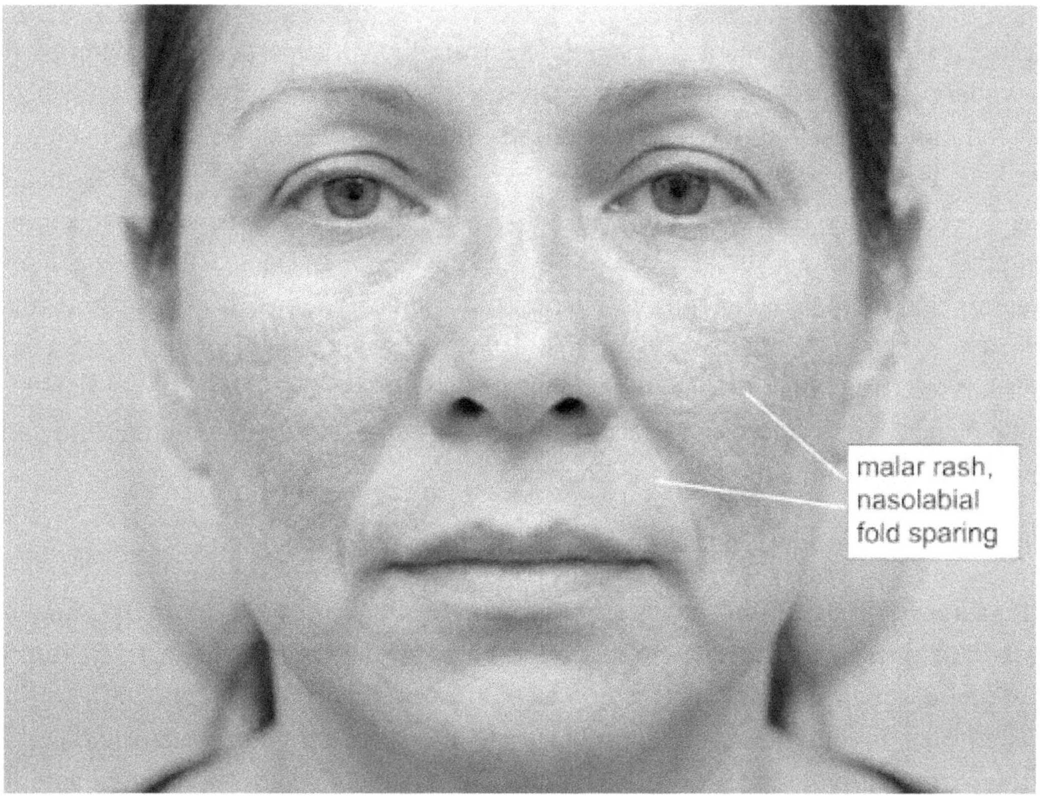

Clinical Presentation and Clinicopathologic Correlation

Clinical Morphology of the Lupus Erythematosus Subtypes

Acute cutaneous lupus erythematosus presents classically as the malar or "butterfly" rash, an erythematous, mildly edematous eruption across the malar eminences and nasal bridge with characteristic sparing of the nasolabial folds, typically occurring in the setting of active systemic disease and correlating with disease flares. Subacute cutaneous lupus erythematosus presents as annular or papulosquamous erythematous plaques favoring sun-exposed skin of the upper trunk and extensor arms, and discoid lupus erythematosus presents as well-demarcated, erythematous, scaly plaques with follicular plugging, favoring the face, scalp, and ears, that heal with scarring, dyspigmentation, and, on the scalp, permanent scarring alopecia, a healing pattern with meaningfully different cosmetic and functional implications than the other lupus subtypes and one that underscores the importance of early, effective treatment in this specific subtype.

Clinical Morphology of Dermatomyositis

Dermatomyositis presents with several distinctive cutaneous findings, Gottron papules (violaceous, flat-topped papules over the extensor finger joints), the heliotrope rash (violaceous discoloration of the upper eyelids, often with associated periorbital edema), and the shawl sign (erythema in a photodistributed pattern across the upper back and shoulders), each of which carries high diagnostic specificity when present, together with proximal muscle weakness reflecting the myositis component of this disease, though a subset of patients present with cutaneous findings alone, termed amyopathic or clinically amyopathic dermatomyositis, without clinically evident muscle involvement at the time of skin diagnosis. Given dermatomyositis's malignancy association discussed in the etiology section, newly diagnosed adult patients warrant age-appropriate cancer screening beyond routine health maintenance, with some authorities recommending more extensive screening, including pelvic and chest imaging, given the specific malignancy associations this disease carries.

Clinical Morphology and Systemic Evaluation for Morphea and Systemic Sclerosis

Morphea presents as one or more well-demarcated, initially erythematous to violaceous plaques that evolve to a central ivory-white, indurated, sclerotic center with a violaceous "lilac ring" border in active lesions, in a plaque, generalized, linear, or deep subtype distribution, the linear subtype carrying particular clinical significance when it crosses a joint or affects a growing child, given the risk of contracture and growth disturbance in these settings. Systemic sclerosis presents with diffuse or acral-predominant skin thickening, Raynaud phenomenon, and characteristic nailfold capillary changes, dilated and dropout capillary loops visible on capillaroscopy, together with a range of internal organ manifestations, pulmonary fibrosis, pulmonary arterial hypertension, renal crisis, and gastrointestinal dysmotility among the most clinically significant, that determine this disease's overall prognosis more than the cutaneous findings alone.

Nailfold Capillaroscopy Examination: Procedure and Findings

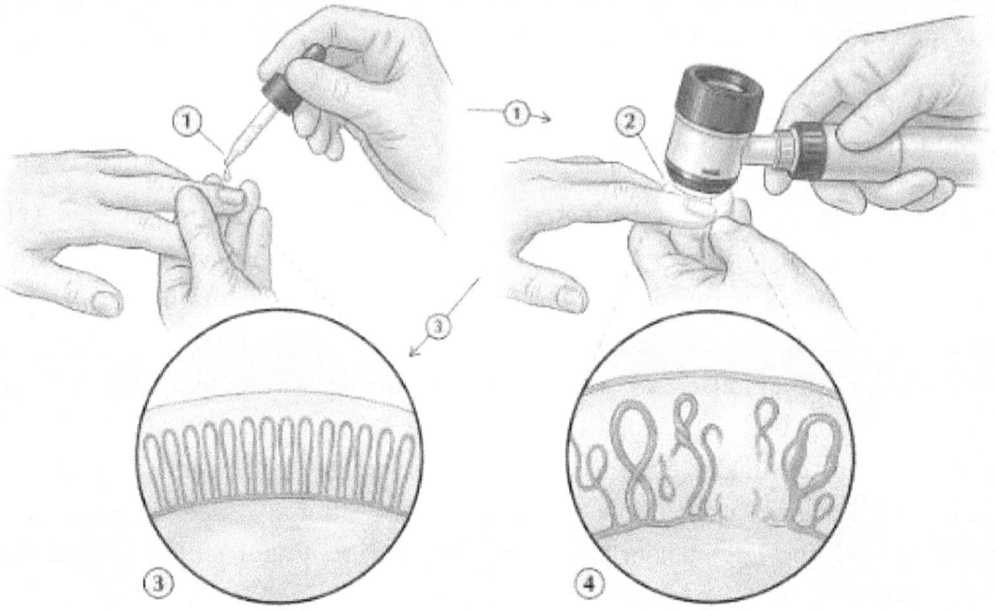

① Immersion oil application
② Dermoscope/capillaroscope positioning at proximal proximal nailfold
③ Normal capillary loop pattern
④ Dilated/dropout capillary pattern

Special Populations: Pediatric and Drug-Induced Disease

Juvenile dermatomyositis, distinct from its adult counterpart, carries a substantially lower malignancy association, closer to that of the general pediatric population, but a comparatively higher risk of calcinosis cutis and, in more severe cases, cutaneous ulceration and lipodystrophy, complications that shape long-term monitoring priorities differently than in adult-onset disease, where malignancy screening dominates the early evaluation period discussed in the prevention and screening section below.

Linear morphea in children carries particular clinical significance beyond its adult counterpart, since lesions crossing a growth plate or joint can produce limb length discrepancy, joint contracture, or, when affecting the face and scalp in the specific en coup de sabre distribution, underlying facial asymmetry and, rarely, central nervous system involvement, making early recognition and aggressive treatment, often with systemic immunosuppression rather than topical therapy alone, more strongly indicated in pediatric linear morphea than in adult-onset plaque morphea. Drug-induced lupus erythematosus, most classically associated with hydralazine, procainamide, and, increasingly recognized, tumor necrosis factor-alpha inhibitors discussed in Chapter 8's biologic therapy context, typically presents with a milder cutaneous and systemic phenotype than idiopathic lupus erythematosus and generally resolves following discontinuation of the culprit medication, paralleling the drug-induced vasculitis discussion in Chapter 9 in both its recognition pattern and management approach.

Cutaneous Manifestations of Limited Systemic Sclerosis (CREST Syndrome)

Limited cutaneous systemic sclerosis, historically termed CREST syndrome for its characteristic constellation of Calcinosis cutis, Raynaud phenomenon, Esophageal dysmotility, Sclerodactyly, and Telangiectasia, presents with more restricted, acral-predominant skin sclerosis relative to diffuse systemic sclerosis, together with a comparatively later onset of internal organ involvement, though pulmonary arterial hypertension, occurring independent of pulmonary fibrosis in this specific subtype, represents an important and potentially underrecognized complication warranting specific screening in limited disease. Calcinosis cutis, firm, whitish, occasionally ulcerating subcutaneous nodules resulting from dystrophic calcium deposition, and cutaneous telangiectasia, most prominent on the face, lips, and hands, are each visually distinctive findings that, together with the digital sclerosis and characteristic facial changes (perioral furrowing, a pinched nasal appearance) of this disease, allow experienced clinicians to recognize limited systemic sclerosis on inspection alone in many cases, even before biopsy or serologic confirmation.

CLINICAL PEARL: A biopsy showing interface dermatitis in a patient with photodistributed skin findings supports lupus erythematosus or dermatomyositis but cannot reliably distinguish between them; Gottron papules, heliotrope rash, and proximal muscle weakness are the clinical findings that most reliably make this distinction, underscoring why clinical photographs and a thorough history are as valuable as the biopsy itself in this specific differential.

Differential Diagnosis and Histologic Mimickers

Lupus Erythematosus Versus Dermatomyositis

As developed above, distinguishing lupus erythematosus from dermatomyositis on histology alone is frequently not possible given their substantial interface dermatitis overlap, and the practical approach relies on integrating the histologic interface pattern with clinical morphology (malar rash and photodistribution favoring lupus; Gottron papules, heliotrope rash, and proximal weakness favoring dermatomyositis) and serologic testing (antinuclear antibody panel and myositis-specific antibodies) discussed in the ancillary studies section below, a diagnostic approach that depends more heavily on this multi-modal correlation than perhaps any other differential in this chapter.

A 58-year-old patient presents with a several-week history of violaceous, flat-topped papules over the extensor metacarpophalangeal and interphalangeal joints, violaceous discoloration of the upper eyelids with mild periorbital edema, and new difficulty rising from a seated position, prompting biopsy of a hand papule given a differential of dermatomyositis versus lupus erythematosus. Pattern assignment identifies an interface dermatitis with vacuolar basal keratinocyte change, a sparse superficial perivascular lymphocytic infiltrate, and notably increased dermal mucin, without significant follicular plugging or the deep periadnexal infiltrate that would be expected in discoid lupus erythematosus. Differential narrowing correlates the histologic findings, which are individually more supportive of dermatomyositis than lupus given the mucin-prominent, plugging-sparse pattern, with the highly specific clinical findings of Gottron papules and the heliotrope rash, together with the patient's new proximal weakness, to favor dermatomyositis over lupus erythematosus. Diagnosis is confirmed with elevated creatine kinase and a positive anti-TIF1-gamma antibody, prompting both systemic immunosuppressive therapy and, given the specific antibody result identified, an expedited age-appropriate malignancy evaluation given this antibody's particularly strong malignancy association among the myositis-specific antibody panel.

Discoid Lupus Erythematosus Versus Lichen Planopilaris and Other Scarring Alopecias

Subacute cutaneous lupus erythematosus's psoriasiform variant can additionally be mistaken clinically for psoriasis given overlapping scaly, erythematous plaque morphology, though the underlying interface dermatitis pattern on biopsy, together with the strong anti-Ro/SSA serologic association and the characteristic photodistribution rather than psoriasis's more typical extensor and scalp predilection, resolves this distinction in the great majority of cases where biopsy is pursued. This distinction carries genuine clinical importance beyond diagnostic precision alone, since the treatment approaches for these two entities, antimalarial and photoprotective strategies for lupus erythematosus versus the biologic and topical vitamin D analog-based approaches more typical of psoriasis management, diverge substantially despite the superficial clinical resemblance.

On the scalp, discoid lupus erythematosus must be distinguished from lichen planopilaris and other primary scarring alopecias, a distinction developed further in the specialized hair and scalp pathology content of this book's later chapters, but relevant here because discoid lupus erythematosus's deep periadnexal lymphocytic infiltrate and follicular plugging, together with increased dermal mucin and a more superficial and deep perivascular infiltrate pattern extending beyond the immediate follicular unit, help distinguish it from the more follicular-centered, less deeply extending lymphocytic infiltrate of lichen planopilaris, though overlap and diagnostic difficulty between these entities is well recognized, particularly in end-stage, burned-out scarring alopecia where the specific inciting process may no longer be histologically apparent.

Neonatal Lupus Erythematosus Versus Other Annular Infantile Eruptions

Neonatal lupus erythematosus's annular, often periorbital cutaneous lesions can resemble other annular infantile eruptions, including annular erythema of infancy and, less commonly, an early presentation of tinea corporis, distinguished from neonatal lupus erythematosus by the biopsy findings, a vacuolar interface dermatitis in neonatal lupus erythematosus that is absent in the other entities, together with maternal anti-Ro/SSA serologic confirmation, which is specific to the neonatal lupus erythematosus diagnosis and absent in its clinical mimickers. Given the cardiac implications discussed in the etiology section, confirming or excluding this diagnosis promptly, through biopsy and maternal serology together, carries meaningfully higher stakes than most other pediatric annular eruption evaluations, justifying an expedited diagnostic approach relative to the more routine timeline appropriate for most other benign infantile dermatoses.

Morphea/Systemic Sclerosis Versus Other Sclerosing Dermatoses

Scleredema, most commonly associated with poorly controlled diabetes mellitus and, less commonly, a preceding streptococcal infection or an underlying paraproteinemia, shows thickened dermal collagen bundles separated by increased interstitial mucin rather than the homogenized, mucin-poor sclerosis of morphea, favoring the upper back, neck, and shoulders in a distribution distinct from morphea's more variable plaque or linear distribution. Scleromyxedema, associated with an underlying paraproteinemia in the great majority of cases, shows a similar increase in dermal mucin together with a proliferation of dermal fibroblasts, producing the characteristic waxy, closely spaced papules of this condition, and warrants hematologic evaluation for an underlying plasma cell dyscrasia given this strong association. Nephrogenic systemic fibrosis, occurring in patients with renal impairment following exposure to certain gadolinium-based contrast agents, shows a proliferation of dermal fibroblasts and thickened collagen bundles with variable mucin, and a history of recent gadolinium-enhanced imaging in a patient with renal impairment presenting with new, rapidly progressive skin thickening should prompt specific consideration of this diagnosis, now substantially less common given modern contrast agent safety protocols but still an important historical and occasionally encountered differential.

Morphea and systemic sclerosis must be distinguished from other sclerosing skin conditions, including scleredema, scleromyxedema, nephrogenic systemic fibrosis, and eosinophilic fasciitis, each of which produces dermal or fascial sclerosis through a distinct mechanism and requires distinct management, making this a clinically important differential despite these entities' comparative rarity relative to morphea itself. Eosinophilic fasciitis in particular, characterized by fascial rather than purely dermal sclerosis, prominent tissue eosinophilia, and a full-thickness biopsy extending to fascia, illustrates why biopsy depth, discussed further in the ancillary studies section, is a critical practical consideration whenever a sclerosing process is being evaluated, since a superficial punch biopsy may fail to capture the fascial involvement that would otherwise distinguish this entity from morphea.

A 42-year-old patient with several months of progressive bilateral forearm swelling, tightness, and mild tenderness following a period of unusually strenuous physical activity presents for biopsy given a differential including morphea, eosinophilic fasciitis, and another sclerosing process. Standard punch biopsy initially performed shows only mild superficial dermal changes without diagnostic sclerosis, prompting a repeat, deeper incisional biopsy extending to fascia given continued clinical suspicion. The deeper specimen identifies thickened, fibrotic fascia with a dense infiltrate rich in eosinophils, extending focally into the overlying deep dermis, a pattern distinct from morphea's more purely dermal, eosinophil-poor sclerosis. Diagnosis of eosinophilic fasciitis is established, prompting systemic corticosteroid therapy and hematology referral to evaluate for an associated hematologic abnormality occasionally reported in this condition, illustrating directly why adequate biopsy depth, extending to fascia when this specific entity is a genuine consideration, is essential for accurate diagnosis rather than a superficial biopsy that would have missed this specific, fascia-centered process entirely.

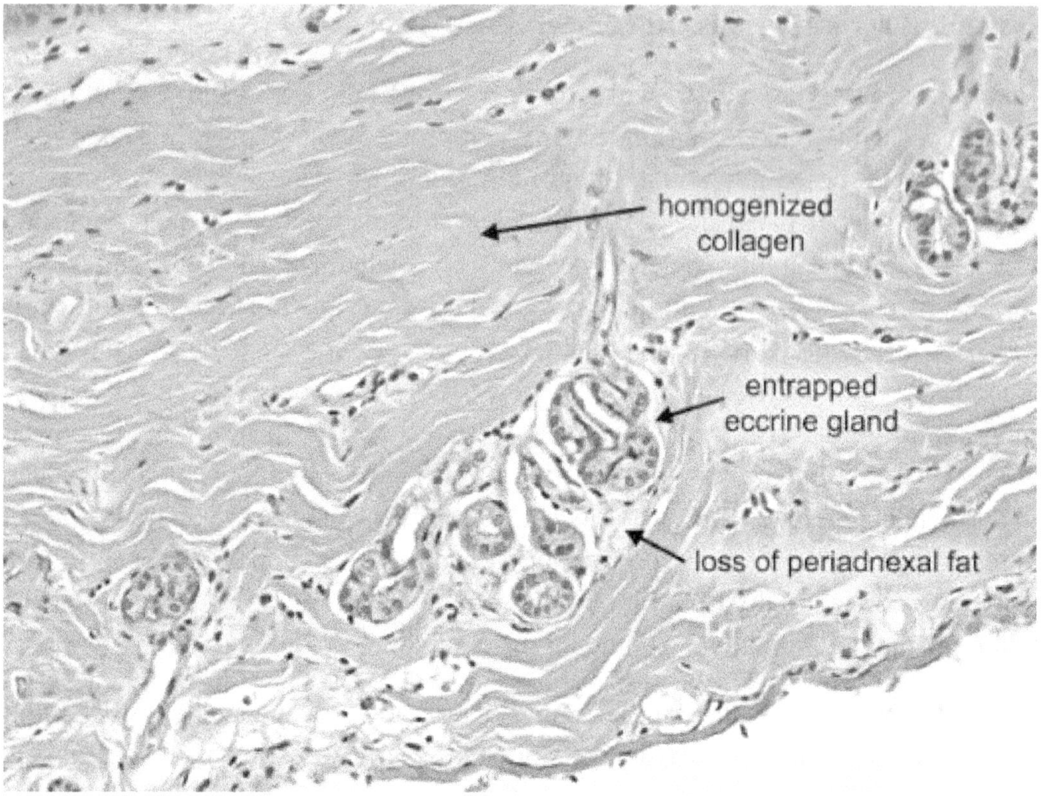

Ancillary Studies

Direct Immunofluorescence: The Lupus Band Test

Direct immunofluorescence of lesional skin in lupus erythematosus, the classic "lupus band test," shows a continuous, granular band of immunoglobulin (typically IgG and IgM) and complement deposition along the dermal-epidermal junction, a finding supportive of but not entirely specific for lupus erythematosus, since a similar band can occasionally be seen in other interface dermatoses and, importantly, can be present in sun-exposed but clinically uninvolved skin in patients with systemic lupus erythematosus, a finding sometimes used as supportive evidence for systemic disease when biopsied from an appropriate control site. Direct immunofluorescence is generally less diagnostically necessary in dermatomyositis, which typically shows a less consistent or absent immunoreactant band, making a positive, well-formed lupus band a point of distinction favoring lupus erythematosus when this specific ancillary study is pursued in an ambiguous interface dermatitis case.

Muscle Enzyme and Imaging Correlation for Dermatomyositis

Pulmonary function testing, including diffusion capacity for carbon monoxide, and high-resolution computed tomography of the chest are essential baseline and monitoring studies for any confirmed systemic sclerosis diagnosis given this disease's substantial pulmonary morbidity, while echocardiography with specific attention to estimated pulmonary artery pressure screens for the pulmonary arterial hypertension that can complicate limited systemic sclerosis independent of interstitial lung disease, as discussed in the clinical presentation section above.

Serum creatine kinase and aldolase levels, together with electromyography and, increasingly, magnetic resonance imaging of the proximal musculature, support the myositis component of a dermatomyositis diagnosis and help distinguish clinically amyopathic dermatomyositis, in which these studies remain normal despite the characteristic cutaneous findings, from disease with subclinical or clinically evident muscle involvement, a distinction that carries direct implications for the intensity and specific composition of the systemic immunosuppressive regimen selected. Muscle biopsy, when pursued, characteristically shows a perifascicular pattern of muscle fiber atrophy and inflammation reflecting the same complement-mediated microangiopathic mechanism discussed in the etiology section, distinguishing dermatomyositis from other inflammatory myopathies on muscle histology in a manner that parallels this chapter's emphasis on integrating multiple diagnostic modalities rather than relying on skin biopsy alone.

Serologic Correlation

Complement levels (C3, C4) and anti-double-stranded DNA antibody titers, when trended serially, provide additional useful information for monitoring systemic lupus erythematosus disease activity, declining complement and rising anti-double-stranded DNA titers correlating with disease flares in many though not all patients, information most directly relevant to the treating rheumatologist but worth understanding as part of the broader clinical context surrounding a cutaneous lupus erythematosus biopsy, particularly when a report is being prepared for a patient with known systemic disease and active monitoring already underway.

A negative antinuclear antibody result does not exclude cutaneous-limited lupus erythematosus, particularly discoid lupus erythematosus without systemic involvement, since this serologic marker is more closely tied to systemic disease activity than to the presence of cutaneous-limited disease, an important point to communicate when a strongly suggestive biopsy is paired with unexpectedly negative initial serologic testing rather than allowing this combination to be misread as excluding the diagnosis.

Antinuclear antibody testing, together with more specific autoantibody panels, anti-double-stranded DNA and anti-Smith for systemic lupus erythematosus, anti-Ro/SSA for subacute cutaneous lupus erythematosus, and myositis-specific antibodies including anti-Jo-1, anti-Mi-2, and anti-TIF1-gamma for dermatomyositis, the last of which carries a particularly strong malignancy association, provides essential complementary information that, combined with the histologic and clinical findings discussed throughout this chapter, establishes the specific final diagnosis in most connective tissue disease cases. Anti-centromere and anti-Scl-70 (anti-topoisomerase I) antibody testing, together with nailfold capillaroscopy, supports the distinction between limited and diffuse systemic sclerosis subtypes once a sclerosing process has been confirmed histologically, extending the diagnostic workup into disease subtyping with direct prognostic implications, given the differing internal organ involvement risk profiles between these subtypes.

CAUTION: A skin biopsy showing dermal sclerosis confirms a sclerosing process but cannot, by itself, distinguish morphea from systemic sclerosis or from the rarer sclerosing mimickers discussed above. Reporting this distinction as though histology alone resolved it risks delaying the systemic evaluation and organ-specific monitoring that a systemic sclerosis diagnosis specifically requires.

Management Implications

Connecting Diagnosis to Treatment Pathway

As with the granulomatous, vasculopathic, and panniculitis patterns discussed in the three preceding chapters, management across this chapter's connective tissue disease spectrum diverges according to the specific diagnosis reached rather than following a single unified treatment algorithm, reinforcing once again why the systematic diagnostic approach this chapter has developed, interface-versus-sclerosis assessment first, mucin and specific histologic clue assessment second, and clinical-serologic correlation throughout, carries direct and substantial consequence for the specific therapy a given patient ultimately receives.

Cutaneous lupus erythematosus is managed with strict photoprotection, topical or intralesional corticosteroids for localized disease, and antimalarial agents, most often hydroxychloroquine, for more extensive or refractory disease, with systemic immunosuppression reserved for patients with concurrent systemic lupus erythematosus; dermatomyositis is managed with systemic corticosteroids and steroid-sparing immunosuppressive agents alongside malignancy screening in adult-onset disease; morphea is managed with topical or intralesional corticosteroids, phototherapy, or systemic immunosuppression for extensive or rapidly progressive disease, particularly the linear subtype in children; and systemic sclerosis is managed with a combination of disease-modifying and organ-specific therapy tailored to the pattern of internal organ involvement identified through the systemic evaluation this diagnosis requires.

Prevention and Screening

Age-appropriate malignancy screening for newly diagnosed adult-onset dermatomyositis patients, as discussed above, typically includes screening beyond routine health maintenance guidelines, with some authorities recommending computed tomography of the chest, abdomen, and pelvis, together with age-appropriate gynecologic and gastrointestinal cancer screening, concentrated within the first one to two years following diagnosis given the temporal clustering of malignancy diagnosis around this window. Pregnant patients with known anti-Ro/SSA or anti-La/SSB antibody positivity, whether or not they carry an established lupus erythematosus diagnosis, warrant serial fetal cardiac monitoring, typically with fetal echocardiography beginning in the second trimester, given the congenital heart block risk discussed earlier in this chapter, a screening practice with genuine potential to identify early, still-treatable conduction abnormality before irreversible complete heart block develops.

Complications and Prognosis

Neonatal lupus erythematosus's cutaneous findings resolve spontaneously without scarring in the great majority of affected infants as maternal antibody clears, but congenital heart block, once established, is generally permanent and frequently requires pacemaker placement, making this complication, rather than the transient cutaneous findings, the primary determinant of long-term morbidity for infants affected by this specific neonatal lupus erythematosus manifestation. Morphea, particularly the linear subtype affecting a growing child, carries a risk of permanent limb length discrepancy, joint contracture, or facial asymmetry when inadequately treated during the active disease phase, underscoring why aggressive early treatment in pediatric linear morphea, discussed in the special populations section above, is weighted more heavily toward preventing irreversible structural complications than toward the cutaneous findings alone.

Discoid lupus erythematosus carries a risk of permanent scarring and dyspigmentation, particularly disfiguring on the face and scalp, making early, effective treatment valuable for limiting these long-term cosmetic and, for scalp disease, functional consequences, while acute and subacute cutaneous lupus erythematosus generally heal without significant scarring, reflecting their comparatively more superficial and less destructive interface pattern. Systemic sclerosis carries the most guarded overall prognosis among the entities in this chapter, driven by internal organ involvement rather than the cutaneous findings themselves, with pulmonary and renal complications historically representing the leading causes of disease-related mortality, underscoring why early recognition and systemic evaluation, rather than treatment of the cutaneous findings in isolation, is the most consequential contribution the dermatopathologist and treating clinician can make to this specific patient's long-term outcome.

Patient Education and Counseling

Patients diagnosed with mixed connective tissue disease or another overlap syndrome benefit from counseling that their condition may not fit neatly into a single named diagnosis, and that ongoing monitoring across multiple organ systems, rather than a single treatment protocol, will likely characterize their long-term care, framing that helps set realistic expectations for a patient population that can otherwise find the absence of a single, clean diagnostic label unsettling. Mothers found to carry anti-Ro/SSA or anti-La/SSB antibodies benefit from clear counseling regarding the congenital heart block risk to future pregnancies and the fetal cardiac monitoring this risk warrants, delivered with appropriate reassurance that the great majority of pregnancies in antibody-positive mothers proceed without this specific complication.

Patients with cutaneous lupus erythematosus benefit from thorough counseling regarding strict, consistent photoprotection, including broad-spectrum sunscreen, protective clothing, and sun avoidance during peak hours, given ultraviolet light's direct role in disease pathogenesis discussed earlier in this chapter, and from understanding that disease flares often correlate directly with sun exposure. Patients newly diagnosed with adult-onset dermatomyositis benefit from clear communication regarding the recommended malignancy screening and its rationale, avoiding either alarming overemphasis or inappropriate minimization of this risk, while patients with morphea or systemic sclerosis benefit from realistic counseling regarding the chronic, often slowly progressive nature of these conditions and the specific systemic monitoring, pulmonary function testing and echocardiography among the most important for systemic sclerosis, that ongoing management requires.

Across every entity in this chapter, patients benefit from understanding that a dermatopathology diagnosis in this disease category typically represents the beginning, rather than the end, of a diagnostic and monitoring process, given how consistently this chapter has emphasized the integration of biopsy findings with clinical, serologic, and, for several entities, radiographic and functional testing, a multidisciplinary care model that most patients navigate most successfully when they understand its rationale from the outset.

THE REACTION PATTERN RECOGNITION SYSTEM — The Connective Tissue Disease Pattern Family

---

The Pattern: The connective tissue disease pattern organized by interface versus sclerosing histology, cutting across mucin assessment: lupus erythematosus (acute, subacute, discoid), dermatomyositis, morphea, and systemic sclerosis.

Histologic Signature: Vacuolar interface change with deep periadnexal infiltrate and follicular plugging defines discoid lupus; interface change with prominent dermal mucin and minimal plugging defines dermatomyositis; homogenized, hypocellular collagen with adnexal entrapment defines morphea and systemic sclerosis, histologically indistinguishable from each other; mucin without interface or sclerosis defines tumid lupus erythematosus.

The Decision: Assess the dermal-epidermal junction first for interface change versus the dermal collagen for sclerosis, then assess mucin as a secondary axis, then correlate with clinical morphology (malar rash, Gottron papules, sclerotic plaque distribution) and targeted serologic testing to reach the specific final diagnosis.

Trap Logic: Lupus and dermatomyositis overlap substantially on histology and require clinical and serologic distinction; morphea and systemic sclerosis are histologically indistinguishable and require clinical distribution, capillaroscopy, and serologic distinction; eosinophilic fasciitis mimics morphea but requires deep, fascia-including biopsy to identify; and a negative antinuclear antibody does not exclude cutaneous-limited lupus erythematosus.

Pattern Anchor: Interface points toward lupus/dermatomyositis and requires clinical-serologic distinction; sclerosis points toward morphea/systemic sclerosis and requires distribution-serologic distinction. Biopsy depth to fascia when eosinophilic fasciitis is a consideration; never assume standard punch depth is adequate for a sclerosing differential; and never assume mucin-rich sclerosis is morphea without excluding scleredema and scleromyxedema first.

Summary and Key Concepts

The connective tissue diseases of the skin are organized around two dominant histologic patterns, interface dermatitis (lupus erythematosus, dermatomyositis) and dermal sclerosis (morphea, systemic sclerosis), with dermal mucin serving as a recurring cross-cutting diagnostic clue.

The three cutaneous lupus erythematosus subtypes, acute, subacute, and discoid, differ in interface intensity, follicular plugging, and infiltrate depth, correlating with differing systemic lupus erythematosus risk that guides the required clinical evaluation, while tumid and neonatal lupus erythematosus extend this spectrum further with mucin-predominant and transient antibody-mediated presentations respectively.

Lupus erythematosus and dermatomyositis overlap substantially on histology and are most reliably distinguished through clinical morphology (Gottron papules, heliotrope rash, proximal weakness) and myositis-specific serologic testing.

Morphea and systemic sclerosis are histologically indistinguishable on skin biopsy alone, making clinical distribution, nailfold capillaroscopy, and centromere/Scl-70 serologic testing essential for this critical distinction given systemic sclerosis's substantially more guarded internal organ prognosis, and requiring careful exclusion of the mucin-rich mimickers scleredema and scleromyxedema.

Adequate biopsy depth, extending to fascia when eosinophilic fasciitis is a consideration, and the lupus band direct immunofluorescence test are the two ancillary techniques most likely to change management across this chapter's differential diagnosis, alongside careful attention to overlap syndromes and neonatal disease that do not fit a single entity cleanly.

CHAPTER 12: INFECTIOUS DERMATOSES: BACTERIAL, FUNGAL, VIRAL, AND PARASITIC

Learning Objectives

1. Classify cutaneous infections by organism class and by predominant histologic reaction: suppurative, granulomatous, vesiculobullous, cytopathic, and eosinophilic hypersensitivity.
2. Identify the histopathologic features and diagnostic criteria of the major bacterial, superficial and deep fungal, herpesvirus, papillomavirus, poxvirus, and parasitic dermatoses.
3. Recognize the histologic clues, including host immune status, that identify a specific organism class even before special stains confirm the diagnosis.
4. Correlate histologic findings across cutaneous infections with clinical presentation, host immune status, and epidemiologic context.
5. Construct a full differential diagnosis distinguishing infectious dermatoses from their inflammatory, autoimmune, and neoplastic mimickers.
6. Select the appropriate special stains, bedside tests, cultures, and molecular studies for a suspected infectious dermatosis.

Definition and Classification

Organizing Cutaneous Infection by Reaction and by Organism

This chapter also carries a distinct clinical urgency relative to several of this book's earlier chapters, since a meaningful subset of the entities discussed here, necrotizing soft tissue infection, disseminated herpesvirus infection in an immunocompromised or neonatal host, and crusted scabies among them, represent genuine diagnostic and treatment emergencies where delay measured in hours to days, rather than the more typical weeks-long evaluation timeline appropriate for many other reaction patterns in this book, can meaningfully affect patient outcome.

Cutaneous infectious disease differs from every other chapter in this book in one fundamental respect: it is organized by causative organism rather than by a single unifying reaction pattern, since bacteria, fungi, viruses, and parasites each provoke histologically distinct tissue responses that in turn overlap substantially with the reaction patterns already developed across this book's earlier chapters, superficial and deep fungal infection producing the granulomatous pattern discussed in Chapter 8, certain bacterial infections producing the vasculopathic pattern discussed in Chapter 9, and specific viral infections producing a distinctive vesiculobullous pattern this chapter introduces in detail. This chapter therefore functions as an integrative capstone for cutaneous infection specifically, applying the diagnostic disciplines already established throughout this book to the organism-specific context that determines both the histologic pattern encountered and the specific ancillary studies required to confirm organism identity.

A second organizing principle, host immune status, cuts across every organism class discussed in this chapter and carries particular diagnostic weight given the immunocompromised-host principle first developed in Chapter 8: an immunocompetent host typically mounts a well-organized, pattern-specific response that aids histologic recognition, while an immunocompromised host may show a blunted, atypical, or minimal tissue response despite substantial organism burden, a principle that applies with equal or greater force to the viral and parasitic infections this chapter adds to the granulomatous and vasculopathic infectious presentations already discussed in earlier chapters.

Classification by Predominant Histologic Reaction

Bacterial infections most often produce a suppurative (neutrophil-rich, abscess-forming) reaction, though certain bacteria, notably mycobacteria discussed in Chapter 8, produce a granulomatous reaction instead; superficial fungal infections produce a comparatively mild, often psoriasiform or spongiotic reaction confined to the stratum corneum and epidermis, while deep fungal infections produce the granulomatous or mixed suppurative-granulomatous reaction already discussed in Chapter 8; viral infections produce a spectrum ranging from the distinctive vesiculobullous, cytopathic pattern of the herpesviruses to the epidermal hyperplasia of human papillomavirus infection to the vasculopathic pattern of certain viral hemorrhagic processes; and parasitic and arthropod-related infections produce a predominantly eosinophil-rich hypersensitivity reaction, developed further throughout this chapter.

Organism Class	Representative Entity	Predominant Reaction	Key Diagnostic Clue
Bacterial (pyogenic)	Impetigo, folliculitis, cellulitis	Suppurative	Neutrophilic infiltrate; organisms on Gram stain
Bacterial (mycobacterial)	Cutaneous tuberculosis, leprosy	Granulomatous	See Chapter 8
Superficial fungal	Dermatophytosis, tinea versicolor	Mild spongiotic/psoriasiform	Hyphae in stratum corneum on PAS-D
Deep fungal	Histoplasmosis, blastomycosis	Granulomatous/suppurative	See Chapter 8
Viral (herpesvirus)	Herpes simplex, varicella-zoster	Vesiculobullous, cytopathic	Multinucleated keratinocytes with margination
Viral (papillomavirus)	Verruca vulgaris, condyloma	Epidermal hyperplasia	Koilocytosis, papillomatosis
Parasitic/arthropod	Scabies, arthropod bite reaction	Eosinophilic hypersensitivity	Organism/mite parts; wedge-shaped eosinophilic infiltrate

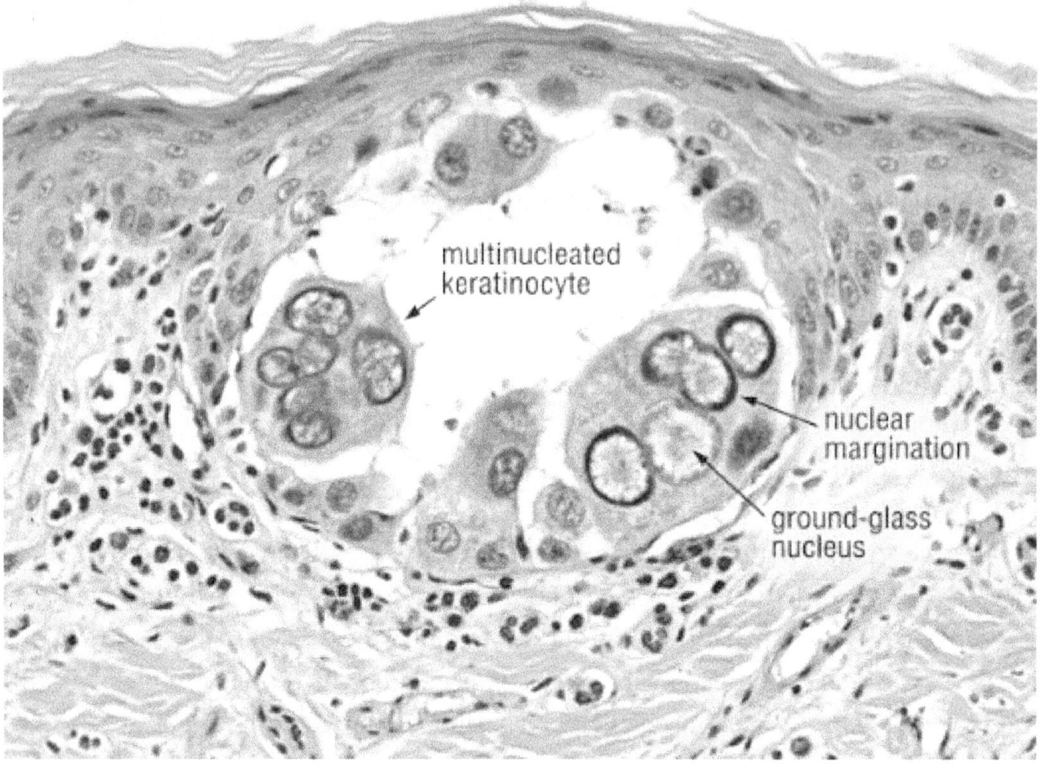

Etiology and Pathogenesis

Mechanisms of Bacterial Skin Infection

The organism-first classification this chapter applies mirrors, at a broader level, the mechanistic organizing principle this book has used since Chapter 3: just as the earlier reaction-pattern chapters trace a specific tissue response back to its underlying immunologic or pathophysiologic mechanism, this chapter traces the tissue response back to the specific causative organism, with the practical consequence that identifying the organism class from the histologic pattern, rather than simply describing the inflammatory pattern in isolation, is what allows the pathologist to direct the clinician toward organism-specific, rather than merely pattern-directed, therapy.

Pyogenic bacterial infections, most often caused by Staphylococcus aureus and Streptococcus pyogenes, invade the skin through a break in the epidermal barrier or through direct follicular involvement, triggering a robust neutrophilic response that, depending on the depth and extent of invasion, produces the clinical and histologic spectrum from superficial impetigo to folliculitis to deeper cellulitis and abscess formation, a spectrum organized principally by the depth of bacterial invasion and the corresponding depth of the resulting suppurative reaction. Toxin-mediated bacterial skin disease, exemplified by staphylococcal scalded skin syndrome, in which exfoliative toxin produced by a often distant staphylococcal infection cleaves desmoglein 1 within the superficial epidermis, illustrates that bacterial skin disease can occur through toxin-mediated mechanisms without requiring direct bacterial invasion of the skin itself, a distinct pathogenesis with direct implications for the histologic findings, superficial intraepidermal cleavage without significant inflammation or organisms within the specimen, discussed further below.

Mechanisms of Superficial Fungal Infection

Dermatophyte species are further classified by their natural reservoir, anthropophilic species adapted to human hosts and typically producing a milder, more chronic infection with less pronounced inflammation, zoophilic species adapted to animal hosts and typically producing a more acute, intensely inflammatory infection when transmitted to an incidental human host, and geophilic species adapted to soil, an ecological classification that correlates meaningfully with the clinical intensity of a given dermatophyte infection and can, together with a directed exposure history including animal contact, help suggest the likely causative organism even before culture confirmation returns.

Dermatophyte fungi, keratinophilic organisms restricted to the non-viable, keratin-containing stratum corneum, hair, and nail, produce their clinical and histologic effects primarily through the host inflammatory response to fungal antigens and metabolic byproducts rather than through direct tissue invasion of viable cells, explaining why dermatophyte infection typically produces a comparatively mild, superficial inflammatory reaction relative to the deep fungal infections discussed in Chapter 8, which do invade viable tissue. Tinea versicolor, caused by Malassezia species, a lipophilic yeast that is part of normal cutaneous flora in most individuals, illustrates a distinct mechanism in which overgrowth of an already-resident organism, rather than new organism acquisition, produces the characteristic hypopigmented or hyperpigmented scaly patches this condition presents with, a mechanism worth distinguishing from the acquired infection model that applies to most other entities in this chapter.

Mechanisms of Viral Skin Infection

Latency, the capacity of herpesviruses to establish a lifelong, non-replicating infection within sensory ganglia following primary infection, with periodic reactivation triggered by stress, ultraviolet exposure, illness, or immunosuppression, is a defining biological feature that distinguishes this viral group from the other viral entities discussed in this chapter and directly explains the recurrent, often lifelong clinical course of both herpes simplex virus and varicella-zoster virus infection, in contrast to the typically non-recurring, self-limited course of a primary human papillomavirus or molluscum contagiosum infection once cleared by the host immune system.

Herpesviruses (herpes simplex virus types 1 and 2, and varicella-zoster virus) directly infect and replicate within keratinocytes, producing characteristic cytopathic effect, including the multinucleation, nuclear molding, and peripheral chromatin margination discussed above, that reflects the virus's direct cytotoxic effect on infected cells, culminating in cell lysis and the formation of the intraepidermal vesicle that defines this infection's clinical and histologic presentation. Human papillomavirus, by contrast, does not produce direct keratinocyte cytolysis but instead induces epidermal hyperproliferation and koilocytic change, vacuolated, atypical-appearing keratinocytes with perinuclear clearing reflecting the virus's productive infection cycle within terminally differentiating keratinocytes, a fundamentally different mechanism from the herpesviruses that explains the two viral groups' substantially different histologic presentations despite both being viral in origin.

Mechanisms of Parasitic and Arthropod-Related Skin Disease

Pediculosis (lice infestation) and cutaneous larva migrans, caused respectively by lice species adapted to specific body regions and by hookworm larvae penetrating the skin of a host in whom they cannot complete their life cycle, round out this chapter's parasitic and arthropod-related entities, each producing a broadly similar eosinophil-rich hypersensitivity histologic pattern to scabies and arthropod bites, though cutaneous larva migrans carries the additional, highly distinctive clinical feature of a serpiginous, migrating track reflecting the larva's subcutaneous movement, a clinical finding sufficiently specific that biopsy is rarely necessary for diagnosis in a patient with an appropriate travel or environmental exposure history.

Scabies, caused by the mite Sarcoptes scabiei var. hominis, results from direct mite burrowing within the stratum corneum, with the resulting clinical eruption reflecting not primarily the mite's physical presence but rather a delayed-type hypersensitivity reaction to mite antigens, mite feces, and mite eggs, explaining why the extensive, pruritic eruption of scabies typically extends well beyond the immediate vicinity of the relatively few mites actually present on a given patient at any one time. Arthropod bite reactions, resulting from a hypersensitivity response to injected salivary antigens during blood feeding by mosquitoes, fleas, bedbugs, and other arthropods, produce a broadly similar eosinophil-rich hypersensitivity pattern to scabies but without the organism itself typically being present within the biopsy specimen, since the arthropod has usually completed feeding and departed before the bite reaction and subsequent biopsy occur.

Mechanisms of Molluscum Contagiosum and Other Poxviruses

Molluscum contagiosum virus, a poxvirus, infects keratinocytes and drives a distinctive pattern of epidermal hyperproliferation with the accumulation of large, eosinophilic cytoplasmic inclusion bodies (Henderson-Patterson bodies) that progressively enlarge and displace the nucleus as infected keratinocytes migrate toward the skin surface, a productive viral replication cycle mechanistically distinct from both the cytolytic herpesvirus mechanism and the koilocytic human papillomavirus mechanism discussed above, despite molluscum's superficial clinical resemblance to a viral wart. This distinct mechanism explains molluscum's characteristic umbilicated, dome-shaped papule morphology, reflecting central expulsion of the virus-laden, degenerating keratinocyte debris through a central pore, a clinical and histologic correlation developed further in the sections below.

Deep and Necrotizing Bacterial Infection

Beyond the superficial pyogenic infections discussed above, certain bacterial pathogens and toxin-mediated mechanisms produce deeper, more destructive tissue injury: Group A Streptococcus and, less commonly, other organisms can produce necrotizing fasciitis, discussed in Chapter 10's infectious panniculitis section, through a combination of direct tissue invasion and exotoxin-mediated tissue destruction, while Vibrio vulnificus and other water-associated organisms produce a rapidly progressive, hemorrhagic, bullous soft tissue infection following exposure to contaminated water or seafood, particularly in patients with underlying liver disease or immunocompromise, illustrating that the epidemiologic exposure history, water or seafood contact specifically in this example, can be as diagnostically important as the histologic findings themselves for certain bacterial pathogens within this chapter's scope.

THE REACTION PATTERN RECOGNITION SYSTEM — Organism Class Recognition Before Special Stain Confirmation

The Pattern: Recognizing the Organism Class from the Histologic Reaction and Host Immune Status Before Special Stains Confirm the Specific Organism

Histologic Signature: A predominantly neutrophilic infiltrate suggests bacterial infection; a granulomatous infiltrate suggests mycobacterial or deep fungal infection (see Chapter 8); multinucleated keratinocytes with cytopathic change suggest herpesvirus; koilocytosis and papillomatosis suggest human papillomavirus; a wedge-shaped, eosinophil-rich infiltrate suggests an arthropod or parasitic hypersensitivity reaction.

The Decision: Assess the dominant inflammatory cell type and any organism-specific cytopathic or structural change first, since this narrows the organism class before special stains are selected, directing fungal stains toward a spongiotic/psoriasiform pattern, Gram stain toward a suppurative pattern, and a search for mite parts or organism fragments toward an eosinophil-rich wedge-shaped infiltrate, then integrate host immune status throughout.

Trap Logic: An immunocompromised host can show a blunted or atypical reaction for any organism class discussed in this chapter, understating the apparent severity of infection; a partially treated bacterial infection may show comparatively sparse neutrophils despite ongoing infection; and herpesvirus cytopathic change can be subtle or focal, requiring examination of multiple levels when clinical suspicion remains high despite an initially unremarkable biopsy.

Pattern Anchor: Match the dominant inflammatory cell and any organism-specific cytopathic change to the organism class first, then confirm with the targeted special stain, culture, or molecular study that class specifically requires. Never default to a broad-spectrum special stain panel without first narrowing the organism class through pattern recognition.

Histopathologic Features and Diagnostic Criteria

Diagnostic Features of Bacterial Skin Infection

Staphylococcal scalded skin syndrome, introduced in the etiology section above, shows superficial intraepidermal cleavage within the granular layer, notably without significant acantholysis at the level of cleavage itself and without organisms or a significant inflammatory infiltrate present within the specimen, since the disease results from a distant toxin-producing infection rather than direct cutaneous bacterial invasion, a histologic pattern that, when recognized, should prompt investigation for the primary infectious source elsewhere in the body, most often the nasopharynx, conjunctiva, or umbilicus in affected neonates, rather than treatment directed at the skin specimen site itself.

Erysipelas, a superficial variant of streptococcal cellulitis involving the upper dermis and superficial lymphatics specifically, presents with sharply demarcated, raised, tender erythema, in contrast to the more poorly demarcated erythema of deeper cellulitis, a clinical distinction reflecting the differing depth of tissue involvement between these two related but histologically and clinically distinguishable streptococcal skin infections.

Impetigo shows a subcorneal or intracorneal pustule with acantholytic keratinocytes and neutrophils, often with visible cocci within the pustule on careful examination or with Gram staining, a superficial process reflecting the typically superficial nature of this specific bacterial infection. Folliculitis shows a neutrophilic infiltrate centered on and often destroying the hair follicle, with organisms, when identifiable, located within the follicular lumen or infundibulum, while cellulitis, less commonly biopsied given its usual clinical diagnosis, shows a diffuse dermal and subcutaneous neutrophilic infiltrate with edema and, in more severe cases, vessel involvement that can approach the vasculopathic pattern discussed in Chapter 9 when the infection produces secondary vascular compromise.

Diagnostic Features of Superficial Fungal Infection

Dermatophyte infection shows a comparatively mild superficial perivascular lymphocytic infiltrate with variable spongiosis, and the diagnostic finding, hyphae within the stratum corneum, is often subtle and easily overlooked on routine hematoxylin and eosin staining, making a PAS-D stain, discussed in Chapter 2 and again in the ancillary studies section below, essential for confident identification in the great majority of cases, a point worth emphasizing given how frequently this diagnosis can be missed without this specific stain. A useful low-power clue supporting dermatophyte infection even before special staining is the "sandwich sign," compact orthokeratosis alternating with a more basket-weave pattern corresponding to the alternating growth phases of the causative organism, a subtle but recognizable pattern that should prompt PAS-D staining whenever identified. Tinea versicolor shows a comparatively mild histologic reaction with characteristic short hyphae and budding yeast forms within the stratum corneum, sometimes described as a "spaghetti and meatballs" pattern, readily identified on PAS-D staining and occasionally visible even on routine hematoxylin and eosin staining given the organism's comparatively larger size and greater abundance relative to dermatophyte hyphae.

Diagnostic Features of Viral Skin Infection

Varicella-zoster virus infection, whether primary varicella or reactivation zoster, shows histology essentially identical to herpes simplex virus infection at the keratinocyte level, and in a biopsy specimen showing intraepidermal vesiculation with the characteristic multinucleated cytopathic change, the distinction between these two herpesviruses rests entirely on clinical distribution and, when needed, the ancillary studies discussed below, rather than on any histologic feature specific to either virus individually, a limitation worth stating plainly in any pathology report addressing this specific differential.

Herpesvirus infection shows the intraepidermal vesicle with acantholysis and the characteristic multinucleated keratinocytes with nuclear molding, peripheral chromatin margination, and ground-glass nuclear appearance discussed above, findings that, while highly suggestive of herpesvirus infection as a class, cannot reliably distinguish herpes simplex virus from varicella-zoster virus on histology alone, a distinction requiring the ancillary studies discussed below when clinically important. Human papillomavirus infection (verruca vulgaris and condyloma acuminatum) shows papillomatosis (undulating epidermal surface), hyperkeratosis, and koilocytosis, vacuolated keratinocytes with perinuclear clearing and peripherally displaced, often irregular nuclei, concentrated in the upper spinous and granular layers, together with, in verruca vulgaris specifically, characteristic vertically oriented, tapering rete ridges at the lesion's lateral margins and prominent hypergranulosis with coarse keratohyalin granules.

Diagnostic Features of Molluscum Contagiosum

Molluscum contagiosum shows a cup-shaped, endophytic epidermal proliferation with large, eosinophilic, glassy cytoplasmic inclusion bodies (Henderson-Patterson bodies) that become progressively larger and more basophilic as infected keratinocytes ascend toward the surface, ultimately discharging through a central pore that corresponds to the clinical umbilication, findings sufficiently distinctive that molluscum contagiosum is rarely a diagnostic challenge once adequately sampled, though a superficial or tangentially sectioned biopsy can occasionally fail to capture the full cup-shaped architecture needed for confident recognition.

Diagnostic Features of Scabies and Arthropod Bite Reactions

Scabies and arthropod bite reactions share a broadly overlapping histologic picture, a superficial and deep perivascular infiltrate rich in eosinophils, often with a wedge-shaped configuration extending from the papillary into the reticular dermis, and, in more indurated or persistent lesions, particularly in the specific entity of a persistent nodular arthropod bite reaction, a component of dermal fibrosis reflecting the chronic, relapsing nature of the hypersensitivity response. Scabies-specific mite parts, ova, or fecal pellets, when identified, definitively confirm the diagnosis over a nonspecific arthropod bite reaction, though as discussed in the ancillary studies section below, their absence does not exclude scabies given the condition's characteristically low organism burden in classic, non-crusted presentations.

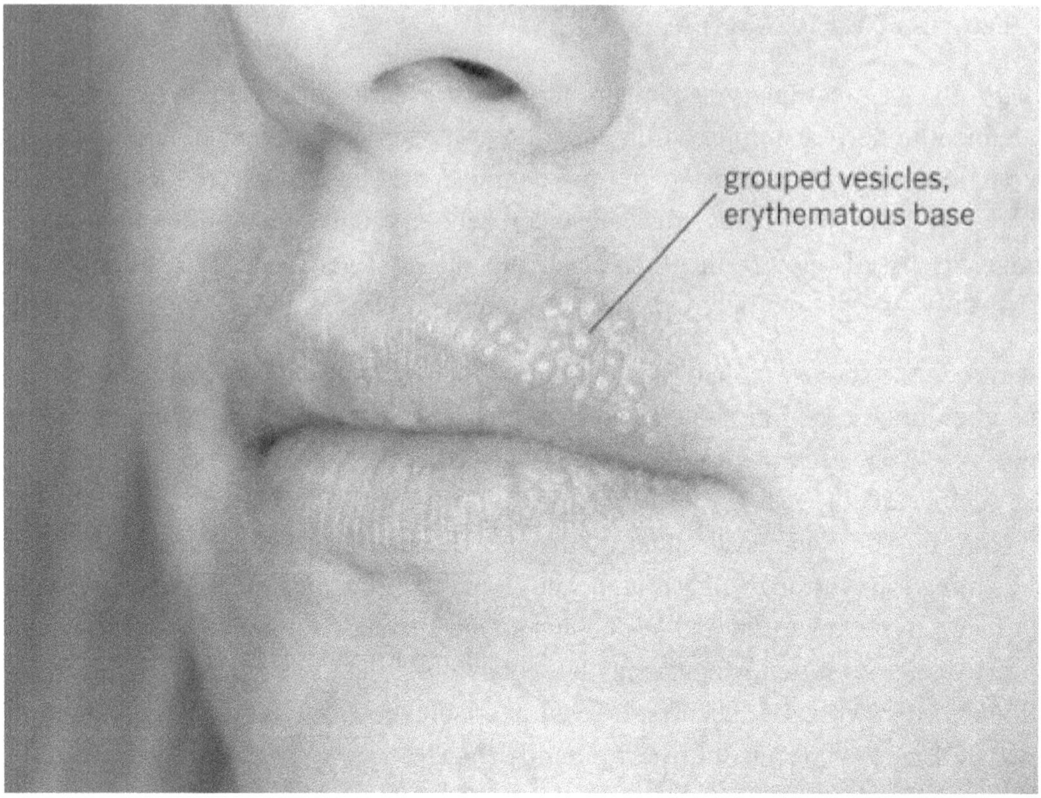

Clinical Presentation and Clinicopathologic Correlation

Clinical Morphology of Bacterial Skin Infection

Bullous impetigo, a distinct clinical variant resulting from localized exfoliative toxin production at the site of infection rather than the more superficial, non-toxin-mediated mechanism of classic non-bullous impetigo, presents with flaccid bullae that rupture to leave a characteristic collarette of scale, and shares its underlying toxin-mediated superficial cleavage mechanism with staphylococcal scalded skin syndrome discussed above, differing principally in the localized rather than generalized extent of toxin effect, itself a reflection of localized infection and toxin production rather than the hematogenous toxin dissemination that characterizes staphylococcal scalded skin syndrome.

Impetigo presents as honey-colored crusted erosions, most common in children, favoring the face and other exposed areas, while folliculitis presents as follicular-centered erythematous papules and pustules that can occur anywhere hair-bearing skin is present, and cellulitis presents as an expanding area of warm, tender, poorly demarcated erythema, typically diagnosed clinically without biopsy but occasionally sampled when the diagnosis is uncertain or when a mimicker, including the lipodermatosclerosis discussed in Chapter 10, is a genuine consideration. Necrotizing soft tissue infection, discussed in Chapter 10's infectious panniculitis section, represents the most urgent bacterial skin and soft tissue presentation, and this chapter's emphasis on rapid organism class recognition, discussed in the rhythm layer above, applies with particular urgency in this specific, life-threatening clinical context.

Clinical Morphology of Fungal and Viral Skin Infection

Tinea capitis, dermatophyte infection of the scalp, carries particular clinical significance among the dermatophyte infections given its capacity to produce scarring alopecia if inadequately treated and its distinct epidemiology, favoring young children and requiring systemic rather than topical antifungal therapy given the difficulty topical agents have penetrating the hair follicle to the depth required for cure, a treatment distinction worth emphasizing whenever this specific dermatophyte infection subtype is diagnosed or suspected.

Dermatophyte infection presents as annular, scaly plaques with an active, often slightly raised border and central clearing, the specific clinical name varying by body site (tinea corporis, tinea pedis, tinea cruris, tinea capitis), while tinea versicolor presents as hypopigmented or hyperpigmented, finely scaly patches favoring the trunk, accentuated by ultraviolet exposure that tans unaffected skin while affected skin remains relatively unchanged. Herpes simplex virus presents as grouped vesicles on an erythematous base, classically perioral or genital and frequently recurrent at the same site given the virus's established latency within sensory ganglia, while varicella-zoster virus presents as either primary varicella (disseminated vesicles in a non-immune host) or herpes zoster (grouped vesicles in a dermatomal distribution reflecting reactivation of latent virus within a single sensory ganglion), a distribution difference with direct diagnostic value even before biopsy is considered.

Special Populations: Immunocompromised Hosts and Disseminated Infection

Immunocompromised patients, extending the principle developed in Chapter 8 and revisited throughout this book, are susceptible to atypical, disseminated, or unusually severe presentations across every organism class discussed in this chapter: disseminated herpes zoster crossing multiple dermatomes, extensive or treatment-resistant dermatophyte infection, and crusted (Norwegian) scabies, a markedly hyperinfested variant showing thick, crusted plaques teeming with mites, occurring specifically in immunocompromised or neurologically impaired patients unable to mount the itch-scratch response that normally limits mite burden in immunocompetent hosts. Crusted scabies carries particular infection control significance given its markedly elevated organism burden and correspondingly higher contagiousness relative to classic scabies, making prompt recognition, appropriate isolation precautions, and coordinated treatment of both the patient and close contacts an important component of managing this specific presentation beyond the individual patient's own treatment.

Clinical Morphology of Molluscum Contagiosum and Arthropod Reactions

Molluscum contagiosum presents as firm, dome-shaped, flesh-colored to pearly papules with a characteristic central umbilication, most common in children and, in adults, associated with sexual transmission when occurring in an anogenital distribution or with immunocompromise when presenting as unusually extensive or persistent disease, a clinical pattern that, together with the biopsy findings discussed above, should prompt consideration of underlying immunosuppression when the presentation is unusually severe. Arthropod bite reactions present as pruritic papules, often grouped or in a linear array reflecting a single feeding episode across adjacent skin, with morphology and distribution varying by the specific arthropod responsible, flea bites favoring the lower legs and ankles, bedbug bites favoring exposed skin during sleep, and mosquito bites occurring wherever skin was exposed during outdoor activity, environmental and exposure history often providing more diagnostically useful information than the biopsy itself for this specific, generally self-limited entity.

Special Populations: Congenital and Perinatal Infection

Congenital syphilis, while caused by a spirochete rather than the organism classes emphasized elsewhere in this chapter, deserves specific mention given its capacity to produce a range of cutaneous findings, including a diffuse maculopapular eruption with characteristic palmoplantar involvement, together with systemic manifestations spanning skeletal, hepatic, and central nervous system involvement, findings that together underscore why any suspected congenital infection warrants a broad, systematic evaluation rather than a skin-limited diagnostic focus alone.

Congenital and perinatal infections carry distinct and often more severe implications than their acquired counterparts: neonatal herpes simplex virus infection, acquired most often through intrapartum exposure to maternal genital herpes, carries substantial morbidity and mortality risk and requires urgent recognition and antiviral treatment given the potential for disseminated, life-threatening disease in the neonate, a risk profile dramatically different from typical recurrent herpes simplex virus infection in an immunocompetent adult. Congenital varicella syndrome, resulting from maternal varicella infection during early pregnancy, produces characteristic cutaneous scarring in a dermatomal distribution together with limb hypoplasia and other congenital anomalies, illustrating that the same virus, varicella-zoster virus, produces dramatically different clinical presentations depending on the timing and context of infection, congenital exposure during organogenesis producing structural anomalies rather than the typical vesicular eruption of postnatally acquired varicella.

CLINICAL PEARL: A biopsy showing multinucleated, cytopathic keratinocytes confirms herpesvirus infection as a class but cannot distinguish herpes simplex virus from varicella-zoster virus; clinical distribution (grouped, recurrent, perioral or genital versus dermatomal) and, when the distinction carries management consequence, immunohistochemistry or molecular testing make this specific determination.

Differential Diagnosis and Histologic Mimickers

Herpesvirus Infection Versus Other Vesiculobullous Processes

Eczema herpeticum, disseminated herpes simplex virus infection superimposed on a background of atopic dermatitis or another disrupted skin barrier condition, represents a distinct and clinically urgent presentation of herpesvirus infection that can be mistaken for a severe flare of the underlying eczematous condition itself, a mistake with meaningful treatment consequence given the need for prompt antiviral therapy rather than escalated topical corticosteroid treatment that would otherwise be appropriate for a straightforward eczema flare. The clinical clue most useful for distinguishing eczema herpeticum from a simple eczema flare is the presence of punched-out erosions and monomorphic vesicles or pustules superimposed on the background dermatitis, a distribution and morphology that should prompt Tzanck smear or biopsy whenever identified in a patient with known atopic dermatitis presenting with acute worsening.

Herpesvirus infection must be distinguished from the autoimmune bullous diseases discussed in this book's earlier chapters and from other acantholytic processes, a distinction made straightforward in most cases by the presence of the characteristic multinucleated, cytopathic keratinocytes that are absent in autoimmune bullous disease, though direct immunofluorescence, when performed, can help resolve genuinely ambiguous cases and additionally excludes a concurrent or superimposed autoimmune bullous process, an occasionally encountered and clinically important overlap scenario in which herpesvirus infection is superimposed on a background autoimmune blistering disease.

Dermatophyte Infection Versus Its Inflammatory Mimickers

Dermatophyte infection's annular, scaly clinical morphology can closely mimic several inflammatory dermatoses discussed elsewhere in this book, including nummular eczematous dermatitis and, particularly when treated with topical corticosteroids that partially suppress the inflammatory response while allowing continued fungal proliferation (tinea incognito), the diagnosis can become genuinely difficult both clinically and histologically, making PAS-D staining an essential, low-cost step for any biopsy of an annular or scaly eruption where dermatophyte infection has not already been confidently excluded by potassium hydroxide preparation or fungal culture. This scenario illustrates directly why this chapter's organizing principle, organism class recognition before assuming an inflammatory diagnosis, carries genuine diagnostic stakes: a biopsy interpreted as spongiotic dermatitis without PAS-D staining performed risks missing an underlying dermatophyte infection that would not respond to, and could be worsened by, topical corticosteroid therapy directed at a presumed inflammatory diagnosis.

A 34-year-old patient presents with a several-week history of an expanding, minimally itchy, annular, scaly plaque on the trunk, previously treated with a topical corticosteroid for presumed nummular eczema without improvement and, if anything, mild worsening and expansion of the affected area. Biopsy is obtained given the atypical treatment response, and initial hematoxylin and eosin sections show a mild superficial spongiotic dermatitis without an obviously specific diagnostic feature, prompting reflexive PAS-D staining given this chapter's emphasis on active fungal exclusion whenever an annular, scaly, treatment-resistant eruption is encountered. PAS-D staining identifies scattered hyphae within the stratum corneum, confirming dermatophyte infection (tinea incognito) rather than the presumed eczematous process, and the corticosteroid-modified presentation is recognized as explaining both the atypical, only mildly inflamed histologic appearance and the lack of response to, and probable worsening from, topical corticosteroid therapy. Diagnosis of tinea incognito is rendered, prompting a switch to appropriate topical or systemic antifungal therapy and illustrating directly why PAS-D staining should be considered routinely, rather than reserved only for clinically obvious fungal presentations, whenever an annular or scaly eruption fails to respond as expected to standard eczema-directed treatment.

Molluscum Contagiosum Versus Other Umbilicated Papules

Molluscum contagiosum's umbilicated papule morphology overlaps clinically with a handful of other umbilicated lesions, including, in an immunocompromised patient, cutaneous cryptococcosis and other deep fungal infections presenting with molluscum-like lesions, a clinically important mimicker given the substantially different management these entities require, making biopsy with special staining a reasonable and prudent step whenever an immunocompromised patient presents with new umbilicated papules rather than assuming a presumptive molluscum contagiosum diagnosis on clinical grounds alone. In an immunocompetent host, this distinction is rarely necessary given molluscum's characteristic appearance and benign course, but the threshold for biopsy should lower substantially whenever immunocompromise, atypical morphology, or a poor treatment response is present.

Verruca Vulgaris Versus Other Papillomatous and Hyperkeratotic Lesions

Verruca vulgaris must be distinguished from seborrheic keratosis and other papillomatous or hyperkeratotic epidermal lesions discussed in this book's later chapters on epidermal neoplasms, a distinction generally made straightforward by the presence of koilocytosis and the characteristic vertically oriented, tapering rete ridge pattern specific to verruca vulgaris, findings absent in seborrheic keratosis's more horizontally oriented, "string sign" architecture. In an immunocompromised patient, atypical, extensive, or treatment-resistant verrucae should additionally prompt consideration of a coexisting or evolving squamous neoplastic process, given human papillomavirus's recognized oncogenic potential in specific high-risk subtypes and in the setting of prolonged immunosuppression, a consideration developed further in this book's later chapters covering epidermal and keratinocytic neoplasms.

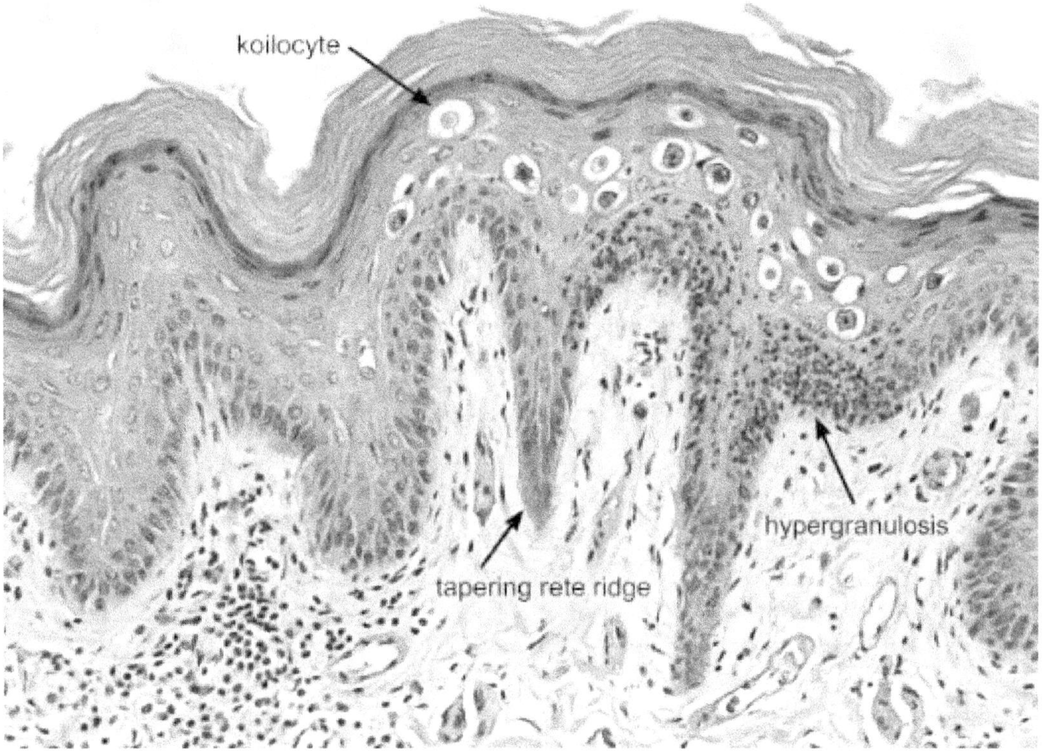

Ancillary Studies

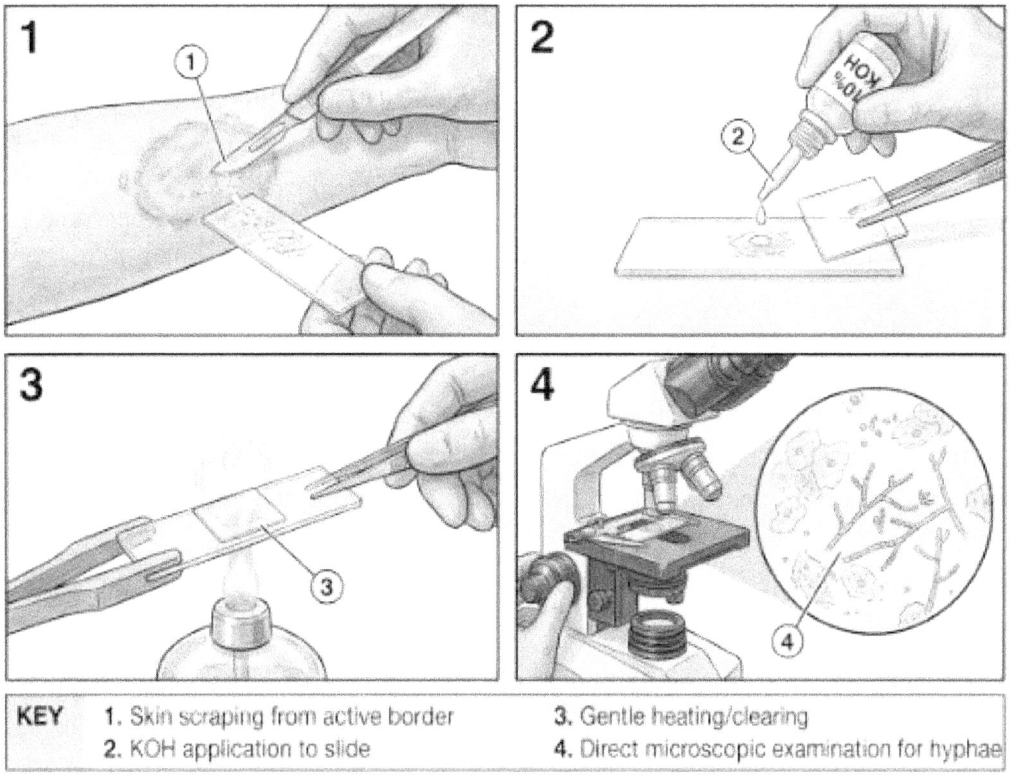

Special Stains and Gram Staining

Blood culture and, when clinically indicated, additional site-specific cultures should be pursued whenever a bacterial skin infection is accompanied by systemic signs of infection, fever, hypotension, or altered mental status, since these findings raise concern for bacteremia or sepsis extending beyond the local cutaneous process, a scenario in which the skin biopsy or culture represents only one component of a broader, systemically directed diagnostic evaluation.

Gram staining identifies and classifies bacteria as gram-positive or gram-negative and by morphology (cocci versus rods), providing rapid, actionable information supporting empiric antimicrobial selection, discussed further in Chapter 10's infectious panniculitis section, while PAS-D and Grocott methenamine silver staining, discussed extensively in Chapter 2 and again in Chapter 8, remain the essential stains for identifying dermatophyte hyphae and other fungal organisms within this chapter's superficial fungal infections, with PAS-D generally preferred for stratum corneum-confined dermatophyte infection given its superior staining of the surrounding keratin architecture relative to Grocott methenamine silver.

Immunohistochemistry and Molecular Studies for Viral Identification

A 3-day-old neonate presents with grouped vesicles on the scalp at the site of a prior fetal scalp electrode, together with lethargy and poor feeding, prompting urgent evaluation given concern for neonatal herpes simplex virus infection given the maternal history of genital herpes simplex virus infection during the pregnancy. Tzanck smear performed at the bedside shows multinucleated giant keratinocytes, providing rapid presumptive confirmation of herpesvirus infection as a class and supporting immediate initiation of empiric intravenous acyclovir while formal skin biopsy and, critically, cerebrospinal fluid and blood polymerase chain reaction testing are pursued to evaluate for disseminated and central nervous system involvement given the substantial morbidity and mortality risk this specific presentation carries in a neonate. Skin biopsy subsequently confirms the characteristic cytopathic changes, and polymerase chain reaction testing identifies herpes simplex virus type 2, confirming disseminated neonatal herpes simplex virus infection, a diagnosis in which the speed of recognition and treatment initiation, achieved here through the rapid bedside Tzanck smear rather than awaiting formal biopsy results, directly and substantially influences long-term neurologic outcome.

Immunohistochemistry using type-specific antibodies, or, increasingly, polymerase chain reaction-based molecular testing, distinguishes herpes simplex virus from varicella-zoster virus when this distinction carries specific management consequence, most often in an immunocompromised or pregnant patient where antiviral treatment selection or infection control precautions differ meaningfully between these two related but distinct herpesviruses. Human papillomavirus subtyping, while not routinely performed on a typical verruca vulgaris biopsy, becomes clinically relevant in the specific context of anogenital lesions and in immunocompromised patients, where identifying a high-risk oncogenic subtype can meaningfully inform the surveillance and management approach beyond simple lesion removal.

Identifying Mite Parts and Confirming Scabies

Dermoscopy, an ancillary technique performed at the bedside rather than in the pathology laboratory, can identify the classic "delta wing jet" sign, corresponding to the mite's pigmented mouthparts and forelegs visible at the end of a burrow, and can additionally guide biopsy or skin scraping toward a site with a higher likelihood of containing an identifiable mite, meaningfully improving the diagnostic yield of subsequent histologic or microscopic examination relative to a randomly selected biopsy site within a broader eczematous or excoriated area.

Confirming scabies histologically requires identifying mite parts, ova, or fecal pellets (scybala) within the stratum corneum, a finding present in only a subset of biopsies given the relatively low mite burden typical of classic (non-crusted) scabies, meaning that a negative biopsy does not exclude the diagnosis and that a strongly suggestive clinical presentation, burrows, characteristic distribution favoring finger webs and flexural surfaces, and a wedge-shaped, eosinophil-rich dermal infiltrate on histology, should support empiric treatment even without directly identified organism parts. Crusted scabies, discussed in the clinical presentation section above, shows markedly more abundant mites, ova, and fecal pellets given this variant's substantially higher organism burden, making histologic confirmation correspondingly more straightforward in this specific, high-risk presentation.

Tzanck Smear and Rapid Bedside Diagnosis

The Tzanck smear, performed by unroofing an intact vesicle and cytologically examining the base for multinucleated giant keratinocytes, provides rapid bedside confirmation of herpesvirus infection as a class, though, paralleling the histologic limitation discussed above, it cannot distinguish herpes simplex virus from varicella-zoster virus, making it most useful as an initial, same-visit screening tool that, when positive, can support immediate empiric antiviral therapy while formal biopsy, culture, or molecular testing, when pursued, provides definitive organism-level confirmation and, when needed, type-specific distinction.

Culture and Susceptibility Testing

Viral culture, historically an important diagnostic modality for herpesvirus infection, has been substantially supplanted by the more sensitive and rapid polymerase chain reaction-based molecular testing discussed above in most clinical settings, though viral culture retains occasional utility when antiviral resistance testing is specifically required, a scenario most relevant in immunocompromised patients with recurrent, treatment-refractory herpesvirus infection.

Bacterial culture with antimicrobial susceptibility testing, submitted at the time of biopsy or through a separate swab whenever purulent material is accessible, provides essential organism-specific and resistance information, particularly important given the rising prevalence of methicillin-resistant Staphylococcus aureus in both community and healthcare settings, information that directly shapes empiric antibiotic selection pending culture results and definitively guides therapy once results return. Fungal culture, while slower than PAS-D staining to return a result, provides organism speciation beyond the genus-level information special stains typically offer, valuable when the specific dermatophyte species influences treatment duration or when an atypical, non-dermatophyte mold is being considered in an unusual or treatment-resistant presentation.

CAUTION: A negative fungal or mite-specific finding on a single biopsy level does not exclude dermatophyte infection or scabies respectively, given both entities' potentially patchy or low organism burden. Examining multiple levels, and maintaining clinical suspicion when the presentation strongly suggests either diagnosis despite an initially unremarkable biopsy, prevents this specific and clinically consequential diagnostic pitfall.

Management Implications

Connecting Diagnosis to Treatment Pathway

The management principles this chapter closes with echo those developed across every infectious entity discussed in this book's earlier chapters, granulomatous mycobacterial and deep fungal disease in Chapter 8, infectious panniculitis in Chapter 10: organism-directed therapy, informed by the specific ancillary studies this chapter's differential requires, consistently outperforms empiric, pattern-directed treatment alone, and the diagnostic urgency this chapter has emphasized for its most severe presentations, necrotizing infection, disseminated neonatal herpes, and crusted scabies, reflects this book's broader, recurring theme that accurate and timely pattern recognition carries direct, measurable consequence for patient outcomes.

Bacterial skin infection is managed with organism-directed topical or systemic antimicrobial therapy, with incision and drainage additionally required for abscess formation; superficial fungal infection is managed with topical or, for more extensive or nail/hair-involving disease, systemic antifungal therapy; herpesvirus infection is managed with antiviral therapy, particularly important and often escalated to intravenous administration in immunocompromised or disseminated presentations; human papillomavirus infection is managed with destructive or immune-modulating therapy directed at the visible lesion, since no currently available therapy eradicates the underlying viral infection itself; and scabies is managed with topical or oral scabicidal therapy applied to the affected patient and close contacts simultaneously, given this infection's high transmissibility within households and other close-contact settings.

Complications and Prognosis

Neonatal herpes simplex virus infection, discussed earlier in this chapter, carries a prognosis directly tied to the speed of diagnosis and treatment initiation, with disseminated or central nervous system disease carrying substantially higher morbidity and mortality than skin-limited disease, underscoring once again this chapter's recurring emphasis on diagnostic urgency for its most severe presentations.

Bacterial skin infection generally carries an excellent prognosis with appropriate antimicrobial therapy, though necrotizing soft tissue infection, discussed in Chapter 10, carries substantial morbidity and mortality risk requiring emergent surgical intervention, underscoring the wide prognostic range this single organism class can produce depending on the depth and extent of tissue involvement. Herpes zoster carries a risk of postherpetic neuralgia, persistent pain in the affected dermatome lasting months to years after the acute eruption resolves, occurring more commonly in older patients and representing a substantial, often underappreciated source of long-term morbidity that vaccination, discussed below, meaningfully reduces. Molluscum contagiosum and verruca vulgaris are generally self-limited in immunocompetent hosts, resolving over months to years even without treatment, though this natural history is substantially prolonged or altered in immunocompromised patients, in whom these entities can become extensive, persistent, and more difficult to treat.

Prevention and Screening

Prenatal screening for maternal genital herpes simplex virus infection and appropriate intrapartum management, including consideration of cesarean delivery in mothers with active lesions at the time of delivery, represents an important preventive measure directly reducing the risk of neonatal herpes simplex virus transmission discussed earlier in this chapter.

Herpes zoster vaccination, recommended for eligible adults, meaningfully reduces the incidence and severity of varicella-zoster virus reactivation and its associated complications, including postherpetic neuralgia, representing genuine primary and secondary prevention opportunity for one of this chapter's most clinically significant viral entities. Human papillomavirus vaccination, most protective when administered before sexual debut, reduces the incidence of the high-risk oncogenic subtypes associated with anogenital and oropharyngeal malignancy, extending this chapter's infectious disease coverage into genuine cancer prevention territory, while patients diagnosed with crusted scabies warrant infection control coordination extending beyond the individual patient, as discussed in the clinical presentation section, given this variant's outsized transmission risk to caregivers and close contacts.

Patient Education and Counseling

Patients with recurrent herpes simplex virus infection benefit from counseling regarding trigger avoidance (ultraviolet exposure, stress, and illness among commonly reported triggers), the availability of suppressive antiviral therapy for patients with frequent recurrences, and the ongoing transmission risk even during asymptomatic periods given this virus's capacity for subclinical viral shedding. Patients diagnosed with scabies and their close contacts benefit from clear, specific counseling regarding simultaneous treatment of all household members and close contacts regardless of symptom status, environmental decontamination of bedding and clothing, and the expected persistence of pruritus for several weeks following successful treatment as a normal post-treatment phenomenon rather than a sign of treatment failure, a distinction that, when not proactively explained, frequently leads to unnecessary repeat treatment courses. Parents of children with molluscum contagiosum benefit from reassurance regarding this condition's generally benign, self-limited course, and from practical counseling regarding measures to reduce autoinoculation and transmission to close contacts, including avoiding shared bathing items and covering lesions during contact sports, without the anxiety that a viral skin infection diagnosis can sometimes provoke in parents unfamiliar with this specific, generally low-stakes entity.

THE REACTION PATTERN RECOGNITION SYSTEM — The Infectious Dermatoses Pattern Family

---

The Pattern: Cutaneous infection organized by organism class (bacterial, fungal, viral, parasitic) and by the resulting histologic reaction (suppurative, granulomatous, vesiculobullous/cytopathic, eosinophilic hypersensitivity), integrating this book's earlier granulomatous and vasculopathic infectious content into a unified organism-first framework.

Histologic Signature: Neutrophilic infiltrate with organisms on Gram stain defines bacterial infection; hyphae in the stratum corneum on PAS-D defines dermatophyte infection; multinucleated, cytopathic keratinocytes define herpesvirus infection; koilocytosis and papillomatosis define human papillomavirus infection; large eosinophilic cytoplasmic inclusions define molluscum contagiosum; wedge-shaped eosinophilic infiltrate with mite parts defines scabies.

The Decision: Identify the dominant inflammatory cell type and any organism-specific cytopathic or structural change first to narrow the organism class, then select the targeted special stain, culture, or molecular study that class specifically requires, then correlate with clinical distribution and host immune status.

Trap Logic: Immunocompromised hosts show blunted or atypical reactions across every organism class, understating apparent severity; dermatophyte infection modified by topical corticosteroids (tinea incognito) can mimic an inflammatory dermatosis and worsen with continued corticosteroid use; a negative biopsy for fungal elements or mite parts does not exclude either diagnosis given patchy or low organism burden; and eczema herpeticum can be mistaken for a simple eczema flare, delaying urgent antiviral therapy.

Pattern Anchor: Match the inflammatory pattern and any cytopathic change to organism class before ordering special stains; actively exclude dermatophyte infection with PAS-D staining whenever an annular, scaly, treatment-resistant eruption is biopsied; never let a single negative special stain level override strong clinical suspicion for fungal or parasitic infection; treat neonatal, disseminated, and necrotizing presentations as diagnostic emergencies.

Summary and Key Concepts

Cutaneous infectious disease is organized by causative organism class, bacterial, fungal, viral, and parasitic, each producing a characteristic histologic reaction that, together with immunohistochemical, molecular, and culture-based ancillary studies, confirms the specific organism responsible.

Host immune status modifies the histologic reaction across every organism class in this chapter, with immunocompromised, neonatal, and congenitally infected patients showing blunted, atypical, disseminated, or structurally distinct presentations that require heightened rather than lowered diagnostic suspicion.

Multinucleated, cytopathic keratinocytes confirm herpesvirus infection as a class but require immunohistochemistry or molecular testing, together with clinical distribution, to distinguish herpes simplex virus from varicella-zoster virus when this distinction carries management consequence.

PAS-D staining should be applied liberally to annular, scaly, or treatment-resistant eruptions given dermatophyte infection's capacity to mimic inflammatory dermatitis, particularly when modified by prior topical corticosteroid use (tinea incognito), and eczema herpeticum should be actively excluded whenever atopic dermatitis worsens acutely with new punched-out erosions.

Scabies confirmation depends on identifying mite parts, ova, or fecal pellets, a finding present in only a subset of biopsies given typically low organism burden, making strong clinical suspicion sufficient grounds for empiric treatment even when histologic confirmation is not achieved.

CHAPTER 13: MELANOCYTIC NEVI AND SIMULATORS OF MELANOMA

Learning Objectives

1. Classify melanocytic proliferations by architectural level (junctional, compound, intradermal) and by growth pattern.
2. Distinguish common acquired nevi from the major nevus variants that clinically or histologically simulate melanoma.
3. Identify the histopathologic features and diagnostic criteria of dysplastic (Clark) nevi, Spitz nevi, and blue nevi.
4. Recognize the specific architectural and cytologic features that distinguish benign melanocytic simulators from melanoma.
5. Construct a systematic differential diagnosis for an ambiguous melanocytic proliferation, including the appropriate use of ancillary studies.
6. Select appropriate immunohistochemical and molecular ancillary studies for diagnostically challenging melanocytic lesions.

Definition and Classification

Melanocytic Proliferations as a Structural Continuum

This chapter opens this book's dedicated coverage of pigmented lesion pathology, the diagnostic discipline most closely associated with dermatopathology in both clinical and public perception, and establishes the structural and cytologic vocabulary that Chapter 14's melanoma coverage builds directly upon. Melanocytic nevi are organized along a developmental continuum reflecting the progressive migration of nevus cells from the dermal-epidermal junction into the dermis over time: junctional nevi, with nevus cells confined to the dermal-epidermal junction; compound nevi, with nevus cells present both at the junction and within the dermis; and intradermal nevi, with nevus cells confined entirely to the dermis, having lost their junctional component as the lesion matures, a progression that in most patients unfolds gradually over years to decades and explains the clinically observed tendency of nevi to become more elevated and less pigmented with age.

This chapter's diagnostic framework rests on a single foundational principle that will recur throughout this chapter and into Chapter 14: benign melanocytic proliferations, regardless of specific subtype, show architectural symmetry, maturation with depth (nevus cells becoming smaller, less pigmented, and more dispersed as they extend deeper into the dermis), and cytologic uniformity, while malignant melanocytic proliferations characteristically show asymmetry, a lack of maturation, and cytologic atypia, a set of contrasting criteria this chapter applies systematically to each nevus subtype's specific simulation of melanoma.

Classification of Nevus Variants Covered in This Chapter

Beyond the common acquired nevus, this chapter covers the specific nevus variants most likely to simulate melanoma clinically, histologically, or both: the dysplastic (Clark) nevus, showing architectural and cytologic atypia that can overlap with melanoma; the Spitz nevus, showing large epithelioid and spindled melanocytes that can be cytologically alarming despite benign behavior in the great majority of cases; the blue nevus, showing deeply pigmented dendritic melanocytes within the dermis that can simulate nodular melanoma clinically; and a group of additional simulators, including the recurrent nevus, the deep penetrating nevus, and the combined nevus, each developed in the sections that follow.

Congenital Melanocytic Nevi

Congenital melanocytic nevi, present at birth or appearing within the first weeks of life, are classified by projected adult size into small (less than 1.5 centimeters), medium (1.5 to 20 centimeters), and large or giant (greater than 20 centimeters) categories, a size-based classification that carries direct prognostic and management significance developed throughout this chapter, since melanoma risk, though low in absolute terms for the great majority of congenital nevi, rises with increasing lesion size and is concentrated disproportionately in the large and giant categories. Congenital nevi are histologically and developmentally distinct from common acquired nevi, reflecting melanocytic proliferation during a specific embryonic developmental window rather than the postnatal, sun-exposure-associated proliferation typical of acquired nevi, a distinction that explains this entity's characteristic histologic extension into deeper dermal and subcutaneous structures discussed in the histopathologic features section below. Small and medium congenital nevi are considerably more common than the large and giant categories and, in the great majority of affected patients, follow a clinical course and carry a risk profile close to that of an acquired nevus, a reassuring distinction this chapter emphasizes explicitly given how frequently the term congenital nevus is, understandably but inaccurately, equated by patients and non-specialist clinicians with the substantially higher-risk giant category alone.

Epidemiology of Nevus Development and Risk Stratification

Total nevus count rises through childhood and adolescence, peaks in early adulthood, and gradually declines thereafter as nevi involute, a trajectory that correlates with, and is used clinically as, a surrogate marker for cumulative and intermittent ultraviolet exposure during the developmentally sensitive early decades of life. Individuals with fair skin phototype, red or blond hair, light-colored eyes, and a tendency to freckle or sunburn rather than tan carry both a higher total nevus count and a disproportionately elevated melanoma risk per nevus, a risk-stratification principle that informs the surveillance intensity discussed in the management implications section below, together with family history of melanoma or of numerous dysplastic nevi, which independently elevates risk beyond phenotype alone and frequently prompts referral for formal total body photography and dermoscopic surveillance.

Entity	Architectural Level	Key Distinguishing Feature	Melanoma Simulation Risk
Common acquired nevus	Junctional, compound, or intradermal	Symmetric, well-circumscribed, matures with depth	Low
Dysplastic (Clark) nevus	Junctional or compound	Architectural disorder, lentiginous junctional component, lamellar fibroplasia	Moderate (architectural/cytologic overlap)
Spitz nevus	Junctional, compound, or intradermal	Large epithelioid/spindled melanocytes, Kamino bodies, maturation with depth	High (cytologic atypia)
Blue nevus	Dermal	Deeply pigmented dendritic melanocytes, dermal-based	Moderate (clinical nodular simulation)
Recurrent (persistent) nevus	Junctional/compound at scar	Melanocytic proliferation confined to scar, no extension beyond	High (mimics melanoma at biopsy site)
Deep penetrating nevus	Dermal, wedge-shaped	Pigmented epithelioid/spindled cells in a symmetric wedge	Moderate (deep extension, cytologic atypia)
Congenital melanocytic nevus	Junctional, compound, or intradermal, extending into deep dermis/subcutis	Adnexal and neurovascular infiltration, single-file dermal dispersion	Low overall; rises with size (highest in giant nevi)
Combined nevus	Compound, with distinct dual components	Two histologically distinct melanocytic populations within one lesion	Moderate (can simulate collision with melanoma)
Halo nevus	Junctional or compound, with lymphocytic infiltrate	Dense band-like lymphocytic infiltrate surrounding regressing nevus cells	Low (must exclude regressing melanoma)

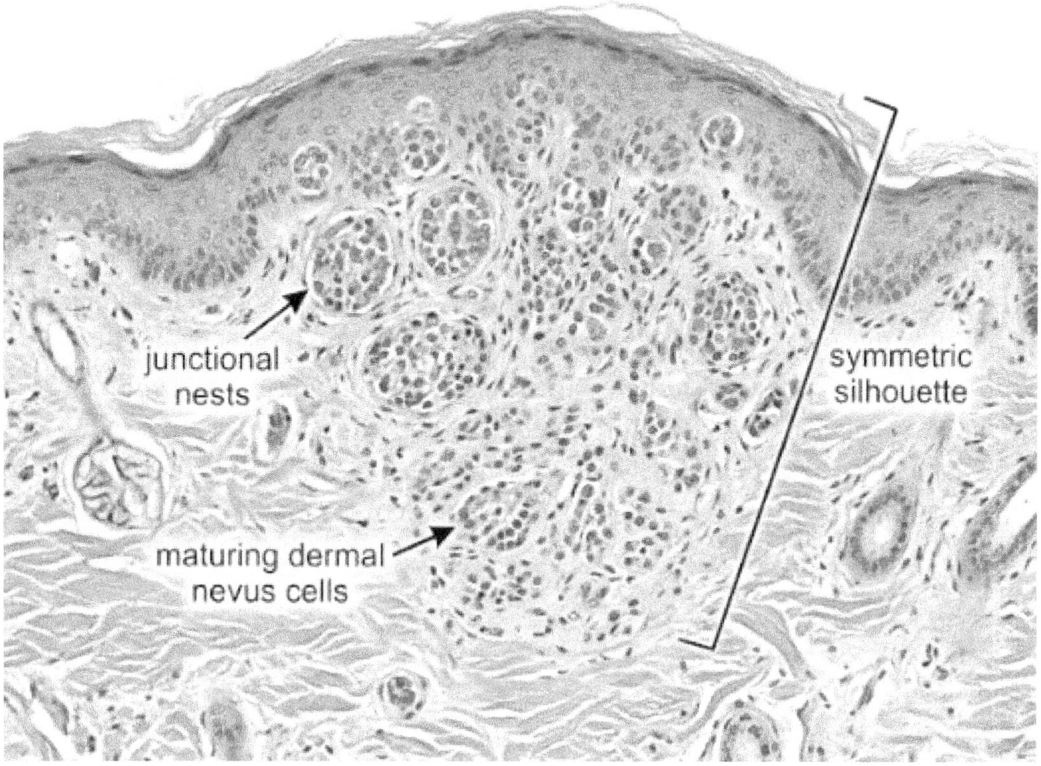

Etiology and Pathogenesis

Mechanisms of Common Acquired Nevus Development

Common acquired nevi arise from clonal proliferation of melanocytes, most often driven by an activating BRAF mutation (most commonly BRAF V600E) that, in the setting of a nevus, triggers oncogene-induced senescence, a protective cellular mechanism that halts further proliferation and explains why the great majority of nevi remain stable, benign lesions throughout life despite harboring a mutation that, in a different cellular context, drives malignant transformation, a phenomenon developed further in Chapter 14's discussion of melanoma pathogenesis. Ultraviolet radiation exposure, particularly intense, intermittent exposure during childhood and adolescence, correlates with total nevus count, explaining the well-established epidemiologic association between high nevus count and increased melanoma risk, though this relationship is understood as a marker of shared ultraviolet exposure and genetic susceptibility rather than direct malignant transformation of individual nevi in the great majority of cases.

Mechanisms of Dysplastic (Clark) Nevus Development

Dysplastic nevi are understood to represent an intermediate point along a biological continuum between common acquired nevi and melanoma, though the great majority of individual dysplastic nevi never progress to melanoma, and current understanding favors dysplastic nevi as both an independent risk marker for melanoma (patients with multiple dysplastic nevi carry elevated overall melanoma risk, often arising at a site distinct from any individual dysplastic nevus) and, less commonly, a direct precursor lesion at the specific site where progression occurs. Familial atypical multiple mole and melanoma syndrome, associated with CDKN2A mutations in a subset of affected families, represents the hereditary extreme of this phenotype, characterized by numerous dysplastic nevi and a markedly elevated lifetime melanoma risk that warrants specific genetic counseling and intensified surveillance protocols discussed in the management implications section below.

Mechanisms of Spitz Nevus Development

Spitz nevi arise from a distinct genetic pathway relative to common acquired and dysplastic nevi, most often driven by kinase fusion events (involving ALK, ROS1, NTRK1, and related kinases) or by HRAS mutations, rather than the BRAF mutations typical of common nevi, a genetically distinct pathway that correlates with this entity's characteristically different cytomorphology, large epithelioid and spindled cells rather than the smaller, more uniform cells of a common nevus, discussed further in the histopathologic features section below. This distinct molecular pathway has increasingly informed the modern classification of Spitz tumors and has become directly relevant to the ancillary molecular testing discussed later in this chapter for diagnostically challenging cases along the Spitz spectrum.

Mechanisms of Blue Nevus Development

Blue nevi arise from melanocytes that fail to complete their normal embryologic migration from the neural crest to the dermal-epidermal junction, remaining instead within the dermis in a dendritic, deeply pigmented form reminiscent of normal dermal melanocytes found in specific anatomic sites (the sacral region in Mongolian spot, for instance), a distinct embryologic origin from the epidermal melanocyte-derived common acquired nevus that explains blue nevi's characteristically dermal-only location without a junctional component, discussed further below. GNAQ and GNA11 mutations, activating mutations in G-protein alpha subunits, have been identified in blue nevi and related dermal melanocytic proliferations, a molecular pathway distinct from both the BRAF pathway of common nevi and the kinase fusion pathway of Spitz nevi, and one shared with uveal melanoma, reflecting these entities' common origin from a similar dermal or extracutaneous melanocytic lineage.

Mechanisms of Congenital Melanocytic Nevus Development

Congenital melanocytic nevi most commonly arise from an activating NRAS mutation acquired during early embryonic melanocyte development, a molecular pathway distinct from the BRAF pathway of common acquired nevi and one that correlates with this entity's characteristic pattern of deep dermal and subcutaneous extension, since the mutation is present in melanocyte precursors before their migration and proliferation throughout the developing dermis is complete, producing a proliferation that is developmentally, rather than simply anatomically, deeper than an acquired nevus. Large and giant congenital nevi carry an associated risk of neurocutaneous melanosis, proliferation of melanocytes within the leptomeninges and central nervous system sharing the same embryonic origin and, in some cases, the same NRAS mutation, a risk that informs the neuroimaging screening discussion in the management implications section below for patients with large or giant congenital nevi, particularly those with numerous satellite nevi, a recognized additional risk marker for this specific complication.

Environmental and Genetic Risk Factors Beyond Ultraviolet Exposure

Beyond ultraviolet exposure and the CDKN2A mutations associated with familial atypical multiple mole and melanoma syndrome discussed above, iatrogenic immunosuppression, in solid organ transplant recipients and patients on long-term immunosuppressive therapy for autoimmune disease, is associated with an increased total nevus count and, in some reports, atypical nevus morphology, a population in whom the surveillance principles discussed throughout this chapter warrant particular vigilance given this population's independently elevated melanoma risk developed further in Chapter 14. Eruptive nevi, the rapid onset of numerous new nevi over a short period, can occur in the setting of immunosuppression, severe systemic illness, blistering disease, or certain chemotherapeutic agents, a phenomenon that, while benign, warrants careful individual lesion assessment given the broader clinical context in which it typically arises.

THE REACTION PATTERN RECOGNITION SYSTEM — Symmetry, Maturation, and Cytologic Uniformity as the Universal Benign Anchor

The Pattern: Symmetry, Maturation with Depth, and Cytologic Uniformity as the Universal Criteria Distinguishing Benign Melanocytic Proliferations from Melanoma

Histologic Signature: A symmetric, well-circumscribed silhouette; nevus cells that progressively decrease in size, pigmentation, and nesting with increasing dermal depth; and cytologically uniform nevus cells without significant nuclear pleomorphism, hyperchromasia, or mitotic activity, particularly in the deep dermal component.

The Decision: Apply these three criteria, symmetry, maturation, cytologic uniformity, to every melanocytic proliferation encountered in this chapter and the next, regardless of specific subtype, as the foundational screening assessment before subtype-specific criteria are applied; a lesion failing one or more of these criteria warrants heightened scrutiny and, frequently, ancillary study support even when a specific benign subtype (Spitz, dysplastic, blue) is otherwise suggested.

Trap Logic: Certain benign nevus variants, most notably the Spitz nevus and the deep penetrating nevus, can show features that individually mimic atypia, large cell size, prominent nucleoli, occasional mitoses in the superficial component, without representing true malignancy, meaning these three criteria must be applied holistically and in the specific context of the suspected subtype rather than mechanically against a single universal threshold.

Pattern Anchor: Symmetric, matures, uniform: benign. Asymmetric, fails to mature, atypical: concerning for melanoma. Every melanocytic lesion in this chapter and the next is assessed against this three-part anchor before any subtype-specific refinement is applied.

Histopathologic Features and Diagnostic Criteria

Diagnostic Features of the Common Acquired Nevus

The common acquired nevus shows nevus cells arranged in well-formed, evenly spaced nests along the dermal-epidermal junction in the junctional and compound subtypes, with a symmetric, dome-shaped or flat silhouette and sharp lateral circumscription, and, in the dermal component of compound and intradermal nevi, progressive maturation with depth as described above, together with cytologically bland, uniform nuclei and rare to absent mitotic figures, particularly in the deep dermal component, where mitotic activity should prompt careful additional evaluation given its comparative rarity in this specific location within a benign nevus.

Diagnostic Features of the Dysplastic (Clark) Nevus

The dysplastic nevus shows architectural disorder, including a lentiginous (single-cell, non-nested) junctional melanocytic proliferation that characteristically extends beyond ("shoulders") the dermal component of the nevus, together with variable cytologic atypia (nuclear enlargement, hyperchromasia, and irregular nuclear contours) and, distinctively, lamellar (concentric, plate-like) fibroplasia surrounding the rete ridges, a stromal response considered a helpful, though not entirely specific, supportive feature for this diagnosis. Dysplastic nevi are graded by the severity of architectural and cytologic atypia, typically as mild, moderate, or severe, a grading system with meaningful, though imperfect, interobserver reproducibility that nonetheless provides clinically useful information regarding the degree of diagnostic concern a given lesion warrants, developed further in the differential diagnosis section below.

Diagnostic Features of the Spitz Nevus

The Spitz nevus shows large epithelioid or spindled melanocytes, often arranged in a wedge-shaped or symmetric dome-shaped silhouette, with abundant eosinophilic to amphophilic cytoplasm and prominent nucleoli, together with characteristic Kamino bodies, eosinophilic, globular deposits of basement membrane material at the dermal-epidermal junction, and, importantly, maturation with depth despite the individual cells' large size and potentially alarming cytologic appearance in isolation. Mitotic figures can be present in a Spitz nevus, particularly in the superficial component, but should be sparse, typically fewer than two per square millimeter, and, critically, absent from the deep or peripheral margin of the lesion, a specific distributional criterion that carries substantial diagnostic weight when distinguishing a Spitz nevus from a Spitzoid melanoma, discussed further in Chapter 14.

Diagnostic Features of the Blue Nevus and Deep Penetrating Nevus

The common (dendritic) blue nevus shows spindled, heavily pigmented dendritic melanocytes admixed with pigment-laden melanophages, situated within the dermis without an epidermal or junctional component, typically arranged in a poorly circumscribed but symmetric band paralleling the epidermal surface, cytologically bland features that distinguish it readily from melanoma once the entity is correctly recognized. The deep penetrating nevus, a related dermal-based entity, shows pigmented epithelioid and spindled melanocytes arranged in a symmetric, wedge-shaped configuration extending from the dermal-epidermal junction into the deep reticular dermis or subcutis, often with perineural and perivascular extension that, while individually concerning in isolation, is an expected architectural feature of this specific benign entity when combined with the lesion's overall symmetric wedge shape and absence of significant cytologic atypia or mitotic activity.

Diagnostic Features of the Congenital Melanocytic Nevus

The congenital melanocytic nevus shows the same junctional-to-compound-to-intradermal architecture as the common acquired nevus, distinguished histologically by its characteristic pattern of adnexal and neurovascular structure infiltration, nevus cells surrounding and extending along hair follicles, sebaceous glands, eccrine ducts, nerves, and vessels, and by a single-file dispersion of nevus cells between individual collagen bundles in the deep dermis, a distinctive splaying pattern not typical of an acquired nevus even when the latter shows deep dermal extension. Congenital nevi frequently extend into the subcutaneous fat and can show a proliferative nodule, a benign, expansile focus within the nevus that can show increased cellularity and occasional mitoses yet remains distinguishable from melanoma arising within a congenital nevus by its overall maintained symmetry and lack of significant cytologic atypia, discussed further in the differential diagnosis section below.

Diagnostic Features of the Combined Nevus and Halo Nevus

The combined nevus shows two histologically distinct melanocytic populations within a single lesion, most commonly a common acquired or Spitz component together with a blue nevus component, a juxtaposition that can produce a clinically and histologically complex, asymmetric-appearing lesion that warrants careful recognition of each individual component's own benign criteria rather than an overall assessment that inappropriately combines the two distinct populations into a single, potentially alarming composite impression. The halo nevus shows a pre-existing nevus, most often a common acquired nevus, surrounded and progressively replaced by a dense, band-like lymphocytic infiltrate reflecting an immune-mediated regression process, with the nevus cells themselves showing degenerative cytologic changes within the inflamed zone that must be distinguished from the cytologic atypia of a genuinely malignant process, a distinction developed in the differential diagnosis section below.

Special Site Nevi: Acral, Genital, and Scalp Locations

Nevi arising at acral sites (palms, soles), genital skin, and the scalp show site-specific histologic features that can mimic the architectural disorder of a dysplastic nevus or, in the case of genital nevi in young patients, cytologic and architectural atypia that can suggest melanoma to an examiner unfamiliar with these site-specific patterns, features that this chapter emphasizes precisely because their misinterpretation is a well-recognized source of diagnostic overcall. Acral nevi characteristically show a lentiginous junctional component with nest formation concentrated along the crista profunda intermedia (the deep, sweat duct-associated ridge), a normal architectural feature of acral skin that must not be mistaken for the shouldering pattern of a dysplastic nevus, while genital and scalp nevi in patients younger than approximately 40 years can show striking architectural disorder and cytologic atypia, so-called atypical genital nevus or atypical nevus of special anatomic sites, that would be classified as at least moderately dysplastic at a non-special site but that behaves in a reliably benign fashion when the specific anatomic site and patient age are correctly incorporated into the diagnostic assessment.

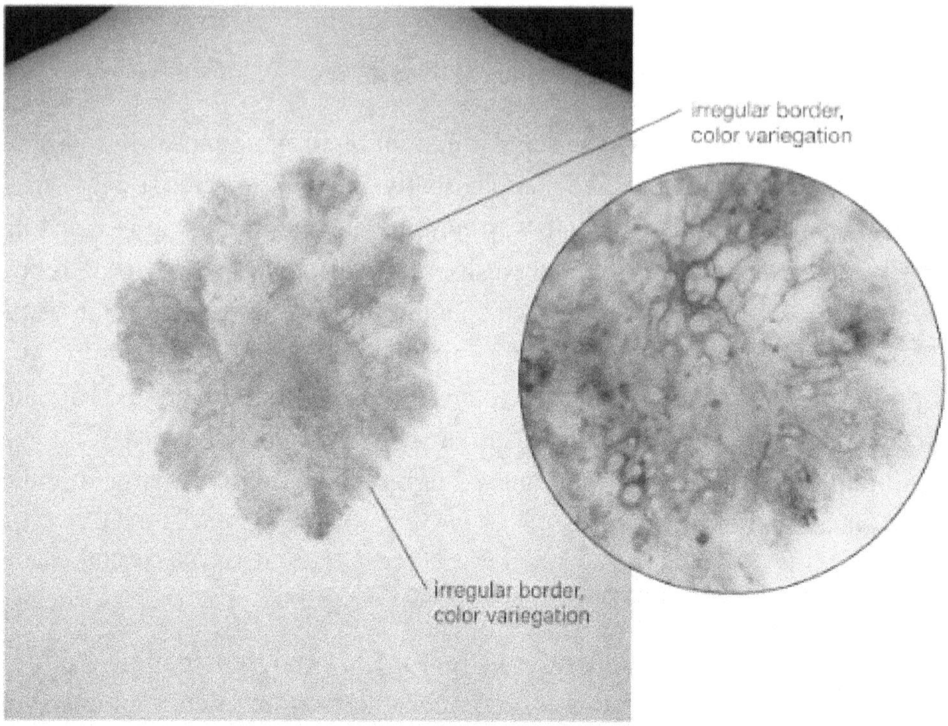

Clinical Presentation and Clinicopathologic Correlation

Clinical Morphology of the Common Acquired and Dysplastic Nevus

Common acquired nevi present as symmetric, well-circumscribed, uniformly pigmented papules or macules, typically appearing during childhood and adolescence and gradually evolving in morphology, from flat and junctional to raised and compound to skin-colored and intradermal, over subsequent decades, a natural evolution that patients and clinicians should understand as expected rather than concerning when it follows this typical, gradual pattern. Dysplastic nevi present with one or more features of the ABCDE criteria (Asymmetry, Border irregularity, Color variegation, Diameter greater than 6 millimeters, Evolution), features that overlap substantially with early melanoma and explain why dysplastic nevi are disproportionately represented among biopsied pigmented lesions, together with a characteristic "fried egg" clinical appearance in some cases, a flat, tan periphery surrounding a more raised, darker central papule.

Clinical Morphology of the Spitz and Blue Nevus

Spitz nevi present classically as a solitary, rapidly growing, pink to red-brown dome-shaped papule or nodule, most common in children and young adults, with the rapid growth phase itself, while alarming to patients and clinicians unfamiliar with this entity's typical natural history, representing an expected feature of this specific benign nevus subtype rather than a sign of malignancy, though this same rapid growth history is precisely what prompts the biopsy that confirms the diagnosis in most cases. Blue nevi present as solitary, deeply pigmented, blue-black to blue-gray papules or nodules, most common on the dorsal hands and feet, scalp, and sacral region, with the distinctive blue-gray color reflecting the Tyndall effect, differential light scattering by dermal melanin as opposed to the browner tones typical of more superficial, epidermal melanin deposition, a color that, given its typical clinical stability and lack of change over time, generally does not raise the same degree of clinical concern as an evolving, variably colored dysplastic nevus or melanoma.

The Recurrent (Persistent) Nevus

The recurrent, or persistent, nevus arises when a previously biopsied nevus, incompletely removed, shows renewed melanocytic proliferation at the biopsy scar site, producing a histologic and, often, clinical picture that can closely mimic melanoma, irregular pigmentation, architectural asymmetry, and, occasionally, mild cytologic atypia within the scar, a diagnostic trap this chapter addresses specifically because of its clinical frequency and the genuine risk of overdiagnosis as melanoma when the history of a prior biopsy at the same site is not communicated to the pathologist. The single most important piece of clinical information for correctly interpreting a recurrent nevus is precisely this prior biopsy history, underscoring once again this book's recurring emphasis on clinicopathologic correlation, since the histologic findings of a recurrent nevus, viewed without this history, can appear genuinely concerning for melanoma arising within a scar.

Clinical Morphology of the Congenital and Combined Nevus

Congenital melanocytic nevi present at birth as tan-to-dark brown patches or plaques, frequently with coarse terminal hair (hypertrichosis) developing over the lesion during infancy and childhood, a clinical feature considered reassuring rather than concerning when it develops uniformly across an otherwise stable lesion. Large and giant congenital nevi, in particular, warrant a structured longitudinal clinical photography protocol from infancy given both the lesion's own evolving surface texture over childhood and the comparatively elevated, though still modest in absolute terms, melanoma risk this specific size category carries, discussed further in the management implications section below. The combined nevus presents clinically as a single lesion with two discernibly different colors or textures, most often a tan-brown papular component adjacent to or overlying a blue-gray nodular component, a biphasic clinical appearance that, when recognized, appropriately lowers rather than raises clinical concern once the two-component pattern is correctly attributed to this specific benign entity.

Special Populations: Pediatric Patients and Pregnancy

Nevi in pregnant patients can show mild enlargement and darkening, particularly during the second and third trimesters, attributed to hormonally mediated melanocyte stimulation, changes that are generally reassuring when uniform, symmetric, and proportionate across the lesion, though any nevus showing markedly asymmetric change, new nodularity, or bleeding during pregnancy warrants the same biopsy threshold applied outside of pregnancy given the absence of evidence that pregnancy itself meaningfully alters appropriate diagnostic thresholds. Halo nevi occur predominantly in children and young adults and are associated with vitiligo in a meaningful minority of affected patients, an association thought to reflect a shared immune-mediated mechanism directed against melanocyte antigens, and multiple halo nevi developing simultaneously or in rapid succession in a child is a recognized, generally reassuring presentation that nonetheless warrants baseline dermatologic examination to exclude an atypical or changing lesion serving as the specific immunologic trigger.

CLINICAL PEARL: A rapidly growing pink papule in a child is the classic presentation of a Spitz nevus, not an urgent melanoma concern; however, this same clinical urgency is precisely why these lesions are biopsied promptly, allowing the maturation and mitotic distribution criteria discussed above to confirm the benign diagnosis rather than requiring watchful observation of a rapidly changing lesion.

Differential Diagnosis and Histologic Mimickers

Dysplastic Nevus Versus Melanoma In Situ

Distinguishing a severely dysplastic nevus from melanoma in situ represents one of the most challenging and consequential differential diagnoses in dermatopathology, resting on the degree and distribution of cytologic atypia (continuous versus discontinuous involvement of the junction, confluence of atypical melanocytes, and the degree of nuclear pleomorphism), the presence or absence of pagetoid (upward) scatter of melanocytes into the epidermis (more characteristic of melanoma though occasionally seen focally in severely dysplastic nevi), and overall architectural symmetry, criteria that, even when carefully applied, produce genuine interobserver variability in a meaningful subset of cases, making this a differential where second opinion consultation is frequently and appropriately sought in clinical practice.

Spitz Nevus Versus Spitzoid Melanoma

As introduced in the histopathologic features section above, distinguishing a Spitz nevus from Spitzoid melanoma depends heavily on architectural symmetry, maturation with depth, and the specific distribution of any mitotic activity (superficial and sparse in Spitz nevus; deep, peripheral, or numerous in Spitzoid melanoma), criteria that, in a genuinely ambiguous case, are supported by the molecular ancillary studies discussed in the ancillary studies section below, given the substantial clinical stakes and diagnostic difficulty this specific differential carries, particularly in adolescent and young adult patients where Spitzoid melanoma, while rare, does occur and carries serious prognostic implications if missed.

A 16-year-old patient presents with a rapidly growing, 8-millimeter, pink-red dome-shaped nodule on the thigh, present for approximately two months, and excisional biopsy is obtained given the lesion's size and growth rate. Pattern assignment identifies a compound proliferation of large epithelioid melanocytes with abundant cytoplasm, prominent nucleoli, and scattered Kamino bodies at the dermal-epidermal junction, with the lesion showing overall symmetry and maturation, smaller, less atypical-appearing cells with increasing depth, and rare mitotic figures confined to the superficial third of the lesion without atypical forms. Differential narrowing weighs the reassuring architectural and maturation features against the individually alarming cytologic appearance of the epithelioid cells, concluding that the overall gestalt, symmetry, maturation, superficially confined sparse mitoses, favors a benign Spitz nevus over Spitzoid melanoma, a conclusion supported by fluorescence in situ hybridization testing showing no evidence of the chromosomal copy number alterations associated with melanoma. Diagnosis of Spitz nevus is rendered, with the report explicitly documenting the specific maturation and mitotic distribution findings that support this benign diagnosis, given how directly this documentation would inform any future comparison should the lesion recur or a new lesion develop at another site.

Congenital Nevus Versus Congenital or Neonatal Melanoma

Congenital melanoma, exceedingly rare, must nonetheless be distinguished from a congenital nevus, particularly a large or giant congenital nevus with an atypical proliferative nodule, resting on the presence of significant cytologic atypia, an elevated and, critically, deep or peripheral mitotic rate, necrosis, and a failure of the expected maturation and adnexal-infiltration pattern described in the histopathologic features section above, features whose presence within a proliferative nodule should prompt strong consideration of melanoma arising within a congenital nevus rather than a benign proliferative nodule, supported by the ancillary studies discussed below when the distinction remains uncertain after careful histologic examination.

Halo Nevus Versus Regressing Melanoma

A halo nevus must be distinguished from a regressing melanoma, since both entities show a pre-existing melanocytic lesion undergoing lymphocyte-mediated destruction; this distinction rests on careful assessment of the residual melanocytes within and adjacent to the inflamed zone for cytologic atypia, since a halo nevus shows bland, degenerating nevus cells consistent with the pre-existing benign lesion, while a regressing melanoma shows atypical melanocytes, often with associated pagetoid scatter and dermal fibrosis with melanophage aggregation, persisting despite the inflammatory infiltrate, together with attention to the patient's age and the lesion's clinical history, since a solitary halo phenomenon developing around a previously stable, typical-appearing nevus in a young patient favors a benign halo nevus, while a halo phenomenon around an atypical, changing, or asymmetric lesion in an older patient warrants heightened concern for regressing melanoma.

A 6-year-old patient presents with a new, symmetric, pale ring of depigmentation surrounding a pre-existing 4-millimeter tan-brown papule on the back, present and stable for approximately one year prior to the halo's appearance, with no other pigmentary or scaling skin changes noted on full skin examination. Pattern assignment identifies a compound nevus with well-formed junctional nesting and dermal maturation, surrounded by a dense, band-like lymphocytic infiltrate closely apposed to the nevus cells, with the nevus cells themselves showing mild cytoplasmic vacuolization and scattered apoptotic changes but no significant nuclear pleomorphism, hyperchromasia, or pagetoid scatter. Differential narrowing weighs the reassuring prior stability of the underlying lesion, the bland cytologic appearance of the residual nevus cells despite the degenerative changes, and the patient's young age against the comparatively rare possibility of a regressing melanocytic malignancy, concluding that the overall histologic and clinical picture is fully consistent with a benign halo nevus undergoing expected immune-mediated regression. Diagnosis of halo nevus is rendered, and the family is counseled that the surrounding nevus, and eventually the halo itself, is expected to fully regress over subsequent months to a few years without intervention, together with baseline examination to exclude vitiligo elsewhere on the skin.

Deep Penetrating Nevus Versus Melanoma

The deep penetrating nevus, given its deep dermal and occasional subcutaneous extension with perineural involvement described in the histopathologic features section above, is distinguished from melanoma primarily by its maintained overall symmetric, wedge-shaped architecture and by the absence of significant cytologic atypia, brisk or atypical mitotic activity, and necrosis, features whose presence should prompt strong consideration of melanoma, occasionally arising within or closely associated with a pre-existing deep penetrating nevus, a rare but recognized scenario in which immunohistochemical proliferation and maturation assessment, together with molecular studies when available, provides valuable supportive evidence for the final diagnostic categorization.

Blue Nevus Versus Nodular Melanoma

Blue nevi must be distinguished from nodular melanoma, particularly the pigmented (melanotic) variant, given both entities' capacity to present as a deeply pigmented dermal nodule; this distinction rests on the blue nevus's characteristic dendritic, spindled melanocyte morphology admixed with pigment-laden melanophages, symmetric silhouette, and, critically, absence of significant cytologic atypia, mitotic activity, or necrosis, features whose presence should prompt strong consideration of melanoma over a blue nevus, a differential further supported by the ancillary studies discussed below when the distinction remains genuinely uncertain after careful histologic examination.

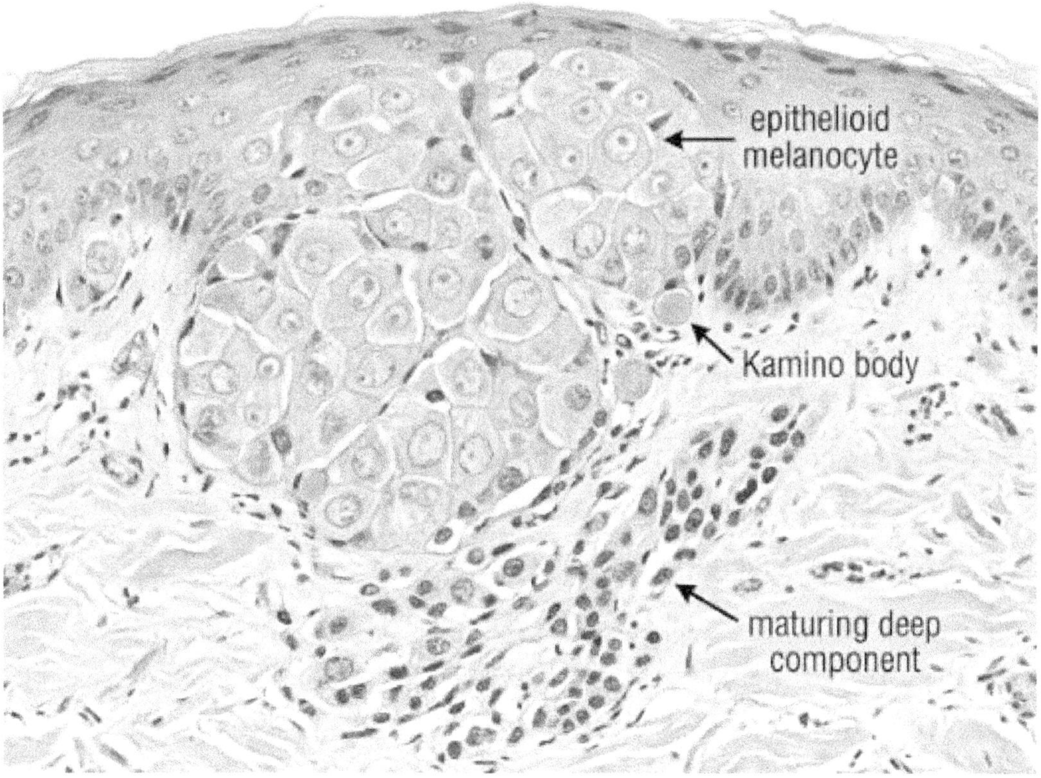

Ancillary Studies

Immunohistochemistry for Melanocytic Lesions

S100, SOX10, Melan-A/MART-1, and HMB-45 immunohistochemistry confirm melanocytic lineage and can highlight the distribution and extent of a melanocytic proliferation, with HMB-45 additionally providing a useful maturation assessment tool in ambiguous cases, since this marker characteristically shows strong staining in the superficial component of a benign nevus with progressive loss of staining in the deeper, more mature component, a maturation gradient that, when lost or reversed (strong deep staining), raises concern for melanoma given this finding's association with a failure of normal maturation. Ki-67 proliferation index, while not specific to melanocytic lesions, can provide supportive information when markedly elevated and, importantly, when elevated proliferation is identified specifically within the deep or peripheral component of a lesion rather than confined to the superficial, expected proliferative zone of a benign nevus.

Molecular Studies for Diagnostically Challenging Lesions

Fluorescence in situ hybridization, using a probe panel targeting chromosomal loci recurrently altered in melanoma (commonly including RREB1, MYB, CCND1, and centromere 6), provides supportive evidence for or against melanoma in genuinely ambiguous melanocytic proliferations, particularly valuable in the Spitz nevus versus Spitzoid melanoma differential discussed above, though this test is best interpreted as one component of the overall diagnostic picture rather than a stand-alone, definitive arbiter given its imperfect sensitivity and specificity. Comparative genomic hybridization and next-generation sequencing-based approaches, increasingly available, provide more comprehensive genomic characterization, including identification of the specific kinase fusion or mutation driving a Spitz tumor, discussed in the etiology section above, information that is refining the classification of borderline Spitzoid melanocytic tumors into more precisely defined risk categories, an active and evolving area of dermatopathology practice.

Dermoscopy as an Ancillary Diagnostic Tool

Dermoscopy, non-invasive surface microscopy performed with a handheld dermatoscope, provides a clinically accessible layer of pattern assessment that complements, but does not replace, histopathologic diagnosis, allowing recognition of specific pigmented-lesion patterns, a regular, symmetric pigment network and comma-shaped vessels favoring a benign nevus; an atypical, disrupted network, irregular streaks, and blue-white structures favoring melanoma, that meaningfully improve the pretest probability assigned to a lesion before biopsy and, in the case of equivocal lesions monitored rather than immediately biopsied, provide an objective, reproducible baseline for detecting the specific morphologic change that would prompt subsequent biopsy. Sequential digital dermoscopic monitoring, photographing a lesion at a fixed interval and comparing images for interval change, is a validated surveillance strategy for selected atypical but not immediately biopsy-warranting lesions, particularly useful in patients with numerous dysplastic nevi where biopsying every atypical-appearing lesion is neither practical nor necessary, provided the patient is a reliable participant in scheduled follow-up.

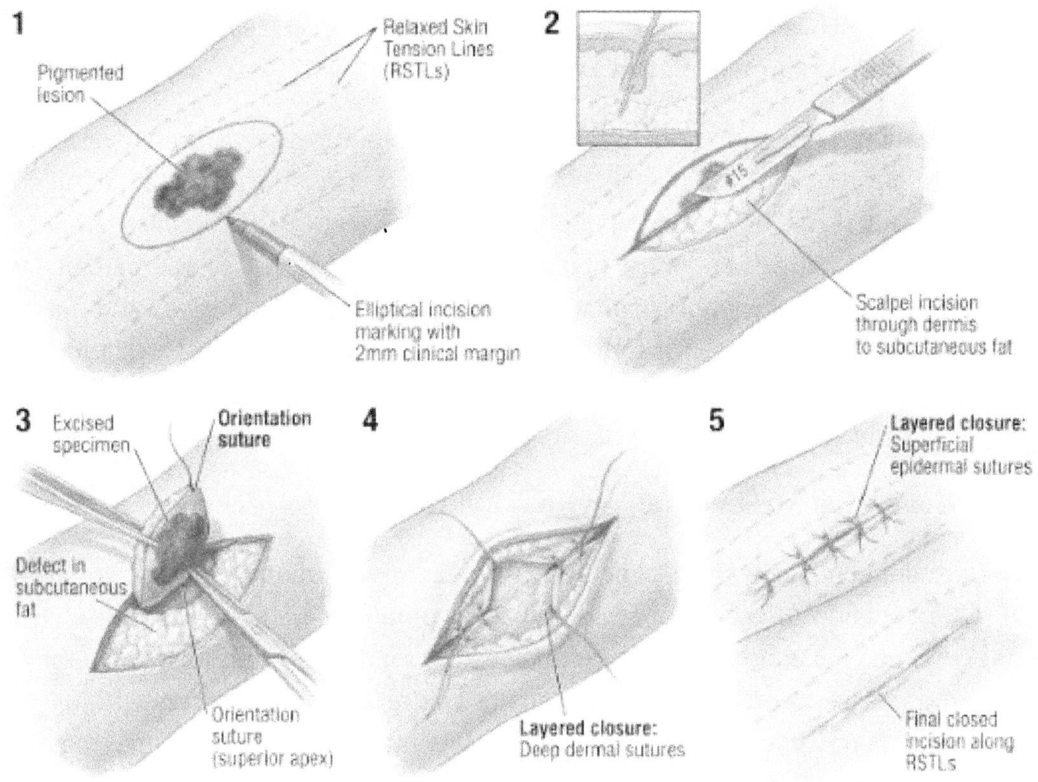

p16 and BAP1 Immunohistochemistry in Selected Diagnostic Scenarios

p16 (CDKN2A gene product) immunohistochemistry, while not routinely required for typical dysplastic or common nevi, can provide supportive information in selected ambiguous lesions, since loss of p16 expression correlates with the CDKN2A pathway alterations more characteristic of melanoma than of benign nevi, though this marker's imperfect specificity means it is interpreted alongside, rather than in place of, the morphologic criteria emphasized throughout this chapter. BAP1 immunohistochemistry is specifically relevant to the BAP1-inactivated melanocytic tumor, a distinct entity showing epithelioid melanocytes with loss of nuclear BAP1 staining, frequently arising in association with a conventional nevus component and, in a subset of patients, marking membership in a hereditary BAP1 tumor predisposition syndrome that also carries elevated risk for uveal melanoma, mesothelioma, and renal cell carcinoma, a finding that, when identified, warrants genetic counseling referral given its implications extending well beyond the cutaneous lesion itself.

CAUTION: A diagnostically ambiguous melanocytic lesion should never be forced into a definitive benign or malignant category when the histologic, immunohistochemical, and molecular findings remain genuinely discordant or insufficient. A descriptive diagnosis ("melanocytic proliferation of uncertain malignant potential") with a recommendation for complete excision and close clinical follow-up is the appropriate, honest response in this specific and clinically important scenario, consistent with the diagnostic honesty principle this book has emphasized throughout.

Management Implications

Connecting Diagnosis to Treatment Pathway

Common acquired nevi require no treatment beyond routine clinical monitoring unless a specific feature prompts biopsy; dysplastic nevi are managed with complete excision when moderately to severely atypical, given the residual risk of an incompletely sampled focus of melanoma, together with enhanced clinical surveillance, including total body photography and dermoscopy, for patients with multiple dysplastic nevi; Spitz nevi are generally managed with complete excision given the diagnostic overlap with melanoma discussed above, ensuring the entire lesion is available for the maturation and margin assessment this diagnosis depends on; and blue nevi generally require no treatment when classic and stable, with excision reserved for atypical, changing, or diagnostically uncertain lesions.

Management of Congenital Melanocytic Nevi and Neurocutaneous Melanosis Risk

Small and medium congenital nevi are generally managed with routine clinical monitoring similar to acquired nevi, with excision reserved for lesions that develop a specific concerning change or that are excised electively for cosmetic or anatomic reasons, most often during childhood when the procedure can be performed with primary closure before the lesion has enlarged proportionately with the growing child. Large and giant congenital nevi warrant referral for baseline magnetic resonance imaging of the neuroaxis when neurocutaneous melanosis risk factors are present, most notably numerous satellite nevi or a posterior axial location, together with staged surgical excision or serial partial excision when feasible, tissue expansion, or, when complete excision is not feasible given lesion size and location, structured long-term surveillance, a management pathway best coordinated through a multidisciplinary team given the complexity and long time horizon these decisions carry.

Complications and Prognosis

The great majority of entities in this chapter carry an excellent prognosis once appropriately diagnosed and, when indicated, excised, reflecting their fundamentally benign biological behavior despite, in several cases, genuinely alarming clinical or histologic features. The primary long-term risk this chapter's entities carry is not from the lesions themselves but from the broader melanoma risk they mark, particularly for patients with multiple dysplastic nevi or a family history consistent with familial atypical multiple mole and melanoma syndrome, reinforcing why this chapter's diagnostic framework serves a risk-stratification function extending well beyond the individual lesion under evaluation. Melanoma risk within a congenital nevus correlates directly with lesion size, low and measured in single-digit percentages over a lifetime for small and medium congenital nevi, but meaningfully elevated, historically estimated in a range extending into the low double digits over a lifetime in some series, for giant congenital nevi, particularly those with numerous satellite lesions, a size-dependent risk gradient that directly informs the surveillance and excision decisions discussed above. Neurocutaneous melanosis, when symptomatic, carries a substantially guarded prognosis given its association with hydrocephalus, seizures, and, in a subset of affected patients, primary central nervous system melanoma, underscoring why baseline neuroimaging and specialist referral are pursued proactively in the specific high-risk congenital nevus population identified above rather than reserved for the development of neurologic symptoms.

Prevention and Screening

Consistent sun protection during childhood and adolescence, broad-spectrum sunscreen, protective clothing, and avoidance of peak-intensity midday sun exposure, remains the single most effective modifiable strategy for reducing lifetime nevus count and, by extension, cumulative melanoma risk, given the disproportionate contribution of early-life intermittent and intense ultraviolet exposure to both outcomes discussed in the etiology section above. Structured surveillance, incorporating periodic full skin examination, dermoscopy, and, for higher-risk patients, total body photography with sequential digital dermoscopic monitoring of specific atypical lesions, is recommended at an interval individualized to overall risk, more frequent for patients with numerous dysplastic nevi, a personal or family history of melanoma, or a diagnosis of familial atypical multiple mole and melanoma syndrome, and less frequent for patients with few, stable, typical-appearing nevi and no elevated risk factors, a risk-stratified approach that avoids both under-surveillance of genuinely high-risk patients and unnecessary over-biopsy of low-risk patients with numerous but individually unremarkable nevi.

Documentation and Reporting Standards

A dermatopathology report for a melanocytic lesion should explicitly document the specific architectural and cytologic features supporting the rendered diagnosis, symmetry, maturation status, mitotic count and distribution, and the presence or absence of pagetoid scatter, rather than a bare categorical diagnosis alone, a documentation standard that serves two related purposes emphasized throughout this book: it allows the referring clinician to correlate the histologic findings with the clinical presentation, and it provides a durable, specific record against which any future biopsy at the same site, most relevant for the recurrent nevus scenario discussed above, or any subsequent second-opinion review can be meaningfully compared. For diagnostically borderline lesions specifically, the report should state explicitly which ancillary studies were performed, their results, and how those results informed the final diagnostic categorization, together with a clear recommendation regarding excision completeness and follow-up interval, ensuring the treating clinician has a complete, actionable picture rather than a diagnostic label alone.

Patient Education and Counseling

Patients with dysplastic nevi benefit from clear counseling regarding the recommended surveillance interval, the rationale for photographic monitoring, and specific instruction on self-examination technique, given this population's elevated overall melanoma risk relative to the general population. Parents of children diagnosed with a Spitz nevus benefit from reassurance regarding this lesion's benign nature despite its rapid growth and concerning initial appearance, while patients with blue nevi benefit from simple counseling that stability over time is the expected and reassuring feature of this diagnosis, with any new change from baseline warranting prompt re-evaluation. Parents of infants with a large or giant congenital nevus benefit from early, structured counseling regarding the surveillance and staged management pathway discussed above, together with practical guidance on sun protection over the nevus itself and connection to peer support resources, given both the long time horizon this diagnosis carries and its potential cosmetic and psychosocial impact through childhood and adolescence.

THE REACTION PATTERN RECOGNITION SYSTEM — The Melanocytic Nevus and Simulator Pattern Family

The Pattern: Benign melanocytic proliferations organized by architectural level and subtype, unified by symmetry, maturation with depth, and cytologic uniformity: common acquired nevus, dysplastic (Clark) nevus, Spitz nevus, blue nevus, recurrent nevus, and deep penetrating nevus.

Histologic Signature: Symmetric nesting with maturation defines the common nevus; lentiginous junctional atypia with lamellar fibroplasia defines the dysplastic nevus; large epithelioid/spindled cells with Kamino bodies and maturation defines the Spitz nevus; dendritic dermal melanocytes with melanophages define the blue nevus.

The Decision: Apply the universal symmetry-maturation-uniformity assessment first, then apply subtype-specific criteria (lentiginous atypia and fibroplasia for dysplastic nevus; mitotic distribution for Spitz nevus; cytologic atypia for blue nevus), escalating to immunohistochemistry and molecular studies when the findings remain genuinely ambiguous.

Trap Logic: Spitz nevi show individually alarming cytology despite benign behavior; recurrent nevi mimic melanoma at a prior biopsy scar without the surgical history; severely dysplastic nevi overlap substantially with melanoma in situ. Always request prior biopsy history and apply subtype-specific criteria rather than generic atypia assessment alone.

Pattern Anchor: Symmetric, matures, uniform: benign, regardless of how alarming individual cytologic features appear in isolation. When these criteria are not clearly met, use ancillary studies and descriptive, uncertainty-acknowledging diagnosis rather than forcing a definitive call.

Summary and Key Concepts

Melanocytic nevi are organized along a junctional-to-compound-to-intradermal developmental continuum, unified by the foundational criteria of symmetry, maturation with depth, and cytologic uniformity that distinguish benign proliferations from melanoma throughout this chapter and into Chapter 14.

Dysplastic (Clark) nevi show lentiginous junctional atypia with shouldering and lamellar fibroplasia, occupying a genuinely challenging diagnostic space that overlaps with melanoma in situ and requires careful architectural and cytologic assessment.

Spitz nevi show individually alarming large epithelioid or spindled melanocytes with Kamino bodies, distinguished from Spitzoid melanoma by symmetry, maturation, and a specific superficial, sparse mitotic distribution rather than cytology alone.

Blue nevi arise from dermal melanocytes that failed normal embryologic migration, presenting as deeply pigmented dermal nodules that must be distinguished from nodular melanoma through cytologic uniformity and absence of atypia, mitoses, or necrosis.

Diagnostically ambiguous melanocytic proliferations warrant fluorescence in situ hybridization or other molecular studies and, when uncertainty persists, an honest descriptive diagnosis with complete excision and close follow-up rather than a forced definitive call.

Congenital, combined, and halo nevi, along with special-site nevi at acral, genital, and scalp locations, each carry distinct histologic features that can mimic melanoma and require site- and context-specific criteria rather than generic atypia assessment.

CHAPTER 14: MELANOMA: DIAGNOSIS, STAGING, AND HISTOLOGIC PITFALLS

Learning Objectives

1. Classify melanoma by major histologic subtype, including superficial spreading, nodular, lentigo maligna, acral lentiginous, desmoplastic, nevoid, and Spitzoid melanoma.
2. Apply the histopathologic criteria distinguishing melanoma from the benign melanocytic simulators introduced in Chapter 13, including asymmetry, lack of maturation, and pagetoid scatter.
3. Determine Breslow depth, ulceration status, and mitotic rate and explain their role in melanoma staging and prognosis.
4. Recognize the specific, deceptive histologic pitfalls associated with nevoid melanoma, desmoplastic melanoma, and melanoma arising in close association with a pre-existing benign nevus.
5. Construct a systematic differential diagnosis for an ambiguous melanocytic proliferation using architectural, cytologic, and ancillary criteria.
6. Connect histopathologic staging parameters directly to the surgical and systemic management pathway, including sentinel lymph node biopsy eligibility and adjuvant therapy selection.

Definition and Classification

Melanoma as the Culmination of This Book's Melanocytic Framework

This chapter builds directly on the diagnostic vocabulary established in Chapter 13, asymmetry, maturation, and cytologic uniformity, applying that same three-part framework in its inverted, malignant form to the definitive diagnosis of melanoma, a malignant proliferation of melanocytes capable of both local invasion and distant metastasis and among the most consequential diagnoses rendered anywhere within dermatopathology practice given the direct and immediate impact an accurate, precisely staged diagnosis has on a patient's surgical management, systemic therapy eligibility, and long-term prognosis. Melanoma is classified into major histologic subtypes reflecting differences in anatomic site, growth pattern, patient age, and underlying molecular pathway, a classification this chapter organizes around because each subtype carries its own characteristic clinical presentation, histologic pitfalls, and, increasingly, molecular signature relevant to targeted systemic therapy selection. This chapter's structure deliberately mirrors Chapter 13's, applying the same seven-part clinical framework, definition, etiology, histopathology, clinical presentation, differential diagnosis, ancillary studies, and management, so the reader carries forward a single, continuous diagnostic method rather than learning an unrelated set of criteria specific to malignancy alone.

Major Histologic Subtypes

Superficial spreading melanoma, the most common subtype in fair-skinned populations, shows a prolonged radial growth phase of pagetoid, intraepidermal melanocyte spread before vertical invasion begins, most often arising on intermittently sun-exposed skin such as the trunk and proximal extremities. Nodular melanoma lacks a substantial radial growth phase, presenting instead with early and often rapid vertical growth and correspondingly greater average Breslow depth at diagnosis, an aggressive natural history discussed further in the clinical presentation section below. Lentigo maligna melanoma arises on chronically sun-damaged skin, most often the head and neck of older patients, evolving from its in situ precursor, lentigo maligna, over a characteristically prolonged radial growth phase measured in years. Acral lentiginous melanoma arises on the palms, soles, and nail apparatus, is not strongly associated with ultraviolet exposure, and, importantly, occurs across all skin types, representing a disproportionately larger fraction of melanoma in patients with darker skin phototypes.

Subtype	Typical Site	Growth Pattern	Molecular Association
Superficial spreading	Trunk, proximal extremities	Prolonged radial phase before vertical invasion	BRAF V600E common
Nodular	Any site	Early, often rapid vertical growth	BRAF or NRAS mutated
Lentigo maligna	Head and neck, chronically sun-damaged skin	Very prolonged radial (in situ) phase	NF1, KIT, BRAF (lower frequency)
Acral lentiginous	Palms, soles, nail apparatus	Variable, often delayed diagnosis	KIT mutations, structural variants; low UV signature
Desmoplastic	Head and neck, sun-damaged skin	Often subtle, deeply infiltrative	NF1 mutations common; low response to some targeted therapies

Epidemiology and Population Risk Distribution

Melanoma incidence has risen steadily over recent decades in fair-skinned populations, a trend attributed predominantly to cumulative ultraviolet exposure patterns and increased detection, though mortality trends have more recently improved, reflecting both earlier detection and the systemic therapy advances discussed in the management implications section below. Melanoma occurs across all skin phototypes, and while overall incidence is markedly lower in patients with darker skin, acral lentiginous melanoma represents a disproportionately larger share of melanoma diagnoses in this population, a distribution associated in multiple studies with more advanced stage at diagnosis, attributed in substantial part to lower index of clinical suspicion, later presentation, and reduced screening access rather than any difference in the fundamental biology of the tumor itself, an equity consideration this chapter emphasizes given its direct bearing on the prevention and screening principles discussed later in this chapter.

Spitzoid Melanoma and Its Relationship to Chapter 13

Spitzoid melanoma, a rare but clinically important subtype showing large epithelioid and spindled melanocytes resembling those of a Spitz nevus, represents the malignant end of the Spitzoid spectrum introduced in Chapter 13's Spitz nevus versus Spitzoid melanoma differential, distinguished by asymmetry, a lack of maturation with depth, deep or peripheral mitotic activity, and, frequently, the specific chromosomal copy number alterations identified by fluorescence in situ hybridization or comparative genomic hybridization discussed in the ancillary studies section below, a subtype this chapter revisits explicitly because its histologic overlap with a benign Spitz nevus is among the most consequential diagnostic challenges in pediatric and young adult dermatopathology.

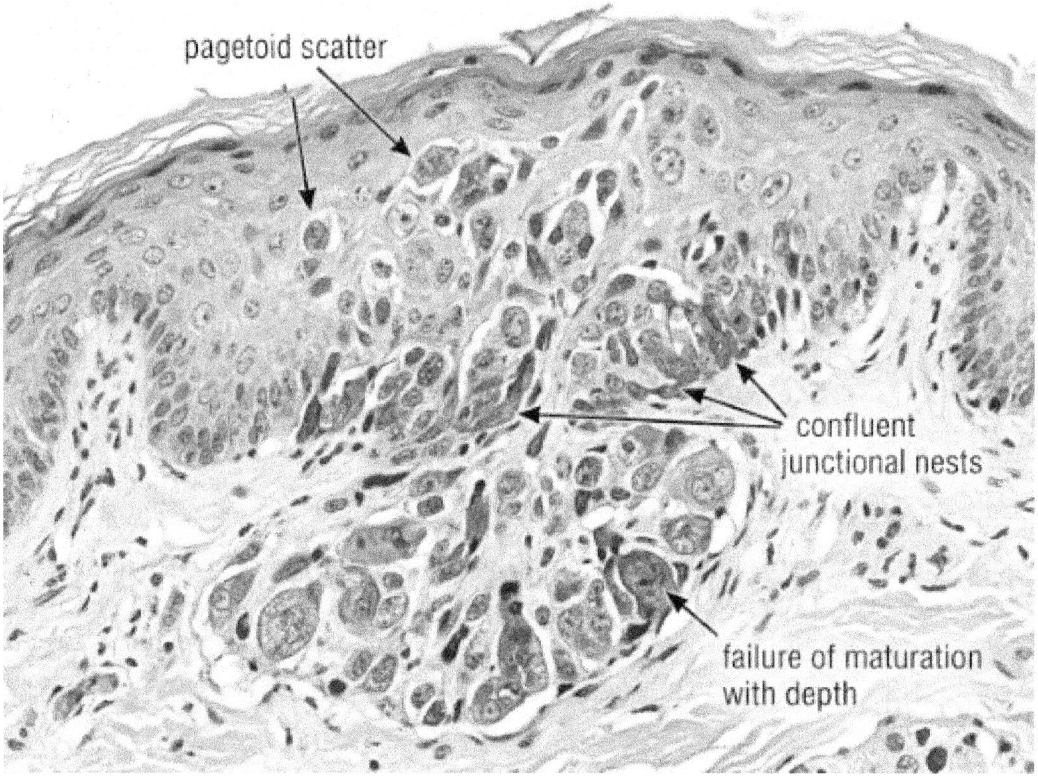

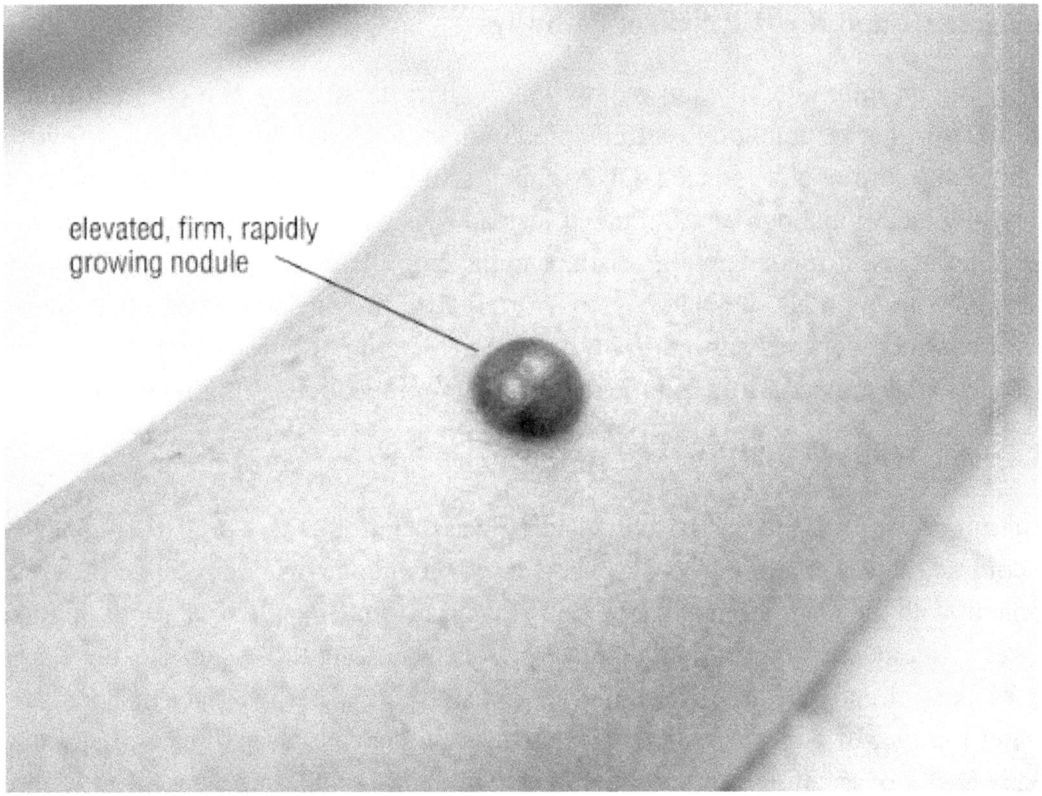

Etiology and Pathogenesis

Molecular Drivers and the Radial-to-Vertical Growth Phase Transition

Melanoma pathogenesis is understood as a multistep progression from normal melanocyte through the radial growth phase, confined to the epidermis and papillary dermis and lacking metastatic competence, to the vertical growth phase, in which a subclone acquires the capacity for dermal invasion, proliferation, and eventual metastasis, a transition driven by the sequential accumulation of oncogenic driver mutations superimposed on the tumor suppressor loss discussed in Chapter 13's dysplastic nevus pathogenesis section. BRAF V600E mutations, present in approximately 40 to 50 percent of cutaneous melanomas overall but concentrated disproportionately in melanomas arising on intermittently sun-exposed skin without chronic sun damage, activate the mitogen-activated protein kinase pathway constitutively and represent the single most therapeutically actionable molecular alteration in melanoma, directly informing the targeted therapy eligibility discussed in the management implications section below. NRAS mutations, present in a smaller but still clinically significant subset, activate the same downstream pathway through a distinct upstream mechanism, while KIT mutations are concentrated in acral, mucosal, and chronically sun-damaged skin melanomas, and NF1 mutations are enriched in desmoplastic melanoma, a site- and subtype-specific molecular landscape this chapter connects directly to the histologic subtype classification above.

Ultraviolet Signature and Non-Ultraviolet Pathways

Melanomas arising on intermittently sun-exposed skin characteristically show a high tumor mutational burden with a UV-signature mutation pattern (predominantly C-to-T transitions at dipyrimidine sites), reflecting cumulative ultraviolet-induced DNA damage, while acral and mucosal melanomas show a comparatively low mutational burden dominated instead by structural chromosomal rearrangements and copy number alterations, a fundamentally distinct mutagenic pathway that explains both this subtype's occurrence in non-sun-exposed sites and its comparatively lower response rate to immune checkpoint inhibitor therapy, which depends substantially on tumor mutational burden and neoantigen load for its mechanism of action, discussed further in the management implications section below.

Melanoma Arising Within a Pre-Existing Nevus

A meaningful minority of melanomas arise in histologic association with a pre-existing nevus, most often a common acquired or, less commonly, a dysplastic or congenital nevus, identifiable by a residual benign nevus component with the maturation and symmetry criteria from Chapter 13 abruptly juxtaposed against an asymmetric, cytologically atypical melanoma component lacking those same features, a juxtaposition this chapter revisits directly in the differential diagnosis section below given its practical diagnostic importance and the risk of either overlooking a small malignant focus within a predominantly benign lesion or, conversely, overcalling a benign nevus component as malignant based on its proximity to a genuinely malignant focus.

Second Primary Melanoma Risk

Patients with a history of one melanoma carry a substantially elevated risk of developing a second, independent primary melanoma relative to the general population, a risk that persists for years after the initial diagnosis and that reflects the same underlying phenotypic and genetic susceptibility factors, high nevus count, fair skin phototype, and cumulative ultraviolet exposure, discussed throughout this chapter and Chapter 13, rather than metastatic spread from the original tumor, a distinction with direct implications for the lifelong surveillance protocol these patients follow after their initial diagnosis and treatment are complete. This elevated second primary risk applies across melanoma subtypes and is a primary driver behind the long-term, often lifelong, dermatologic surveillance recommendation extended to melanoma survivors regardless of their initial stage at diagnosis, discussed further in the prevention and screening section below.

Genetic Predisposition Syndromes and Hereditary Melanoma

Beyond the sporadic BRAF, NRAS, KIT, and NF1 mutations discussed above, a meaningful minority of melanoma arises in the setting of a defined hereditary predisposition syndrome, most commonly familial atypical multiple mole and melanoma syndrome associated with germline CDKN2A mutations, introduced in Chapter 13, and, less commonly, germline CDK4 mutations producing a phenotypically similar syndrome, BAP1 tumor predisposition syndrome, also introduced in Chapter 13 in the context of the BAP1-inactivated melanocytic tumor, and germline pathogenic variants in POT1 and other telomeremaintenance genes, each syndrome carrying implications for family screening and genetic counseling referral that extend well beyond the individual melanoma diagnosis under evaluation. Patients presenting with multiple primary melanomas, melanoma at a young age, or a strong family history of melanoma or pancreatic cancer, the latter specifically associated with CDKN2A-related familial atypical multiple mole and melanoma syndrome, warrant consideration of germline genetic testing referral, a consideration this chapter connects directly to the patient education and counseling discussion at this chapter's close.

THE REACTION PATTERN RECOGNITION SYSTEM — Asymmetry, Failure of Maturation, and Cytologic Atypia as the Universal Malignant Anchor

---

The Pattern: Asymmetry, Failure of Maturation with Depth, and Significant Cytologic Atypia as the Criteria Confirming Melanoma Across Every Histologic Subtype

Histologic Signature: A poorly circumscribed, asymmetric silhouette; melanocytes that fail to decrease in size and pigmentation with increasing dermal depth or that show increasing atypia at the deep or lateral margin; confluent rather than discrete nesting; and pagetoid (upward) scatter of atypical melanocytes into the epidermis.

The Decision: Apply the inverse of Chapter 13's benign anchor to every ambiguous melanocytic proliferation: asymmetry rather than symmetry, failure of maturation rather than maturation, and cytologic atypia rather than uniformity, escalating to the ancillary studies detailed below whenever these criteria are present but not unequivocal, given the substantial clinical consequences of both under- and overdiagnosis in this specific diagnostic category.

Trap Logic: Nevoid melanoma deceptively resembles a benign nevus at low magnification despite malignant behavior; desmoplastic melanoma can show minimal cytologic atypia within a densely fibrotic, paucicellular stroma; and melanoma can arise focally within an otherwise benign-appearing nevus. Each of these traps demands specific subtype-aware scrutiny beyond a single low-magnification gestalt impression.

Pattern Anchor: Asymmetric, fails to mature, atypical: melanoma, regardless of how deceptively bland or nevus-like the overall low-power impression initially appears. When in doubt, examine the deep and lateral margins specifically for the persistence or worsening of atypia that a benign nevus would not show.

Histopathologic Features and Diagnostic Criteria

Core Architectural and Cytologic Criteria

Melanoma shows asymmetry and poor lateral circumscription, confluent rather than well-spaced junctional nesting, pagetoid scatter of melanocytes into the upper epidermis (a feature particularly prominent in superficial spreading melanoma), and, critically, a failure of the normal maturation pattern with increasing dermal depth, melanocytes remaining large, pigmented, and cytologically atypical rather than progressively smaller, less pigmented, and more uniform, the inverse of the benign maturation criterion established in Chapter 13. Cytologic atypia, nuclear enlargement, irregular nuclear contours, hyperchromasia, and prominent, often eosinophilic nucleoli, together with an elevated and, importantly, deep or peripheral rather than exclusively superficial mitotic rate, further supports the diagnosis, with atypical mitotic figures carrying particular diagnostic weight when identified.

Breslow Depth, Ulceration, and Mitotic Rate

Breslow depth, measured in millimeters from the granular layer of the epidermis (or, in an ulcerated tumor, from the base of the ulcer) to the deepest point of tumor invasion, is the single most powerful prognostic parameter in melanoma and the primary determinant of American Joint Committee on Cancer T category, requiring careful, reproducible measurement technique using a calibrated ocular micrometer perpendicular to the skin surface at the point of greatest depth. Ulceration, full-thickness epidermal loss overlying the tumor with an associated host response, and mitotic rate, reported as mitoses per square millimeter in the area of highest mitotic density, both carry independent prognostic significance and are reported alongside Breslow depth in every invasive melanoma pathology report, together with additional parameters including lymphovascular invasion, perineural invasion, tumor-infiltrating lymphocyte density and pattern, and the presence or absence of regression, each developed further in the ancillary studies and management implications sections below.

Nevoid and Desmoplastic Melanoma: Deceptive Histologic Patterns

Nevoid melanoma shows a deceptively bland, nevus-like low-magnification silhouette, small, relatively uniform-appearing melanocytes arranged in a superficially nevus-like architecture, that on closer inspection shows subtle but genuine departures from a benign nevus: mild but present asymmetry, incomplete or absent maturation, an elevated mitotic rate including mitoses in the deep component, and, often, a slightly expansile, pushing rather than infiltrative deep border, features that demand deliberate, systematic scrutiny precisely because this subtype's overall gestalt is designed by its deceptive nature to reassure an examiner relying on gestalt alone. Desmoplastic melanoma shows sparse, spindled melanocytes with minimal cytologic atypia embedded within a densely fibrotic, collagenous stroma, frequently with a lymphoid aggregate at the base of the lesion and, in the pure desmoplastic subtype, an epidermal component that can be minimal or entirely absent, features that together produce a low cellularity, scar-like histologic appearance that is a well-recognized and clinically significant source of both delayed diagnosis and diagnostic difficulty.

Regression, Tumor-Infiltrating Lymphocytes, and Lymphovascular Invasion

Regression, partial or complete replacement of the tumor by fibrosis, melanophage aggregation, and a lymphocytic infiltrate, reflects host immune-mediated tumor destruction and, when extensive, can obscure the original Breslow depth, requiring the pathologist to note the presence and extent of regression explicitly, since regressed melanoma has historically been associated with a modestly less favorable prognosis when regression is extensive, attributed to the possibility of a deeper original tumor component no longer measurable at the time of biopsy. Tumor-infiltrating lymphocyte density and pattern (brisk, non-brisk, or absent) and the presence of lymphovascular or perineural invasion each carry additional prognostic and, in some cases, sentinel lymph node biopsy risk-stratification significance, with a brisk tumor-infiltrating lymphocyte response associated with a more favorable outcome and documented lymphovascular invasion associated with an increased risk of nodal and distant metastatic spread.

Melanoma In Situ Versus Invasive Melanoma

Melanoma in situ shows the full asymmetry, confluence, and cytologic atypia criteria of invasive melanoma but confined entirely to the epidermis without dermal invasion, a distinction with direct staging and management consequences, since melanoma in situ requires narrower excision margins and does not warrant sentinel lymph node biopsy, developed further in the management implications section below. Distinguishing melanoma in situ from an early, minimally invasive melanoma requires careful, systematic examination of the entire dermal-epidermal junction for even a single focus of dermal invasion, since even a minimal Breslow depth carries materially different staging and management implications, underscoring the diagnostic precision this specific distinction demands.

Perineural and Angiotropic Spread Patterns

Perineural invasion, tumor cells tracking along a peripheral nerve, is reported specifically because its presence is associated with an increased risk of local recurrence and, in some anatomic sites, warrants consideration of a wider surgical margin or adjuvant radiation therapy, a finding that carries particular significance in desmoplastic melanoma, described above, where neurotropism is a characteristic and comparatively frequent feature. Angiotropism, tumor cells arranged along the external surface of vessel walls without frank intravascular invasion, is a distinct and increasingly recognized pattern associated with local and in-transit metastatic spread through a mechanism resembling extravascular migratory metastasis, a finding this chapter notes specifically because it can be present even in the absence of classic lymphovascular invasion and, when identified, should be documented in the pathology report given its independent association with regional recurrence risk.

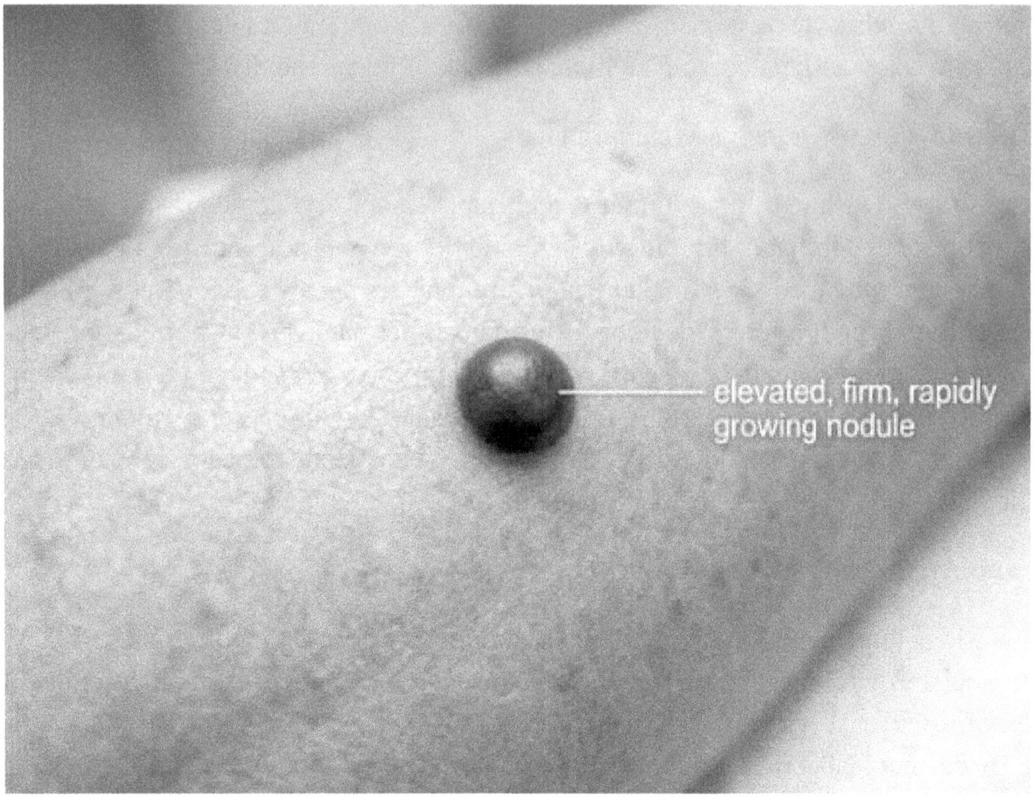

Clinical Presentation and Clinicopathologic Correlation

The ABCDE Criteria and the Ugly Duckling Sign

Melanoma classically presents with one or more of the ABCDE criteria, Asymmetry, Border irregularity, Color variegation, Diameter greater than 6 millimeters, and Evolution (change in size, shape, or color over time), with evolution increasingly recognized as among the most sensitive individual criteria, since a changing lesion, even one otherwise unremarkable in appearance, warrants biopsy consideration given how directly this feature captures the biological behavior distinguishing melanoma from the vast majority of stable benign nevi. The ugly duckling sign, a lesion that appears clinically distinct from a given patient's other nevi, complements the ABCDE criteria by leveraging the observation that an individual patient's nevi tend toward a consistent personal phenotype, making a lesion that departs from this pattern disproportionately more likely to represent melanoma even when it does not independently meet full ABCDE criteria.

Subtype-Specific and Amelanotic Presentations

Nodular melanoma frequently lacks the classic ABCDE features given its comparatively symmetric, uniformly pigmented, rapidly enlarging papulonodular presentation, better captured by an alternative mnemonic, Elevated, Firm, and Growing, that this chapter emphasizes specifically because reliance on ABCDE criteria alone risks delayed recognition of this aggressive subtype. Amelanotic melanoma, lacking clinically visible pigmentation entirely, presents as a pink to red papule, nodule, or plaque that can closely mimic a wide range of benign and inflammatory entities, basal cell carcinoma, pyogenic granuloma, or an inflamed cyst among them, a presentation this chapter emphasizes because the absence of pigmentation should never be used to exclude melanoma from a differential diagnosis for a new, changing, or bleeding lesion regardless of color.

Mucosal and Ocular Melanoma

Mucosal melanoma, arising on oral, nasal, anorectal, or vulvovaginal mucosa, and ocular (uveal) melanoma, arising from the choroid, ciliary body, or iris, share the same fundamental melanocytic origin as cutaneous melanoma but follow distinct molecular pathways, uveal melanoma in particular characterized by GNAQ and GNA11 mutations shared with the blue nevus lineage discussed in Chapter 13, and distinct clinical behavior, including a comparatively higher rate of hematogenous rather than lymphatic metastatic spread for uveal melanoma, differences this chapter notes specifically because these subtypes fall outside the ultraviolet-associated cutaneous melanoma framework this chapter otherwise emphasizes and are managed through largely separate, subspecialized clinical pathways in ophthalmology and otolaryngology.

Special Populations: Pediatric and Pregnant Patients

Melanoma in children and adolescents is rare and disproportionately represents the Spitzoid melanoma subtype discussed above, a population in whom the Spitz nevus versus Spitzoid melanoma differential from Chapter 13 carries particularly high stakes given both the rarity of genuine pediatric melanoma and the comparatively common occurrence of benign but cytologically alarming Spitz nevi in this same age group. Melanoma diagnosed during pregnancy does not appear to carry an independently worse prognosis when matched for stage at diagnosis, though the physiologic pigmentary changes of pregnancy discussed in Chapter 13 can complicate timely clinical recognition, and management, including surgical excision and, when indicated, sentinel lymph node biopsy using appropriately modified radiotracer protocols, generally proceeds without substantial delay given the established safety of these interventions during pregnancy.

CLINICAL PEARL: A lesion that a patient describes as new, changing, or simply different from their other moles, the ugly duckling sign, warrants biopsy consideration regardless of whether it independently satisfies full ABCDE criteria, since this comparative, patient-specific assessment captures a meaningful fraction of melanomas that would otherwise be missed by rigid criteria application alone.

Lentigo Maligna: A Distinct Clinical Course

Lentigo maligna, the in situ precursor of lentigo maligna melanoma, presents as a slowly enlarging, irregularly pigmented macule or patch on chronically sun-damaged skin, most often the malar cheek, nose, or temple of an older patient, following a clinical course measured in years rather than months, a comparatively indolent evolution that this chapter emphasizes because it can, paradoxically, delay biopsy given the lesion's slow change and frequent resemblance to a benign solar lentigo, a resemblance developed further in the differential diagnosis section below. Biopsy of a suspected lentigo maligna should sample the area of greatest clinical concern, most pigmented, most irregular, or most recently changed, given this entity's tendency toward patchy, non-uniform involvement across a broad clinical field, a sampling consideration with direct implications for the completeness and reliability of the histopathologic assessment.

Differential Diagnosis and Histologic Mimickers

Melanoma Versus the Benign Simulators of Chapter 13

Every benign entity developed in Chapter 13, the dysplastic nevus, Spitz nevus, blue nevus, deep penetrating nevus, and recurrent nevus, represents a specific, named differential consideration against melanoma, distinguished by the systematic application of this chapter's asymmetry-failure of maturation-atypia framework against Chapter 13's symmetry-maturation-uniformity framework, an inverse pairing this book has built deliberately across these two consecutive chapters to reinforce melanocytic pattern recognition as a single continuous diagnostic skill rather than two unrelated bodies of knowledge, with the specific ancillary studies discussed below available whenever this framework does not resolve a genuinely ambiguous lesion.

Melanoma Arising Within a Pre-Existing Nevus

As introduced in the etiology section above, melanoma arising within a pre-existing nevus requires careful, deliberate mapping of the lesion at low magnification to identify the specific transition zone between the benign nevus component, showing the expected symmetry and maturation, and the malignant component, showing asymmetric growth, failure of maturation, and cytologic atypia typically concentrated at one pole or margin of the overall lesion, a mapping exercise that both confirms the malignant diagnosis and, importantly, informs the Breslow depth measurement, which is taken from the malignant component specifically rather than from the overall lesion including its benign nevus remnant.

A 58-year-old patient presents with a longstanding pigmented lesion on the back that the patient reports has darkened and developed an irregular border over the preceding four months, with dermoscopy showing an atypical pigment network at the lesion's periphery and a structureless blue-black area centrally. Pattern assignment identifies a compound melanocytic proliferation with a peripheral zone showing well-formed, symmetric nesting and dermal maturation consistent with a pre-existing common acquired nevus, abruptly transitioning at the lesion's central and one lateral margin to a zone of confluent, asymmetric junctional nesting with prominent pagetoid scatter, cytologic atypia, and melanocytes persisting without maturation to a measured depth of 1.4 millimeters into the reticular dermis, with two mitotic figures identified per square millimeter and no ulceration. Differential narrowing confirms melanoma arising in association with a pre-existing nevus, with Breslow depth measured specifically from the malignant component at the point of deepest invasion, corresponding to American Joint Committee on Cancer pathologic T2a. Diagnosis of invasive melanoma, superficial spreading type, arising in association with a pre-existing melanocytic nevus, is rendered, with the report documenting Breslow depth, mitotic rate, ulceration status, and margin status to directly inform the surgical and sentinel lymph node biopsy discussion detailed in the management implications section below.

Spitzoid Melanoma Versus Spitz Nevus

Building directly on Chapter 13's treatment of this differential, Spitzoid melanoma is distinguished from a Spitz nevus by asymmetry, a lack of maturation with depth, mitotic figures identified in the deep or peripheral component of the lesion rather than confined to the superficial third, and, frequently, a greater overall size and a wider range of patient age at presentation than the classic pediatric and young adult Spitz nevus population, criteria that in a genuinely ambiguous case are supported by fluorescence in situ hybridization or comparative genomic hybridization, since Spitzoid melanoma more consistently shows the copy number alterations characteristic of melanoma while a benign Spitz nevus, including its variant showing an isolated 11p gain, typically does not.

A 45-year-old patient presents with a 12-millimeter, variably pigmented, asymmetric papule on the shoulder with a reported six-month growth history, larger and more irregular than the classic pediatric Spitz nevus presentation. Pattern assignment identifies a compound proliferation of large epithelioid melanocytes with Kamino body-like eosinophilic globules at the junction, but with notable asymmetry, confluent junctional nesting extending beyond the dermal component, and melanocytes persisting without maturation into the deep reticular dermis, where three mitotic figures per square millimeter are identified, including one atypical form. Differential narrowing weighs the Spitzoid cytomorphology against the asymmetry, failure of maturation, and deep mitotic activity, concluding that the overall pattern favors Spitzoid melanoma over a benign Spitz nevus, a conclusion supported by comparative genomic hybridization showing multiple chromosomal copy number alterations inconsistent with a benign Spitz nevus. Diagnosis of Spitzoid melanoma is rendered, with Breslow depth measured at 1.8 millimeters, and the case is referred for wide local excision and sentinel lymph node biopsy discussion consistent with this chapter's management implications section below.

Desmoplastic Melanoma Versus Scar and Neurofibroma

Given desmoplastic melanoma's low cellularity and dense fibrotic stroma described in the histopathologic features section above, this entity is readily mistaken for a scar, particularly at a site of prior trauma or biopsy, or for a neural tumor such as neurofibroma, given shared spindled morphology and, in some cases, overlapping S100 immunoreactivity; distinguishing features include a lymphoid aggregate at the base of the lesion, an overlying junctional melanocytic component (present in the mixed but often absent in the pure desmoplastic subtype), and, on immunohistochemistry, more consistent and diffuse S100 and SOX10 positivity than the patchier staining typical of neurofibroma, together with a low but present proliferation index inconsistent with a mature scar.

Lentigo Maligna Versus Solar Lentigo and Pigmented Actinic Keratosis

Lentigo maligna must be distinguished from a solar lentigo, a benign, uniform proliferation of hyperpigmented but non-atypical basal keratinocytes without an increase in melanocyte density, and from pigmented actinic keratosis, which shows keratinocytic rather than melanocytic atypia; lentigo maligna itself shows an increased density of atypical melanocytes, often with confluence and nesting, extending along the basal layer of a chronically sun-damaged epidermis, frequently with striking extension down adnexal structures, hair follicles and eccrine ducts in particular, a distribution that can complicate margin assessment and is discussed further in the management implications section below given its relevance to the surgical approach this specific subtype requires. Given the subtle, patchy nature of early lentigo maligna and its substantial overlap with the background melanocytic hyperplasia of chronically sun-damaged skin, this specific differential is one where immunohistochemical melanocyte density assessment, discussed in the ancillary studies section below, is used more routinely than in most other melanocytic differentials.

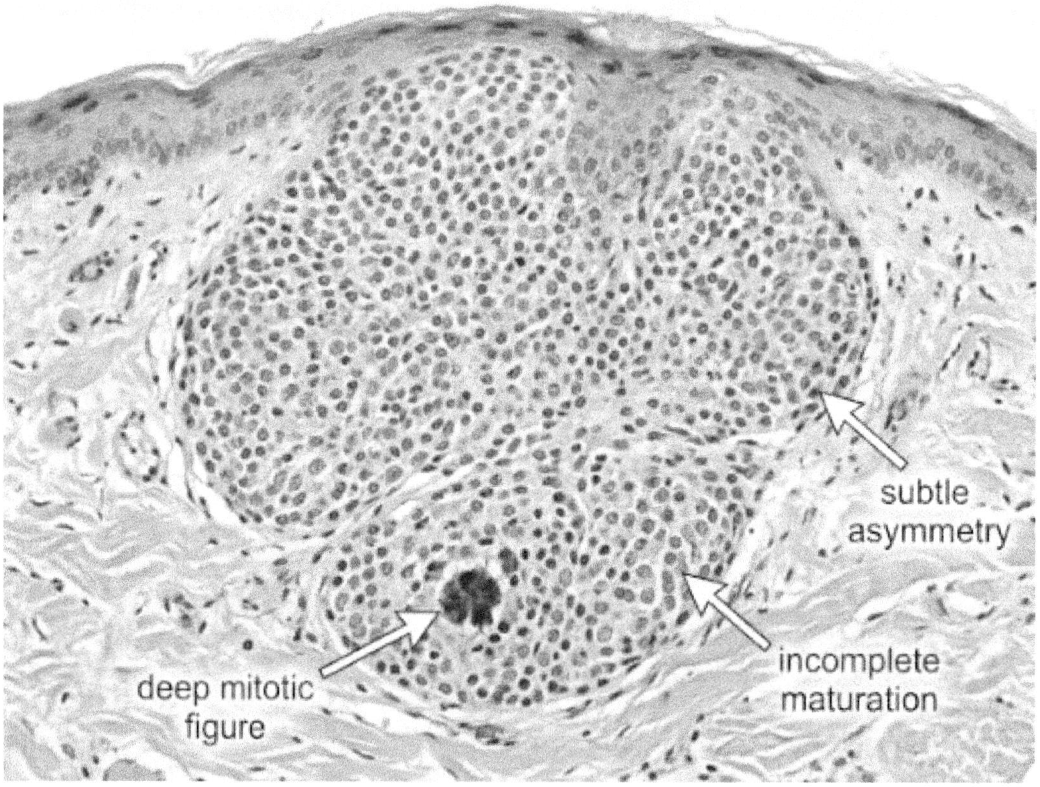

Ancillary Studies

Melanocyte Density Assessment for Lentigo Maligna

Melan-A/MART-1 immunohistochemistry, in addition to its role confirming melanocytic lineage broadly, is used specifically in the lentigo maligna differential discussed above to quantify melanocyte density along the basal layer, since lentigo maligna characteristically shows a markedly increased density of basal melanocytes, frequently confluent or approaching confluence, relative to the sparse, evenly spaced melanocyte population of chronically sun-damaged but non-neoplastic skin, a quantitative assessment that meaningfully improves diagnostic reproducibility in this specific, subtle differential and is also frequently used intraoperatively to assess margin clearance during staged excision of lentigo maligna, discussed further in the management implications section below.

Immunohistochemistry in Diagnostically Challenging Melanoma

S100, SOX10, Melan-A/MART-1, and HMB-45 confirm melanocytic lineage as in Chapter 13, with HMB-45's maturation gradient assessment carrying particular value in melanoma, where its persistence of strong staining into the deep component, rather than the expected superficial-to-deep loss of staining seen in a benign nevus, supports a failure-of-maturation pattern consistent with malignancy. Ki-67 proliferation index is frequently and diffusely elevated in melanoma, including within the deep dermal component, a pattern distinct from the confined, superficial proliferative zone typical of a benign nevus, providing valuable supportive evidence particularly in the nevoid melanoma scenario discussed above, where low-power morphology alone can be misleadingly reassuring.

Molecular and Staging-Relevant Ancillary Studies

Fluorescence in situ hybridization and comparative genomic hybridization, introduced in Chapter 13 for the Spitz nevus differential, apply equally to genuinely ambiguous melanocytic lesions in this chapter's differential, identifying the chromosomal copy number alterations characteristic of melanoma when morphology alone remains insufficient. BRAF mutation testing, performed on confirmed invasive or metastatic melanoma tissue, does not contribute to the initial diagnosis itself but is essential for subsequent systemic therapy selection, since BRAF V600E-mutant melanoma is eligible for targeted BRAF and MEK inhibitor combination therapy, a molecular result this chapter connects directly to the management implications discussed below. Sentinel lymph node biopsy, while a surgical rather than a purely histologic ancillary study, is itself subjected to detailed histopathologic and immunohistochemical evaluation for micrometastatic disease, with even minimal tumor deposits identified by immunohistochemistry carrying independent staging and prognostic significance.

Gene Expression Profiling and Prognostic Molecular Testing

Gene expression profiling assays, analyzing the expression pattern of a defined panel of genes within the primary tumor, have been developed as an adjunct prognostic tool intended to refine risk stratification beyond Breslow depth and ulceration alone, particularly for the intermediate-thickness melanoma population where sentinel lymph node biopsy results alone leave some prognostic uncertainty, though these assays remain an adjunct to, rather than a replacement for, the established histopathologic staging parameters detailed throughout this chapter, and their optimal role in routine clinical decision-making continues to be refined as further validation data accumulates. Germline genetic testing, distinct from the somatic BRAF mutation testing performed on tumor tissue, is pursued specifically in the hereditary melanoma scenario discussed in the etiology section above, using peripheral blood or saliva rather than tumor tissue, a testing pathway coordinated through genetic counseling given its implications for the patient's family members.

KEY POINT: Breslow depth, ulceration status, and mitotic rate together determine American Joint Committee on Cancer T category, which in turn determines both surgical margin width and sentinel lymph node biopsy eligibility, meaning the precision and completeness of the histopathologic report directly and immediately shapes the surgical management this patient receives.

Multidisciplinary Tumor Board Correlation

Diagnostically or prognostically complex melanoma cases, including nevoid melanoma, melanoma arising within a pre-existing nevus, Spitzoid melanoma, and cases with discordant ancillary study results, benefit from multidisciplinary tumor board discussion integrating the dermatopathologist's histologic and immunohistochemical findings with the treating dermatologist's or surgical oncologist's clinical assessment and, when relevant, the medical oncologist's perspective on systemic therapy implications, a collaborative review process this book has emphasized at multiple points as the appropriate response to genuine diagnostic uncertainty rather than a forced, unilateral final call. Second-opinion dermatopathology review, whether formally requested through tumor board or obtained through direct pathologist-to-pathologist consultation, is particularly valuable for thin melanomas with borderline Breslow depth measurements near a staging threshold, given how directly small measurement differences at these thresholds can alter the sentinel lymph node biopsy recommendation and overall management pathway.

Management Implications

Staging, Surgical Margins, and Sentinel Lymph Node Biopsy

American Joint Committee on Cancer staging integrates Breslow depth and ulceration status (T category), regional lymph node involvement identified clinically or by sentinel lymph node biopsy (N category), and distant metastasis (M category) into an overall stage that directly determines the management pathway: wide local excision with margins determined by Breslow depth (generally 0.5 to 1 centimeter for in situ disease, 1 centimeter for tumors up to 1 millimeter, and up to 2 centimeters for thicker tumors), sentinel lymph node biopsy offered for tumors generally exceeding 0.8 millimeters in depth or showing high-risk features such as ulceration at lesser depths, and completion lymph node dissection or systemic therapy considered when sentinel node involvement or higher-stage disease is identified.

Staged Excision for Lentigo Maligna and Lentigo Maligna Melanoma

Given the frequently indistinct clinical margins and adnexal extension of lentigo maligna discussed in the differential diagnosis and ancillary studies sections above, staged excision techniques, examining the complete peripheral margin histologically, whether by frozen section, permanent section staged excision, or Mohs micrographic surgery with melanocyte-specific immunohistochemical staining, are frequently preferred over standard excision with a fixed margin for this specific subtype, given evidence of improved margin control and reduced local recurrence relative to standard excision, particularly on cosmetically and functionally sensitive head and neck sites where this subtype most often arises.

Systemic Therapy: Immunotherapy and Targeted Therapy

Immune checkpoint inhibitor therapy, targeting programmed cell death protein 1 or its ligand, alone or in combination with cytotoxic T-lymphocyte-associated protein 4 blockade, has transformed the management of advanced and high-risk resected melanoma, with response rates and durability that depend substantially on tumor mutational burden, itself linked to the ultraviolet signature pathway discussed in the etiology section above, explaining the comparatively lower response rates observed in acral and mucosal melanoma relative to melanoma arising on intermittently sun-exposed skin. BRAF and MEK inhibitor combination therapy provides an alternative or sequential systemic therapy pathway specifically for BRAF V600E or V600K-mutant melanoma identified by the molecular testing discussed above, with adjuvant systemic therapy, either checkpoint inhibitor or, for BRAF-mutant disease, targeted therapy, now a standard consideration for resected stage IIB through stage IV melanoma given demonstrated reduction in recurrence risk.

Special Considerations in Metastatic and Unresectable Disease

For patients presenting with unresectable locoregional or distant metastatic disease, systemic therapy, immune checkpoint inhibition or, for BRAF-mutant disease, targeted therapy as discussed above, generally represents the primary treatment modality, with surgical resection, radiation therapy, and, for isolated in-transit or unresectable cutaneous metastases, intralesional oncolytic viral therapy reserved for specific clinical scenarios where they offer meaningful additional benefit. Response to systemic therapy in the metastatic setting is monitored through a combination of clinical examination and cross-sectional imaging, with tissue biopsy of a progressing or new lesion sometimes required to distinguish true progression from pseudoprogression, an inflammatory response pattern that can transiently mimic tumor growth on imaging in patients receiving immune checkpoint inhibitor therapy, a distinction with direct implications for whether therapy is continued or changed.

Complications and Prognosis

Prognosis in melanoma correlates directly and powerfully with the histopathologic staging parameters detailed throughout this chapter, with five-year survival exceeding 99 percent for thin, node-negative melanoma but falling substantially with increasing Breslow depth, presence of ulceration, and, most significantly, regional or distant metastatic spread, a prognostic gradient that underscores why early detection, developed in the prevention and screening section below, and precise, complete histopathologic staging together represent the two most powerful levers available for improving melanoma outcomes at a population level. Local recurrence, in-transit metastasis (tumor deposits between the primary site and the regional lymph node basin), and regional or distant metastatic spread each represent recognized patterns of disease progression that inform the surveillance protocols patients follow after initial treatment, with surveillance intensity and duration individualized to the initial stage at diagnosis.

Approximate Stage	Key Defining Features	Approximate 5-Year Survival
Stage 0 (in situ)	Confined to epidermis, no dermal invasion	Approaches 100%
Stage I	Thin, node-negative, no or minimal ulceration	Greater than 95%
Stage II	Thicker primary, node-negative	Approximately 80-90%, varies by substage
Stage III	Regional lymph node or in-transit involvement	Approximately 40-80%, varies substantially by substage
Stage IV	Distant metastatic spread	Improving with systemic therapy but remains substantially lower than earlier stages

These approximate survival figures, drawn from population-level staging data, are presented to illustrate the overall prognostic gradient this chapter's staging parameters produce rather than as a precise individual prognostic tool, since actual outcomes for an individual patient are further modified by tumor subtype, anatomic site, patient age and comorbidity, treatment response, and the systemic therapy advances discussed above, which have measurably improved outcomes for stage III and IV disease relative to the outcomes reflected in older staging cohorts.

Prevention and Screening

Population-level prevention builds directly on the sun protection principles established in Chapter 13, with the added emphasis, specific to melanoma, on total body skin examination performed by a trained clinician at a risk-stratified interval and structured patient self-examination education using the ABCDE criteria and ugly duckling sign discussed above. High-risk populations, patients with familial atypical multiple mole and melanoma syndrome, numerous dysplastic nevi, a personal or strong family history of melanoma, or a history of prior melanoma, warrant more intensive surveillance, including dermoscopy and, in selected cases, total body photography with sequential digital monitoring as introduced in Chapter 13, given this population's substantially elevated absolute risk of developing a subsequent primary melanoma.

Patient and clinician education regarding the specific presentations of nodular and amelanotic melanoma, which do not reliably follow classic ABCDE criteria as discussed in the clinical presentation section above, represents an important and specific component of melanoma prevention and early detection efforts, given evidence that these particular subtypes are disproportionately associated with delayed diagnosis and correspondingly greater Breslow depth at the time of biopsy.

Occupational and recreational ultraviolet exposure counseling, including specific discussion of indoor tanning device avoidance given the well-established, dose-dependent association between indoor tanning and melanoma risk, particularly when initiated during adolescence or young adulthood, represents an additional targeted prevention opportunity this chapter emphasizes given indoor tanning's status as a modifiable exposure distinct from ambient environmental ultraviolet radiation. Community and primary care-based skin cancer screening initiatives, while carrying an ongoing debate regarding optimal population-level screening frequency and cost-effectiveness, have demonstrated value in selected high-risk populations when paired with clear referral pathways to dermatology for lesions identified as concerning, reinforcing the collaborative, multidisciplinary detection pathway this chapter has emphasized throughout.

Melanoma in Immunosuppressed Patients

Solid organ transplant recipients and other chronically immunosuppressed patients carry an elevated melanoma risk together with a documented tendency toward thicker tumors at diagnosis and a comparatively less favorable prognosis stage for stage, attributed both to altered tumor immune surveillance and, in some studies, to a lower index of clinical suspicion and delayed biopsy in this specific population, findings that inform the more intensive dermatologic surveillance protocols this population typically follows and that warrant explicit consideration whenever a pigmented or amelanotic lesion in a transplant recipient shows any of the ABCDE or evolution features discussed in the clinical presentation section above. Response to immune checkpoint inhibitor therapy is generally attenuated in immunosuppressed patients, particularly transplant recipients maintained on immunosuppressive regimens, given this therapy's fundamental mechanism of restoring T-cell mediated antitumor immunity, a consideration that shapes systemic therapy selection and, in some cases, prompts coordinated discussion between oncology and transplant medicine regarding immunosuppression adjustment.

Patient Education and Counseling

Patients newly diagnosed with melanoma benefit from clear, structured counseling regarding what their specific Breslow depth, ulceration status, and stage mean for their surgical plan, sentinel lymph node biopsy recommendation, and, when relevant, systemic therapy eligibility, delivered in terms that connect the pathology report's technical parameters directly to the concrete management decisions those parameters drive, an explanatory bridge this chapter has built throughout to reinforce the direct, consequential link between accurate histopathologic diagnosis and patient outcome that defines this chapter's place at the center of dermatopathology practice. Melanoma survivors and their first-degree relatives benefit from specific counseling regarding the elevated second primary and, for relatives, first primary melanoma risk discussed above, together with structured guidance on lifelong self-examination technique, sun protection, and the recommended clinical surveillance interval, delivered with an emphasis on sustainable, long-term habits rather than a one-time set of instructions given the lifelong duration of this elevated risk.

THE REACTION PATTERN RECOGNITION SYSTEM — The Melanoma Diagnostic and Staging Pattern Family

---

The Pattern: Melanoma organized by histologic subtype and unified by asymmetry, failure of maturation with depth, and cytologic atypia, the direct inverse of Chapter 13's benign anchor: superficial spreading, nodular, lentigo maligna, acral lentiginous, desmoplastic, and nevoid melanoma.

Histologic Signature: Confluent nesting with pagetoid scatter and persistent atypia with depth defines the common subtypes; sparse spindled cells in dense fibrotic stroma defines desmoplastic melanoma; deceptively bland small-cell architecture with subtle asymmetry and deep mitoses defines nevoid melanoma.

The Decision: Apply the universal asymmetry-failure of maturation-atypia assessment first, then measure Breslow depth, ulceration, and mitotic rate to stage the tumor, escalating to immunohistochemistry, molecular studies, and BRAF mutation testing when morphology alone is insufficient or when systemic therapy selection requires it, and route diagnostically complex cases to multidisciplinary tumor board.

Trap Logic: Nevoid melanoma mimics a benign nevus at low power; desmoplastic melanoma mimics a scar or neurofibroma; melanoma can arise focally within an otherwise benign nevus requiring careful transition-zone mapping. Amelanotic and nodular melanoma frequently fail to meet classic ABCDE criteria clinically, and lentigo maligna can be mistaken for a benign solar lentigo given its slow, patchy evolution.

Pattern Anchor: Asymmetric, fails to mature, atypical: melanoma. Breslow depth, ulceration, and mitotic rate, measured precisely and reported completely, directly determine surgical margins, sentinel lymph node biopsy eligibility, and systemic therapy pathway. When morphology alone leaves genuine uncertainty, escalate to ancillary studies and multidisciplinary review rather than a forced unilateral call.

Summary and Key Concepts

Melanoma is classified into superficial spreading, nodular, lentigo maligna, acral lentiginous, desmoplastic, and nevoid subtypes, each with a characteristic site, growth pattern, and molecular association including BRAF, NRAS, KIT, and NF1 mutations.

The universal diagnostic criteria for melanoma, asymmetry, failure of maturation with depth, and cytologic atypia, represent the direct inverse of Chapter 13's benign melanocytic anchor and apply across every histologic subtype.

Breslow depth, ulceration status, and mitotic rate are the core histopathologic parameters determining American Joint Committee on Cancer staging, surgical margin width, and sentinel lymph node biopsy eligibility.

Nevoid melanoma and desmoplastic melanoma represent specific, deceptive histologic pitfalls, a nevus-like low-power appearance and a scar-like paucicellular fibrotic stroma respectively, that demand deliberate, systematic scrutiny beyond gestalt impression.

BRAF mutation testing informs targeted systemic therapy eligibility, while tumor mutational burden, linked to the ultraviolet signature pathway, influences immune checkpoint inhibitor response across melanoma subtypes.

Lentigo maligna and lentigo maligna melanoma follow a distinct, often prolonged clinical course on chronically sun-damaged skin and frequently require staged excision techniques and melanocyte density immunohistochemistry given their indistinct clinical margins.

Second primary melanoma risk, hereditary predisposition syndromes, and elevated risk in immunosuppressed patients each inform the lifelong, individualized surveillance protocols that follow an initial melanoma diagnosis or high-risk phenotype. Multidisciplinary tumor board review supports diagnostically complex cases.

CHAPTER 15: EPIDERMAL AND KERATINOCYTIC NEOPLASMS

Learning Objectives

1. Classify keratinocytic proliferations systematically across the full benign-to-malignant spectrum, including seborrheic keratosis, actinic keratosis, squamous cell carcinoma in situ, invasive squamous cell carcinoma, keratoacanthoma, and basal cell carcinoma.
2. Identify the specific histopathologic features and diagnostic criteria distinguishing each keratinocytic entity, including the major basal cell carcinoma subtypes and their distinct growth patterns.
3. Recognize the specific, deceptive histologic pitfalls associated with keratoacanthoma, irritated seborrheic keratosis, and pseudoepitheliomatous hyperplasia.
4. Construct a systematic, stepwise differential diagnosis for an ambiguous keratinocytic proliferation using architectural, cytologic, and ancillary immunohistochemical criteria.
5. Select appropriate immunohistochemical studies, including BerEP4, to distinguish basal cell carcinoma from squamous cell carcinoma and its various histologic mimickers.
6. Connect histopathologic risk stratification directly to the surgical and topical management pathway for keratinocytic neoplasms, including the specific role of Mohs micrographic surgery.
7. Recognize the deceptively bland or clinically confounded presentations of verrucous carcinoma and Marjolin ulcer, and explain why each carries a well-documented risk of delayed diagnosis.

Definition and Classification

Keratinocytic Proliferations as the Most Common Skin Neoplasms

This chapter addresses the keratinocytic proliferations that, in aggregate, constitute the most frequently biopsied and most commonly diagnosed neoplasms in dermatopathology practice, ranging from the entirely benign seborrheic keratosis through the premalignant actinic keratosis to invasive squamous cell carcinoma and basal cell carcinoma, the two most common malignancies in humans. This chapter's organizing framework differs somewhat from the reaction-pattern-based organization of earlier chapters in this book, instead following the biological continuum from benign keratinocytic proliferation through premalignant change to invasive carcinoma that defines this specific tumor family, a continuum that the named feature's Rhythm Layer callouts translate into a parallel decision framework emphasizing architectural depth of atypia as the unifying diagnostic axis. Despite this organizational shift, this chapter retains the same seven-part clinical structure, definition, etiology, histopathology, clinical presentation, differential diagnosis, ancillary studies, and management, used throughout this book, so the diagnostic method the reader has practiced across the melanocytic chapters carries forward directly into the keratinocytic tumor family covered here.

Classification of Entities Covered in This Chapter

This chapter covers seborrheic keratosis, a benign proliferation of basaloid keratinocytes entirely unrelated to sun exposure or malignant potential; actinic keratosis, a premalignant proliferation of atypical keratinocytes confined to the lower epidermis on chronically sun-damaged skin; squamous cell carcinoma in situ (Bowen disease), showing full-thickness epidermal atypia without dermal invasion; invasive squamous cell carcinoma; keratoacanthoma, a rapidly growing, crateriform keratinocytic proliferation with a distinctive natural history; and basal cell carcinoma, subclassified into nodular, superficial, infiltrative, and morpheaform (sclerosing) patterns, each carrying distinct management implications developed in the management implications section below.

Entity	Epidermal Involvement	Key Distinguishing Feature	Malignant Potential
Seborrheic keratosis	Exophytic, entirely epidermal	Horn (pseudohorn) cysts, basaloid cells, stuck-on silhouette, no atypia	None
Actinic keratosis	Lower epidermal atypia	Parakeratosis alternating with orthokeratosis over follicles, basal layer atypia	Premalignant (low per-lesion risk)
Squamous cell carcinoma in situ	Full-thickness epidermal atypia	No dermal invasion, atypia extends to the granular layer	Premalignant/in situ
Invasive squamous cell carcinoma	Dermal invasion	Atypical keratinocytes with keratinization actively invading the dermis	Malignant, metastatic potential
Keratoacanthoma	Crateriform, exo/endophytic	Central keratin-filled crater, glassy cytoplasm, rapid triphasic growth	Low-grade malignant/regressing variant of SCC
Basal cell carcinoma	Dermal-based basaloid nests	Peripheral palisading, retraction artifact, mucinous stroma	Malignant, rarely metastatic

Epidemiology of Keratinocytic Carcinoma

Basal cell carcinoma and squamous cell carcinoma, together termed keratinocytic (non-melanoma skin) carcinoma, represent the most commonly diagnosed malignancy in fair-skinned populations worldwide, with incidence rising steadily with age and cumulative ultraviolet exposure and a lifetime risk for fair-skinned individuals measured in a substantial fraction of the population, an epidemiologic burden that, despite these tumors' generally favorable prognosis relative to melanoma, makes keratinocytic carcinoma diagnosis and management among the highest-volume components of routine dermatopathology and dermatologic surgical practice. Basal cell carcinoma outnumbers squamous cell carcinoma by a ratio of approximately three or four to one in most fair-skinned populations, though this ratio narrows considerably, and squamous cell carcinoma can predominate, in immunosuppressed patients, a population-specific shift discussed further in the etiology and clinical presentation sections below given its direct clinical significance for surveillance intensity in this group.

Special Variants: Verrucous Carcinoma and Marjolin Ulcer

Verrucous carcinoma, a distinct, well-differentiated squamous cell carcinoma variant most common on the plantar foot, oral mucosa, and anogenital skin, shows a deceptively bland, exophytic, church-spire architecture with bulbous, pushing rather than infiltrative deep margins and minimal cytologic atypia, a histologic gentleness that belies this tumor's locally destructive behavior and that represents a well-recognized diagnostic pitfall this chapter addresses specifically in the differential diagnosis section below. Marjolin ulcer, squamous cell carcinoma arising within a chronic wound, burn scar, or area of long-standing lymphedema or osteomyelitis, follows a distinct pathogenic pathway driven by chronic inflammation and impaired immune surveillance rather than ultraviolet exposure, typically presenting after a latency period measured in years to decades from the original injury and carrying a comparatively more aggressive clinical course than ultraviolet-associated squamous cell carcinoma, a distinct etiology this chapter notes given its relevance to any biopsy obtained from a chronic, non-healing wound.

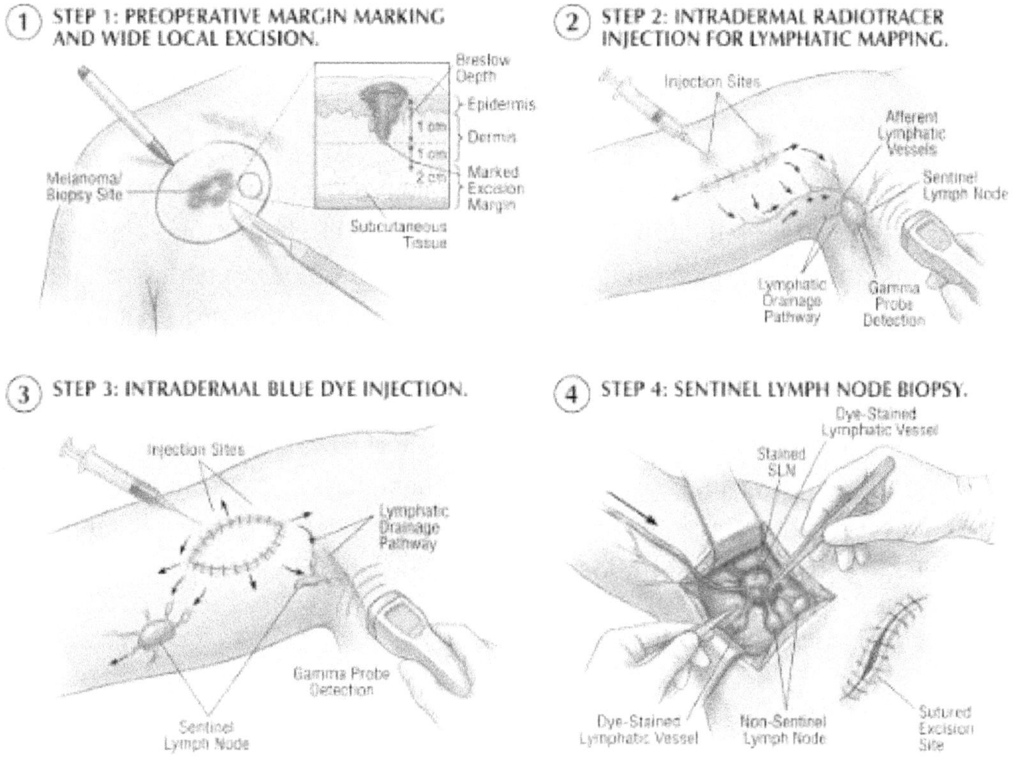

Etiology and Pathogenesis

Molecular Drivers of Seborrheic Keratosis

Seborrheic keratoses harbor activating FGFR3 and PIK3CA mutations in a substantial proportion of lesions, alterations in growth factor signaling pathways distinct from the ultraviolet-associated mutational spectrum driving the premalignant and malignant keratinocytic entities covered later in this chapter, a molecular distinction consistent with this entity's characteristic occurrence independent of cumulative sun exposure and its complete lack of malignant potential. The sign of Leser-Trelat, the abrupt eruptive onset of numerous seborrheic keratoses, has been associated in case reports with an underlying internal malignancy, most often gastrointestinal adenocarcinoma, through a paraneoplastic mechanism thought to involve circulating growth factors, an association this chapter notes given its potential clinical significance despite the entity's own uniformly benign nature.

Ultraviolet-Driven Field Cancerization

Actinic keratosis, squamous cell carcinoma in situ, and invasive squamous cell carcinoma occupy sequential points along a single ultraviolet radiation-driven carcinogenic continuum, field cancerization, in which cumulative ultraviolet exposure produces widespread TP53 mutations across a broad field of chronically sun-damaged skin, with individual keratinocyte clones progressively acquiring additional driver mutations, in genes including CDKN2A, NOTCH1, and components of the RAS-MAPK pathway, as they progress from actinic keratosis through in situ to invasive carcinoma, a stepwise molecular progression that explains both the frequent clinical finding of multiple actinic keratoses within a single anatomic field and the recognized, though individually low, per-lesion risk of any single actinic keratosis progressing to invasive squamous cell carcinoma.

Hedgehog Pathway Activation in Basal Cell Carcinoma

Basal cell carcinoma is driven predominantly by aberrant activation of the Hedgehog signaling pathway, most commonly through loss-of-function mutations in the PTCH1 tumor suppressor gene or, less commonly, activating mutations in SMO, alterations that produce constitutive, ligand-independent pathway activation and drive the characteristic basaloid keratinocyte proliferation of this tumor, a molecular pathway directly targeted by the Hedgehog pathway inhibitor systemic therapies discussed in the management implications section below for advanced or metastatic disease. Gorlin syndrome (nevoid basal cell carcinoma syndrome), associated with germline PTCH1 mutations, produces numerous basal cell carcinomas beginning at a young age together with characteristic extracutaneous findings including odontogenic keratocysts and palmar pitting, a hereditary syndrome this chapter notes given its implications for genetic counseling and lifelong dermatologic surveillance.

Arsenic and Other Chemical Carcinogen Exposure

Notably, chronic arsenic exposure, historically through contaminated well water, certain occupational exposures, or, in earlier decades, arsenic-containing medications, is an established, non-ultraviolet risk factor for both squamous cell carcinoma and basal cell carcinoma, characteristically producing multiple lesions and, distinctively, tumors that can arise on non-sun-exposed skin including the palms and soles, a distribution this chapter notes because it should prompt consideration of arsenic or other chemical carcinogen exposure history when keratinocytic carcinoma or its precursor lesions, including arsenical keratoses, a specific palmoplantar hyperkeratotic lesion, arise at these atypical, non-sun-exposed sites. Coal tar, polycyclic aromatic hydrocarbon, and ionizing radiation exposure represent additional recognized, non-ultraviolet etiologic pathways for keratinocytic carcinoma, each relevant to a specific occupational or medical exposure history that, when present, is documented as part of the complete clinicopathologic correlation this book emphasizes throughout.

Human Papillomavirus Association With Squamous Cell Carcinoma

A subset of cutaneous squamous cell carcinoma, particularly at genital, periungual, and, in immunosuppressed patients, more widespread cutaneous sites, is associated with high-risk human papillomavirus infection, a distinct etiologic pathway from the ultraviolet-driven field cancerization discussed above and one that carries specific relevance for the immunosuppressed patient population discussed further in the clinical presentation section below, given both this population's disproportionately elevated squamous cell carcinoma incidence and the specific human papillomavirus-associated verrucous and warty histologic patterns that can occur in this context. High-risk human papillomavirus subtypes, most notably HPV-16, drive malignant transformation through viral E6 and E7 oncoprotein-mediated degradation of the p53 and retinoblastoma tumor suppressor proteins respectively, a mechanism distinct from, but functionally convergent with, the direct TP53 mutation pathway that ultraviolet radiation drives in the field cancerization model, both pathways ultimately disabling the same core tumor suppressor checkpoint despite their different molecular starting points.

Immunosuppression and Keratinocytic Carcinoma Risk

Solid organ transplant recipients carry a markedly elevated risk of keratinocytic carcinoma, particularly squamous cell carcinoma, which can occur at a risk many-fold higher than the general population and, distinct from the general population pattern, frequently outnumbers basal cell carcinoma in this specific group, an inverted ratio directly relevant to the epidemiology discussed above and attributed to a combination of impaired T-cell mediated tumor immune surveillance, cumulative immunosuppressive drug exposure, and, in a subset of cases, the human papillomavirus association discussed further below. Squamous cell carcinoma arising in solid organ transplant recipients tends toward a more aggressive clinical course, including higher rates of local recurrence, regional metastasis, and multiplicity, findings that directly inform the substantially more intensive dermatologic surveillance protocols this population follows relative to immunocompetent patients, discussed further in the prevention and screening section below.

THE REACTION PATTERN RECOGNITION SYSTEM — Depth and Completeness of Keratinocytic Atypia as the Universal Staging Anchor

The Pattern: Depth and Completeness of Keratinocytic Atypia as the Single Axis Distinguishing Benign, Premalignant, and Malignant Keratinocytic Proliferations

Histologic Signature: No atypia (seborrheic keratosis); atypia confined to the lower third of the epidermis with sparing of the upper layers (actinic keratosis); full-thickness epidermal atypia without invasion (squamous cell carcinoma in situ); and atypical keratinocytes breaching the basement membrane into the dermis (invasive squamous cell carcinoma).

The Decision: Assess every keratinocytic proliferation in this chapter along this single depth-of-atypia axis before applying entity-specific criteria: does atypia exist at all, how much of the epidermal thickness does it involve, and has the basement membrane been breached, a sequential assessment that directly determines whether the lesion is benign, premalignant, in situ, or invasive.

Trap Logic: Irritated seborrheic keratosis can show reactive atypia and squamous eddies mimicking squamous cell carcinoma; keratoacanthoma shows a deceptively organized, symmetric architecture despite representing a variant of squamous cell carcinoma; and basal cell carcinoma, an entirely distinct basaloid rather than squamous lineage, must not be assessed along this same keratinocytic atypia axis.

Pattern Anchor: No atypia: benign. Lower-third atypia: actinic keratosis. Full-thickness atypia, no invasion: in situ. Atypia breaching the basement membrane: invasive. This single depth-of-atypia axis governs every keratinocytic diagnosis in this chapter.

Histopathologic Features and Diagnostic Criteria

Seborrheic Keratosis Histologic Variants

Beyond the classic acanthotic pattern described below, seborrheic keratosis shows several recognized histologic variants, including the hyperkeratotic variant, showing prominent church-spire hyperkeratosis with comparatively less basaloid proliferation; the reticulated (adenoid) variant, showing thin, interconnecting strands of basaloid epithelium; the clonal variant, showing well-demarcated nests of basaloid cells within the epidermis that can superficially mimic Bowen disease or, in heavily pigmented lesions, a melanocytic proliferation at low magnification; and the irritated variant, discussed in the differential diagnosis section below given its overlap with squamous neoplasia, each variant sharing the fundamental horn cyst formation and stuck-on architecture that anchor this entity's benign diagnosis regardless of which specific variant is present.

Diagnostic Features of Seborrheic Keratosis and Actinic Keratosis

Seborrheic keratosis shows an exophytic, sharply demarcated proliferation of small, uniform basaloid keratinocytes with a stuck-on silhouette (the lesion's base remaining at the same horizontal level as the adjacent normal epidermis rather than extending downward), numerous horn (pseudohorn) cysts, and squamous eddies (whorled keratinocyte aggregates) in the irritated variant, without cytologic atypia or dermal invasion at any point. Actinic keratosis shows atypical, hyperchromatic basal keratinocytes with loss of normal polarity confined to the lower third of an otherwise acanthotic epidermis, characteristically alternating parakeratosis (overlying the atypical epidermis) with orthokeratosis (overlying the spared follicular ostia), a distinctive alternating pattern that provides a helpful low-magnification diagnostic clue, together with solar elastosis in the underlying dermis reflecting the chronic ultraviolet damage that drives this entity's pathogenesis.

Diagnostic Features of Verrucous Carcinoma

Verrucous carcinoma shows a markedly acanthotic, papillomatous epidermis with a church-spire architecture of broad, blunt rete ridges, extensive hyperkeratosis with keratin-filled crypts, and minimal cytologic atypia throughout, distinguishing features that, taken in isolation at low magnification, can appear deceptively similar to a benign verruca or to pseudoepitheliomatous hyperplasia discussed in the differential diagnosis section below; the key diagnostic feature is instead found at the tumor's deep margin, which shows bulbous, pushing rather than infiltrative extension into the deep dermis or subcutis, a pattern requiring adequate biopsy depth to appreciate and, correspondingly, a well-recognized source of false-negative or equivocal superficial biopsies in this specific entity.

Diagnostic Features of Squamous Cell Carcinoma In Situ and Invasive Squamous Cell Carcinoma

Squamous cell carcinoma in situ (Bowen disease) shows full-thickness epidermal replacement by atypical, disorganized keratinocytes with loss of normal maturation, frequent mitotic figures at all levels including the upper epidermis, and multinucleated keratinocytes, without invasion through the basement membrane, while invasive squamous cell carcinoma shows this same atypical keratinocyte population breaching the basement membrane and infiltrating the dermis as irregular nests, cords, or single cells, frequently with individual cell keratinization (keratin pearl formation) and a desmoplastic or inflammatory stromal response, with the degree of differentiation, well, moderately, or poorly differentiated, assessed by the proportion of the tumor showing recognizable squamous differentiation and keratinization.

Depth of Invasion and Tumor Thickness in Squamous Cell Carcinoma

Analogous to the Breslow depth measurement central to melanoma staging in Chapter 14, tumor thickness and depth of invasion (specifically, invasion beyond the subcutaneous fat) are measured and reported for invasive squamous cell carcinoma, given their independent association with local recurrence and metastatic risk, together with the degree of histologic differentiation, well-differentiated tumors showing abundant keratinization and minimal atypia, poorly differentiated tumors showing scant keratinization with marked atypia and a correspondingly less favorable prognosis, and perineural invasion, discussed further below, each parameter contributing to the overall risk stratification that determines the surgical and adjuvant treatment approach detailed in the management implications section.

Diagnostic Features of Keratoacanthoma

Keratoacanthoma shows a distinctive crateriform architecture, a central keratin-filled crater flanked by symmetric, buttressing epidermal lips, composed of large keratinocytes with abundant glassy, eosinophilic (ground-glass) cytoplasm, minimal cytologic atypia relative to conventional squamous cell carcinoma, and a pushing, well-circumscribed rather than infiltrative deep border, features that together with this entity's characteristic natural history, discussed in the clinical presentation section below, place it along the spectrum of well-differentiated squamous cell carcinoma while carrying a comparatively more favorable behavior in the great majority of cases.

Diagnostic Features of the Basal Cell Carcinoma Subtypes

Nodular basal cell carcinoma shows large, well-circumscribed dermal nests of basaloid keratinocytes with peripheral palisading and retraction artifact as described above, while superficial basal cell carcinoma shows smaller, multifocal basaloid buds arising from and confined to the undersurface of the epidermis without significant dermal extension, an architectural distinction with direct treatment implications given superficial basal cell carcinoma's amenability to topical and superficially destructive therapies discussed in the management implications section below. Infiltrative basal cell carcinoma shows small, irregular, angulated basaloid nests and cords infiltrating between collagen bundles without the well-organized peripheral palisading of the nodular subtype, while morpheaform (sclerosing) basal cell carcinoma shows thin, single-cell-width strands of basaloid cells embedded within a densely sclerotic, fibrotic stroma, an architecture that, similar to desmoplastic melanoma discussed in Chapter 14, can be sparsely cellular and easily underestimated on a small biopsy, both infiltrative and morpheaform patterns extending significantly beyond their apparent clinical margins and carrying meaningfully higher local recurrence rates than the nodular or superficial subtypes.

Perineural and Perivascular Invasion Assessment

Perineural invasion, tumor cells surrounding or infiltrating a peripheral nerve, is reported explicitly whenever identified in either squamous cell carcinoma or basal cell carcinoma, given its status as a high-risk feature that independently elevates local recurrence and, for squamous cell carcinoma specifically, metastatic risk, with involvement of a named or large-caliber nerve carrying particular clinical significance given the associated risk of clinically silent proximal tumor extension along the nerve sheath beyond the visible tumor margin. This finding directly informs both the surgical approach, favoring Mohs micrographic surgery or wide excision with clear margins, and, in selected high-risk cases, the consideration of adjuvant radiation therapy discussed in the management implications section below.

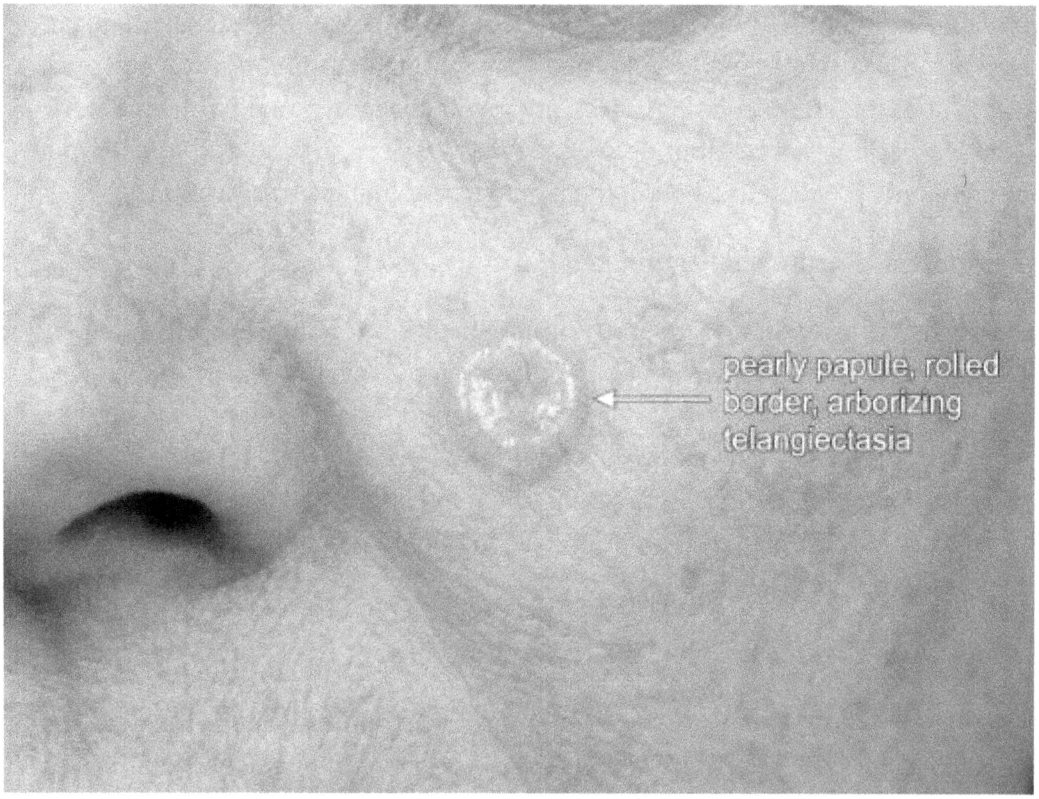

Clinical Presentation and Clinicopathologic Correlation

Clinical Morphology of Seborrheic Keratosis and Actinic Keratosis

Seborrheic keratoses present as well-demarcated, tan-to-brown, waxy or verrucous papules and plaques with a characteristic stuck-on appearance, most common on the trunk and face of middle-aged and older patients, typically multiple and increasing in number with age, a benign, cosmetically motivated diagnosis in the great majority of presentations that nonetheless warrants biopsy when a lesion shows atypical features, rapid change, or bleeding, given the entity's occasional clinical overlap with pigmented basal cell carcinoma or, less commonly, melanoma. Actinic keratoses present as ill-defined, rough, scaly, erythematous papules or patches on chronically sun-exposed skin, the face, scalp, forearms, and dorsal hands in particular, often more easily palpated than visualized given their subtle color contrast with surrounding sun-damaged skin, a tactile "sandpaper" quality that is itself a useful clinical screening sign.

Clinical Morphology of Basal Cell Carcinoma Subtypes

Nodular basal cell carcinoma, the most common subtype, presents as a pearly, translucent papule or nodule with rolled, raised borders and prominent overlying arborizing telangiectasias, frequently with central ulceration in more advanced lesions, most common on the head and neck. Superficial basal cell carcinoma presents as a well-demarcated, erythematous, scaly patch or thin plaque, most common on the trunk, that can closely mimic an inflammatory dermatosis such as nummular eczema or psoriasis clinically, while infiltrative and morpheaform (sclerosing) basal cell carcinoma present as ill-defined, scar-like, indurated plaques with subtle or absent surface changes, a deceptively subtle clinical presentation that correlates directly with these subtypes' more aggressive, deeply infiltrative histologic growth pattern developed in the differential diagnosis and management implications sections below. Pigmented basal cell carcinoma, a clinical rather than histologic variant that can occur across the nodular, superficial, or infiltrative subtypes, shows brown-to-black pigmentation admixed with the otherwise classic pearly, telangiectatic morphology, a presentation that carries genuine clinical overlap with nodular melanoma and pigmented seborrheic keratosis and that this chapter notes specifically as a recognized source of clinical diagnostic uncertainty resolved definitively by biopsy.

Clinical Presentation of Squamous Cell Carcinoma In Situ and Genital Involvement

Squamous cell carcinoma in situ (Bowen disease) presents as a well-demarcated, erythematous, scaly patch or thin plaque, often larger and more sharply demarcated than a typical actinic keratosis, most common on sun-exposed skin of older patients but also occurring on genital skin, where it is termed erythroplasia of Queyrat when involving the glans penis, a genital presentation this chapter notes specifically given its association with high-risk human papillomavirus infection discussed in the etiology section above and the correspondingly important role of colposcopic or penoscopic examination and, when appropriate, human papillomavirus testing in the complete evaluation of genital squamous neoplasia. Squamous cell carcinoma in situ can be mistaken clinically for a persistent inflammatory dermatosis, particularly psoriasis or chronic eczema, when it presents as a solitary, treatment-resistant scaly patch, a clinical overlap that underscores the importance of biopsying any persistent, solitary scaly lesion that fails to respond to appropriate topical anti-inflammatory therapy within an expected timeframe.

The Distinctive Natural History of Keratoacanthoma

Keratoacanthoma presents with a characteristic triphasic natural history: a proliferative phase over three to eight weeks producing rapid growth to a dome-shaped nodule with a central keratin plug, a mature phase of relative stability, and, in a substantial proportion of untreated lesions, a spontaneous involution phase over subsequent months leaving a depressed, atrophic scar, a natural history that historically supported observation as a management option but that in current practice is generally superseded by treatment given both the difficulty of reliably distinguishing keratoacanthoma from conventional squamous cell carcinoma on biopsy and the cosmetic and functional consequences of the scarring that follows even spontaneous involution.

Clinical Presentation of Verrucous Carcinoma

Verrucous carcinoma presents as a slowly enlarging, exophytic, cauliflower-like or warty mass, most often on the plantar foot, where it is frequently and understandably mistaken clinically for a benign plantar wart, a misattribution that, combined with this tumor's deceptively bland histology described above, is a well-recognized contributor to delayed diagnosis and, correspondingly, more extensive local tissue destruction by the time an accurate diagnosis is established, underscoring why any large, longstanding, or treatment-resistant verrucous lesion, particularly on the plantar foot or anogenital skin, warrants biopsy rather than continued empiric wart treatment.

Special Populations: Organ Transplant Recipients

Consistent with the elevated and inverted basal cell carcinoma to squamous cell carcinoma ratio discussed in the etiology section above, solid organ transplant recipients frequently present with numerous, sometimes hundreds over a post-transplant lifetime, keratinocytic carcinomas, most often on chronically sun-exposed skin, with individual lesions sometimes showing atypical, more aggressive clinical morphology, deeper induration, more rapid growth, or a warty, human papillomavirus-associated appearance, that in an immunocompetent patient would be less immediately concerning, findings that support this population's markedly lowered biopsy threshold and the specialized, high-volume dermatologic surveillance clinics many transplant centers maintain specifically for this purpose.

CLINICAL PEARL: A rapidly growing, dome-shaped nodule with a central keratin-filled crater developing over just weeks strongly suggests keratoacanthoma, but this diagnosis should be confirmed histologically and managed with treatment rather than watchful waiting alone, given the genuine difficulty of reliably excluding conventional squamous cell carcinoma on clinical grounds.

Differential Diagnosis and Histologic Mimickers

Keratoacanthoma Versus Conventional Squamous Cell Carcinoma

Distinguishing keratoacanthoma from conventional, well-differentiated squamous cell carcinoma rests on the crateriform architecture, symmetric buttressing epidermal lips, and glassy cytoplasm characteristic of keratoacanthoma against the more haphazard, infiltrative architecture and greater cytologic atypia typical of conventional squamous cell carcinoma, criteria that, in practice, produce genuine diagnostic overlap in a meaningful minority of cases, given which some pathologists favor a unified diagnostic terminology, keratoacanthoma-type well-differentiated squamous cell carcinoma, that acknowledges this overlap directly rather than forcing every lesion into one category or the other, a terminology choice this chapter notes as an area of ongoing practice variation rather than settled consensus.

Irritated Seborrheic Keratosis Versus Squamous Cell Carcinoma

Irritated or inflamed seborrheic keratosis can show squamous eddies, reactive cytologic atypia, and increased mitotic activity that superficially resembles squamous cell carcinoma in situ, distinguished by the overall maintained stuck-on architecture, horn cyst formation, and the basaloid, rather than atypical squamous, character of the proliferating cells outside the reactive squamous eddies themselves, together with the absence of the full-thickness, disorganized atypia and abnormal mitoses characteristic of genuine squamous cell carcinoma in situ.

A 71-year-old patient presents with a rapidly growing, 1.5-centimeter, dome-shaped nodule with a central keratin plug on the dorsal forearm, present for approximately five weeks. Pattern assignment identifies a symmetric, crateriform epidermal proliferation with buttressing epidermal lips, composed of large keratinocytes with abundant glassy eosinophilic cytoplasm and minimal cytologic atypia, together with a well-circumscribed, pushing deep border and a mixed inflammatory infiltrate at the base including eosinophils. Differential narrowing weighs the symmetric crateriform architecture and glassy cytoplasm, favoring keratoacanthoma, against residual concern given the entity's overlap with well-differentiated squamous cell carcinoma, concluding that the overall architectural and cytologic picture is most consistent with keratoacanthoma. Diagnosis of keratoacanthoma, keratoacanthoma-type squamous cell carcinoma, is rendered given the practice pattern discussed above, and complete surgical excision is recommended given the diagnostic overlap with conventional squamous cell carcinoma and the scarring that would otherwise follow spontaneous involution.

Actinic Keratosis Versus Early Squamous Cell Carcinoma In Situ

Distinguishing a severely atypical (hypertrophic or bowenoid) actinic keratosis from early squamous cell carcinoma in situ rests on whether the atypical keratinocyte population remains confined to the lower epidermis with preserved maturation in the upper layers, favoring actinic keratosis, or extends full-thickness with complete loss of normal maturation, favoring squamous cell carcinoma in situ, a distinction that can be genuinely difficult on a small or tangentially sectioned biopsy and that carries direct management significance given the different treatment approaches, field-directed topical therapy for actinic keratosis versus definitive surgical or ablative treatment for confirmed in situ disease, discussed in the management implications section below.

Verrucous Carcinoma Versus Verruca Vulgaris and Pseudoepitheliomatous Hyperplasia

Verrucous carcinoma, given its deceptively bland cytology described in the histopathologic features section above, must be distinguished both from a benign verruca vulgaris, showing the characteristic koilocytic change, vertical tiers of parakeratosis, and papillomatous architecture of a human papillomavirus-associated wart without verrucous carcinoma's bulbous, pushing deep margin, and from pseudoepitheliomatous hyperplasia, a reactive, non-neoplastic epidermal proliferation that can occur overlying an underlying inflammatory or infectious process (deep fungal infection, granular cell tumor, or a chronic ulcer among recognized triggers) and that can appear alarmingly atypical and infiltrative-appearing on a superficial biopsy despite its entirely benign, reactive nature, a mimicker this chapter emphasizes because recognizing its association with an underlying trigger, rather than the epidermal changes alone, is often the key to avoiding a false-positive malignant diagnosis.

A 68-year-old patient presents with a 2-centimeter, scaly, erythematous, well-demarcated plaque on the lower leg, present and slowly enlarging over approximately eight months, clinically favored as either superficial basal cell carcinoma or an inflammatory dermatosis such as nummular eczema. Pattern assignment identifies multifocal small basaloid buds arising from the undersurface of the epidermis, each showing peripheral palisading and retraction artifact, confined to the papillary dermis without deeper extension, with no infiltrative or morpheaform component identified after examination of multiple levels. Differential narrowing confirms superficial basal cell carcinoma over an inflammatory dermatosis given the unequivocal basaloid palisading and retraction artifact, and over the deeper nodular or infiltrative subtypes given the confinement of tumor buds to the papillary dermis alone. Diagnosis of superficial basal cell carcinoma is rendered, with the report noting the absence of any deeper or infiltrative component given its direct relevance to the topical or superficially destructive treatment options discussed in the management implications section below, which are specifically appropriate for this confirmed superficial-only subtype.

Basal Cell Carcinoma Versus Trichoepithelioma and Other Follicular Tumors

Basal cell carcinoma must be distinguished from trichoepithelioma and other benign follicular neoplasms sharing a basaloid cytomorphology, a differential developed more fully in Chapter 16's coverage of adnexal neoplasms, resting on basal cell carcinoma's characteristic peripheral palisading with retraction (clefting) artifact between tumor nests and the surrounding stroma, mucinous stromal change, and an infiltrative or destructive growth pattern, against trichoepithelioma's more organized, symmetric architecture with papillary mesenchymal bodies and horn cyst formation resembling follicular differentiation, a distinction with direct management consequences given the two entities' entirely different malignant potential. On a small or superficial biopsy lacking the deep architectural context needed to assess this distinction directly, immunohistochemistry, discussed in the ancillary studies section below, together with clinical correlation regarding lesion growth rate and destructive behavior, frequently becomes the deciding factor, underscoring why this specific differential is one where obtaining an adequately deep and representative biopsy specimen carries particular diagnostic importance.

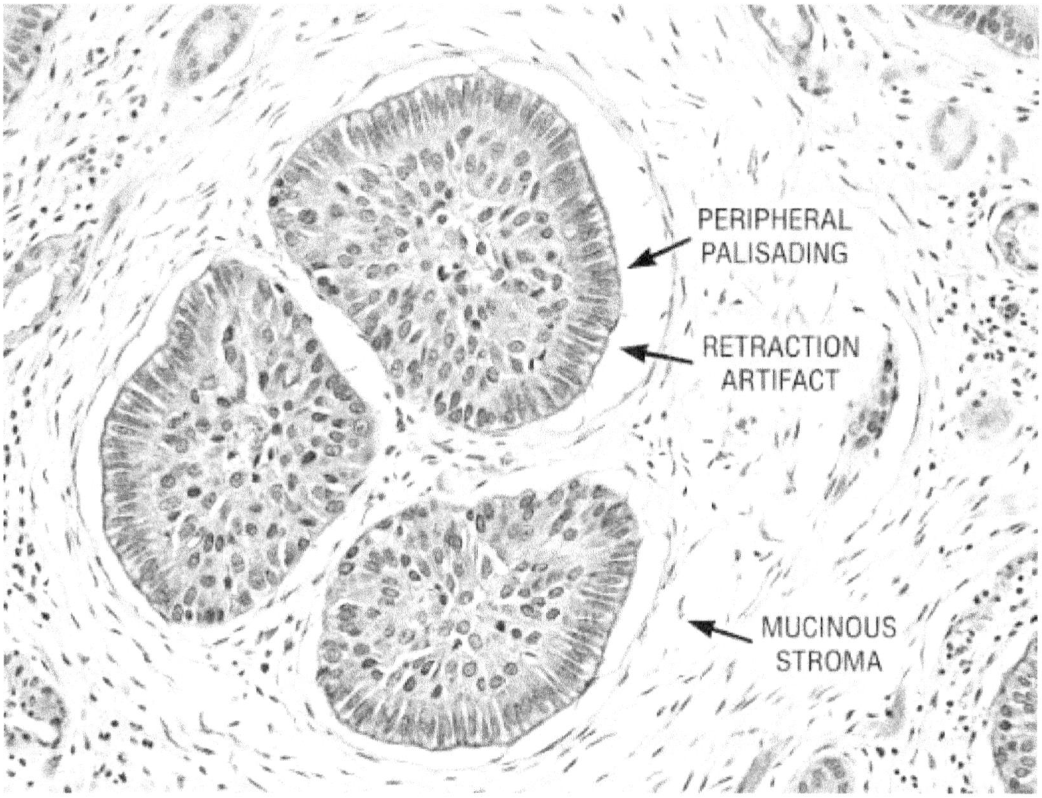

Ancillary Studies

Pigmented Lesion Overlap and Confirmatory Melanocytic Markers

For pigmented basal cell carcinoma or a heavily pigmented irritated seborrheic keratosis showing genuine clinical overlap with a melanocytic neoplasm, as discussed in the clinical presentation section above, S100, SOX10, or Melan-A/MART-1 immunohistochemistry, the same melanocytic lineage markers introduced in Chapters 13 and 14, can be used to confirm that any pigmented or dendritic cell population within the lesion represents incidental melanophages or colonizing benign melanocytes rather than a genuine melanocytic proliferation, a confirmatory step that, together with the basaloid or squamous architectural features already discussed, resolves this specific pigmented-lesion overlap definitively.

Immunohistochemistry Distinguishing Basal Cell Carcinoma From Squamous Cell Carcinoma

BerEP4 immunohistochemistry shows strong, diffuse membranous staining in basal cell carcinoma with characteristic absence or marked reduction in squamous cell carcinoma, providing a useful distinguishing marker in ambiguous basaloid proliferations, while p63 and CK5/6 stain both entities given their shared keratinocytic lineage and are therefore more useful for confirming epithelial origin broadly than for distinguishing between these two specific entities. Ki-67 proliferation index is typically elevated in both squamous cell carcinoma and basal cell carcinoma relative to benign keratinocytic proliferations, providing supportive rather than specific diagnostic information, most useful when distinguishing a genuinely atypical proliferation from a reactive or irritated benign process such as the irritated seborrheic keratosis discussed above.

p53 and Immunohistochemical Assessment of Field Cancerization

p53 immunohistochemistry can highlight the extent of ultraviolet-associated keratinocyte mutation across a field of chronically sun-damaged skin, showing patchy to widespread nuclear staining in actinic keratosis and squamous cell carcinoma in situ that extends beyond the area of overt histologic atypia, a finding that provides useful supportive context for the field cancerization concept discussed in the etiology section above though it is not routinely required for the diagnosis of any individual, histologically unambiguous lesion in this chapter's differential.

Immunohistochemistry Supporting the Verrucous Carcinoma and Pseudoepitheliomatous Hyperplasia Differential

Ki-67 proliferation index and p53 immunohistochemistry can provide supportive, though not definitive, evidence in the verrucous carcinoma versus pseudoepitheliomatous hyperplasia differential discussed above, with a markedly elevated and full-thickness Ki-67 proliferative pattern favoring a genuine neoplastic process over reactive pseudoepitheliomatous hyperplasia, which typically retains a more confined, basally oriented proliferative zone despite its alarming architectural complexity; however, given the substantial overlap that can exist even with immunohistochemical support, this differential more than most in this chapter depends on adequate biopsy depth and clinical correlation, including identification of an underlying trigger for pseudoepitheliomatous hyperplasia, rather than immunohistochemistry as a stand-alone arbiter.

Molecular Testing and Emerging Biomarkers

Tumor mutational burden in keratinocytic carcinoma, particularly ultraviolet-associated squamous cell carcinoma, is among the highest of any solid tumor type, a molecular characteristic that underlies the meaningful response rates observed with immune checkpoint inhibitor therapy in advanced, unresectable, or metastatic squamous cell carcinoma discussed in the management implications section below, though routine molecular profiling is not required for the diagnosis or initial management of the great majority of localized, surgically resectable tumors covered in this chapter. PD-L1 expression testing, while more established in other solid tumor contexts, has a more limited and evolving role in guiding keratinocytic carcinoma immunotherapy decisions, with treatment eligibility currently determined predominantly by disease stage and resectability rather than a specific biomarker threshold.

KEY POINT: BerEP4 immunohistochemistry is the single most useful ancillary marker for distinguishing basal cell carcinoma from squamous cell carcinoma or its mimickers in a genuinely ambiguous basaloid proliferation, given its strong positivity in basal cell carcinoma and characteristic negativity or marked reduction in squamous lineage tumors.

Management Implications

Risk Stratification and Surgical Margins

As with the staging framework detailed for melanoma in Chapter 14, this risk stratification is a direct product of the histopathologic parameters this chapter has emphasized throughout, meaning report completeness and precision translate immediately into surgical decision-making. Squamous cell carcinoma and basal cell carcinoma are risk-stratified by tumor size, anatomic location, histologic subtype, depth of invasion, and the presence of high-risk features including perineural invasion, poor differentiation, and prior treatment failure, a stratification that directly determines the treatment modality selected: standard surgical excision with margins determined by risk category for low-risk tumors, and Mohs micrographic surgery, offering complete margin assessment with maximal tissue conservation, preferentially selected for high-risk tumors, tumors in cosmetically or functionally sensitive locations, recurrent tumors, and the infiltrative and morpheaform basal cell carcinoma subtypes discussed above given their characteristic subclinical extension beyond apparent clinical margins.

Topical and Field-Directed Therapy for Actinic Keratosis

Individual actinic keratoses are treated with cryotherapy or, for numerous lesions within a single field of cancerization, field-directed topical therapy, including topical 5-fluorouracil, imiquimod, or photodynamic therapy, treatment approaches that target the entire affected field rather than individual clinically apparent lesions alone, an approach directly informed by the field cancerization concept discussed in the etiology section above, since subclinical atypical keratinocyte clones throughout the treated field, not just the visible actinic keratoses, are addressed by field-directed therapy in a way that lesion-by-lesion cryotherapy alone cannot achieve.

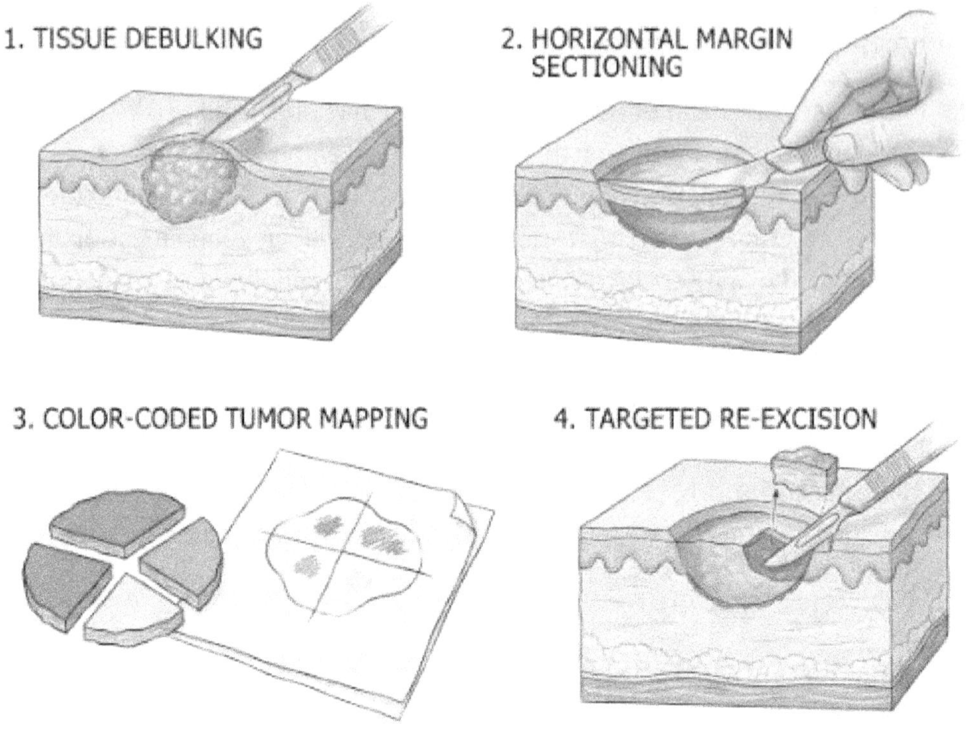

Systemic Therapy for Advanced and Metastatic Disease

Hedgehog pathway inhibitor therapy, targeting the SMO protein directly downstream of the PTCH1 alterations discussed in the etiology section above, is approved for locally advanced or metastatic basal cell carcinoma not amenable to surgery or radiation, providing a targeted systemic therapy option specific to this tumor's defining molecular pathway. Immune checkpoint inhibitor therapy, targeting programmed cell death protein 1, is approved for locally advanced or metastatic squamous cell carcinoma not amenable to curative surgery or radiation, with response rates benefiting from this tumor's characteristically high tumor mutational burden discussed in the ancillary studies section above, together providing meaningful systemic therapy options for the comparatively small subset of keratinocytic carcinoma patients whose disease has progressed beyond the reach of surgical or radiation-based local therapy.

Complications and Prognosis

Basal cell carcinoma carries an excellent prognosis with appropriate treatment and an exceedingly low metastatic rate, though local tissue destruction, particularly for neglected or recurrent infiltrative and morpheaform subtypes, can produce substantial functional and cosmetic morbidity given this tumor's tendency toward deep, locally destructive growth in cosmetically and functionally sensitive head and neck locations. Squamous cell carcinoma carries a generally favorable prognosis for low-risk tumors but a meaningfully elevated metastatic risk for high-risk tumors, those showing perineural invasion, poor differentiation, deep invasion, or arising in an immunosuppressed patient, a risk stratification that directly informs the surveillance intensity and, in selected high-risk cases, adjuvant radiation therapy or sentinel lymph node biopsy consideration these patients receive.

Verrucous carcinoma and Marjolin ulcer each carry a comparatively more guarded local prognosis than typical ultraviolet-associated keratinocytic carcinoma, verrucous carcinoma given its tendency toward extensive local destruction before diagnosis despite a comparatively low metastatic rate, and Marjolin ulcer given both its more aggressive intrinsic biology and its frequent late-stage presentation, together underscoring why the deceptively bland or confounded clinical presentations these two specific entities share, discussed throughout this chapter, carry disproportionate practical significance for long-term patient outcome relative to their comparative rarity.

Risk Category	Key Features	Typical Management
Low-risk squamous cell carcinoma	Small, well-differentiated, no perineural invasion, primary tumor	Standard excision with clear margins
High-risk squamous cell carcinoma	Large, poorly differentiated, perineural invasion, recurrent, or immunosuppressed host	Mohs micrographic surgery; consider adjuvant radiation
Nodular/superficial basal cell carcinoma	Well-circumscribed, low-risk location	Standard excision, electrodesiccation and curettage, or topical/superficial therapy for superficial subtype
Infiltrative/morpheaform basal cell carcinoma	Ill-defined margins, high-risk location, recurrent	Mohs micrographic surgery preferred

Documentation and Reporting Standards

A dermatopathology report for a keratinocytic neoplasm should explicitly document histologic subtype, degree of differentiation for squamous cell carcinoma, depth of invasion, and the presence or absence of perineural or lymphovascular invasion, together with margin status when the specimen is an excision rather than an initial diagnostic biopsy, a documentation standard that, consistent with the reporting principles emphasized in Chapters 13 and 14, directly informs the risk stratification and surgical planning detailed in this section rather than leaving these consequential management decisions to inference from a bare categorical diagnosis alone.

Prevention and Screening

Consistent with the field cancerization mechanism discussed throughout this chapter, sun protection remains the primary modifiable prevention strategy for the entire keratinocytic tumor spectrum, together with regular dermatologic skin examination for patients with substantial cumulative sun exposure, fair skin phototype, or a history of prior keratinocytic carcinoma, a population that carries an elevated risk of developing additional lesions and benefits from structured, ongoing surveillance analogous to the melanoma surveillance protocols discussed in Chapter 14.

Chemoprevention with oral nicotinamide (vitamin B3) has demonstrated a modest but reproducible reduction in the incidence of new keratinocytic carcinoma and actinic keratosis in high-risk, immunocompetent patients with a history of multiple prior lesions, an inexpensive, low-risk adjunct to sun protection and surveillance that this chapter notes given its increasing incorporation into the prevention discussion for this specific high-risk population, though it has not been established as effective in solid organ transplant recipients, a population in whom the immunosuppression-driven risk pathway discussed in the etiology section above appears to operate largely independent of the mechanism nicotinamide is thought to address.

Multidisciplinary Considerations for Marjolin Ulcer and Chronic Wound-Associated Carcinoma

Squamous cell carcinoma arising within a chronic wound or burn scar, Marjolin ulcer as introduced in the definition and classification section above, warrants coordinated management between dermatopathology, surgical oncology, and, frequently, wound care or plastic surgery specialists, given this entity's comparatively more aggressive natural history, its tendency toward delayed diagnosis given the confounding presence of a pre-existing chronic wound, and the frequently more extensive surgical planning, occasionally including amputation for long-standing lower extremity lesions, that this presentation can require relative to squamous cell carcinoma arising on otherwise normal skin. Any chronic wound that fails to heal within an expected timeframe, shows new heaped-up or friable tissue, or begins to bleed or enlarge should be biopsied to exclude Marjolin ulcer, a threshold this chapter emphasizes given the well-documented pattern of delayed recognition this specific presentation carries in clinical practice.

Patient Education and Counseling

Patients newly diagnosed with a keratinocytic carcinoma benefit from counseling regarding their specific risk stratification, the rationale for the selected surgical or topical treatment approach, and the recommended surveillance interval given the meaningfully elevated risk of developing additional keratinocytic tumors after an initial diagnosis, together with practical, sustainable sun protection guidance framed around this population's demonstrated, ongoing risk rather than a one-time educational intervention. Organ transplant recipients and other chronically immunosuppressed patients benefit from specific, structured counseling regarding their substantially elevated risk and the intensive surveillance schedule this risk warrants, delivered, when possible, in coordination with the transplant or immunosuppression-managing team so that dermatologic surveillance is integrated into this population's broader long-term care plan rather than treated as a separate, easily deprioritized concern.

THE REACTION PATTERN RECOGNITION SYSTEM — The Keratinocytic Neoplasm Staging Pattern Family

---

The Pattern: Keratinocytic proliferations organized along a single depth-of-atypia continuum from benign through premalignant to invasive: seborrheic keratosis, actinic keratosis, squamous cell carcinoma in situ, invasive squamous cell carcinoma, keratoacanthoma, and basal cell carcinoma.

Histologic Signature: No atypia with horn cysts defines seborrheic keratosis; lower-third atypia with alternating parakeratosis defines actinic keratosis; full-thickness atypia without invasion defines in situ disease; dermal invasion defines invasive carcinoma; peripheral palisading with retraction artifact defines basal cell carcinoma; bland, church-spire architecture with a bulbous pushing base defines verrucous carcinoma.

The Decision: Assess depth and completeness of keratinocytic atypia first, then apply entity-specific criteria including crateriform architecture for keratoacanthoma and basaloid palisading for basal cell carcinoma, escalating to BerEP4 and other immunohistochemistry when the basaloid-versus-squamous distinction remains genuinely ambiguous, and confirm adequate biopsy depth whenever verrucous carcinoma or Marjolin ulcer is a clinical consideration.

Trap Logic: Irritated seborrheic keratosis mimics squamous cell carcinoma in situ; keratoacanthoma overlaps substantially with well-differentiated squamous cell carcinoma; infiltrative and morpheaform basal cell carcinoma present with deceptively subtle, scar-like clinical morphology despite aggressive local growth; verrucous carcinoma mimics a benign wart clinically and pseudoepitheliomatous hyperplasia both histologically and clinically.

Pattern Anchor: No atypia: benign. Lower-third atypia: actinic keratosis. Full-thickness, no invasion: in situ. Invasion present: malignant. Peripheral palisading with retraction: basal cell carcinoma, an entirely distinct basaloid lineage from the keratinocytic atypia axis governing the rest of this chapter. Verrucous carcinoma and Marjolin ulcer require deliberate deep sampling and clinical context, respectively, given their deceptively bland or confounded presentations.

Summary and Key Concepts

Keratinocytic proliferations are organized along a single depth-of-atypia continuum: no atypia in seborrheic keratosis, lower-third atypia in actinic keratosis, full-thickness atypia without invasion in squamous cell carcinoma in situ, and dermal invasion in invasive squamous cell carcinoma.

Keratoacanthoma represents a distinctive, rapidly growing, crateriform variant along the well-differentiated squamous cell carcinoma spectrum, with genuine, well-recognized histologic overlap that has led some pathologists toward unified keratoacanthoma-type squamous cell carcinoma terminology.

Basal cell carcinoma, an entirely distinct basaloid lineage driven by Hedgehog pathway activation, is subclassified into nodular, superficial, infiltrative, and morpheaform patterns, each carrying distinct clinical presentation and management implications.

BerEP4 immunohistochemistry is the key ancillary marker distinguishing basal cell carcinoma from squamous cell carcinoma and its mimickers, given strong positivity in basal cell carcinoma and characteristic negativity in squamous lineage tumors.

Risk stratification by tumor size, location, histologic subtype, and high-risk features including perineural invasion directly determines the surgical approach, with Mohs micrographic surgery preferentially selected for high-risk and infiltrative or morpheaform tumors.

Verrucous carcinoma and Marjolin ulcer represent distinct, non-ultraviolet-driven squamous cell carcinoma presentations, arising respectively from a deceptively bland exophytic tumor and from chronic wound- or scar-associated malignant transformation, each carrying a well-recognized risk of delayed diagnosis.

Solid organ transplant recipients and other immunosuppressed patients carry a markedly elevated, often inverted-ratio keratinocytic carcinoma risk favoring squamous over basal cell carcinoma, warranting substantially more intensive dermatologic surveillance than the general population, ideally coordinated with the managing transplant team.

CHAPTER 16: ADNEXAL NEOPLASMS: FOLLICULAR, SEBACEOUS, AND SWEAT GLAND ORIGIN

Learning Objectives

1. Classify cutaneous adnexal neoplasms systematically by line of differentiation: follicular, sebaceous, eccrine, and apocrine, using each entity's signature recapitulated structure.
2. Identify the specific histopathologic features distinguishing trichoepithelioma, pilomatricoma, tricholemmoma, syringoma, poroma, spiradenoma, cylindroma, hidradenoma, and the sebaceous neoplasm spectrum.
3. Recognize the specific histologic pitfalls distinguishing trichoepithelioma from basal cell carcinoma, poroma from porocarcinoma, and microcystic adnexal carcinoma from its benign sclerosing mimickers.
4. Connect specific adnexal neoplasms to their associated hereditary tumor predisposition syndromes, including Brooke-Spiegler, Cowden, and Muir-Torre syndrome.
5. Select appropriate immunohistochemical and mismatch repair protein studies for diagnostically ambiguous or syndromically significant adnexal neoplasms, including the trichoepithelioma and Muir-Torre screening panels.
6. Connect adnexal neoplasm diagnosis directly to surgical management planning and, when a hereditary syndrome is identified or suspected, systemic malignancy screening and genetic counseling referral.
7. Identify microcystic adnexal carcinoma's deceptively bland superficial appearance and explain why adequate biopsy depth is essential to establishing this specific diagnosis.

Definition and Classification

Adnexal Neoplasms Organized Systematically by Line of Differentiation

Cutaneous adnexal neoplasms recapitulate, to varying degrees of completeness, the normal structures of the pilosebaceous unit and the eccrine and apocrine sweat glands, and this chapter organizes its coverage by line of differentiation, follicular, sebaceous, eccrine, and apocrine, a classification framework that mirrors the normal embryologic and adult adnexal anatomy and that provides the most reliable scaffold for recognizing the sometimes bewildering diversity of benign and malignant tumors this specific tumor family encompasses. Within each line of differentiation, this chapter addresses the benign entities most frequently encountered in routine dermatopathology practice together with their corresponding malignant counterparts, emphasizing throughout the specific architectural and cytologic features that distinguish true adnexal differentiation from the keratinocytic and basaloid tumors covered in Chapter 15, a distinction that in practice represents one of the most common sources of diagnostic difficulty this chapter addresses directly. Familiarity with normal adult and developing adnexal histology, the hair follicle with its bulb, matrix, and outer and inner root sheaths, the holocrine sebaceous gland, and the coiled eccrine secretory unit with its straight and coiled ductal segments, is assumed throughout this chapter as the anatomic foundation against which each neoplasm's specific recapitulated differentiation is recognized and named.

Follicular, Sebaceous, and Sweat Gland Entities Covered Comprehensively in This Chapter

Follicular differentiation entities include trichoepithelioma, trichofolliculoma, tricholemmoma, and pilomatricoma, each recapitulating a distinct component of the normal hair follicle. Sebaceous differentiation entities span a benign-to-malignant spectrum from sebaceous hyperplasia and sebaceous adenoma through sebaceoma to sebaceous carcinoma. Eccrine differentiation entities include syringoma, eccrine poroma, eccrine spiradenoma, and cylindroma, together with their malignant counterparts, porocarcinoma and malignant spiradenoma/cylindroma, while apocrine differentiation entities include apocrine hidrocystoma and hidradenoma papilliferum, each developed in the sections that follow. This chapter follows the same seven-part clinical structure used throughout this book, definition, etiology, histopathology, clinical presentation, differential diagnosis, ancillary studies, and management, so the systematic diagnostic method the reader has applied to the melanocytic and keratinocytic tumor families in prior chapters extends directly to this comparatively lower-volume but diagnostically demanding adnexal tumor family.

Entity	Line of Differentiation	Key Distinguishing Feature	Malignant Potential
Trichoepithelioma	Follicular	Horn cysts, papillary mesenchymal bodies, symmetric architecture, CYLD pathway	None (benign)
Pilomatricoma	Follicular (hair matrix)	Basaloid cells transitioning to shadow (ghost) cells, calcification, CTNNB1 pathway	Low (rare pilomatrical carcinoma)
Tricholemmoma	Follicular (outer root sheath)	Clear cell change, peripheral palisading, thickened basement membrane, PTEN pathway	None (benign)
Syringoma	Eccrine duct	Comma-shaped (tadpole) ducts confined to superficial dermis	None (benign)
Eccrine poroma	Eccrine duct	Broad anastomosing bands of cuboidal	Low (porocarcinoma transformation)

		poroid cells extending from epidermis	
Spiradenoma/cylindroma	Eccrine (secretory coil)	Basaloid nests in jigsaw-puzzle pattern with hyaline basement membrane material, CYLD pathway	Low (malignant transformation reported)
Sebaceous neoplasm spectrum	Sebaceous	Sebocytes with multivacuolated, scalloped nuclei; increasing atypia and infiltration with malignancy	Variable (adenoma to carcinoma)
Microcystic adnexal carcinoma	Eccrine/follicular (mixed)	Deeply infiltrative small ducts and keratinizing cysts, deceptively bland cytology	Malignant, locally aggressive, low metastatic risk
Apocrine hidrocystoma	Apocrine	Simple unilocular cystic space with bilayered, decapitation-secreting epithelium	None (benign)
Hidradenoma papilliferum	Apocrine	Bilayered papillary architecture closely resembling an intraductal papilloma	None (benign)

Microcystic Adnexal Carcinoma: A Deceptively Bland Malignancy

Microcystic adnexal carcinoma warrants separate emphasis within this chapter given its combination of deceptively bland cytology and deeply, extensively infiltrative growth, a combination that makes this entity one of the most consequential diagnostic pitfalls in adnexal pathology, showing mixed eccrine ductal and follicular differentiation and infiltrating well beyond its clinically apparent margin into the deep dermis, subcutis, and, characteristically, along nerves, a growth pattern developed further in the histopathologic features and differential diagnosis sections below given its direct relevance to both accurate diagnosis and the extensive surgical planning this tumor requires.

Epidemiology of Adnexal Neoplasms Across Clinical Practice Settings

Benign adnexal neoplasms in aggregate are considerably more common than their malignant counterparts, which collectively represent a small minority of cutaneous malignancy relative to the keratinocytic and melanocytic tumors covered in Chapters 13 through 15, a comparative rarity that, paradoxically, makes accurate recognition of malignant adnexal entities, sebaceous carcinoma and porocarcinoma in particular, more diagnostically challenging given the correspondingly lower baseline clinical and pathologic familiarity these entities receive relative to their higher-volume keratinocytic and melanocytic counterparts. Most adnexal neoplasms in this chapter arise sporadically without an identifiable hereditary syndrome, though, as this chapter emphasizes throughout, a meaningful minority serve as the first diagnostic clue to an underlying hereditary tumor predisposition syndrome, making pattern recognition, multiplicity assessment, and appropriate ancillary testing referral a genuinely high-stakes component of adnexal neoplasm diagnosis despite these tumors' overall rarity.

Hidradenoma and Additional Sweat Gland Entities of Clinical Relevance

Beyond the core eccrine and apocrine entities introduced above, this chapter also addresses nodular hidradenoma (clear cell hidradenoma), a well-circumscribed dermal tumor showing solid and cystic areas composed of polygonal and clear cells with ductal differentiation, and hidradenoma papilliferum, an apocrine-derived tumor arising almost exclusively on anogenital skin and showing a well-circumscribed, papillary, cystic architecture lined by a bilayered epithelium closely resembling an intraductal papilloma of the breast, an anatomic and histologic parallel reflecting the embryologic relationship between anogenital apocrine glands and mammary tissue, together with the mixed tumor (chondroid syringoma), a biphasic neoplasm combining epithelial ductal structures with a chondromyxoid stromal component, most common on the head and neck.

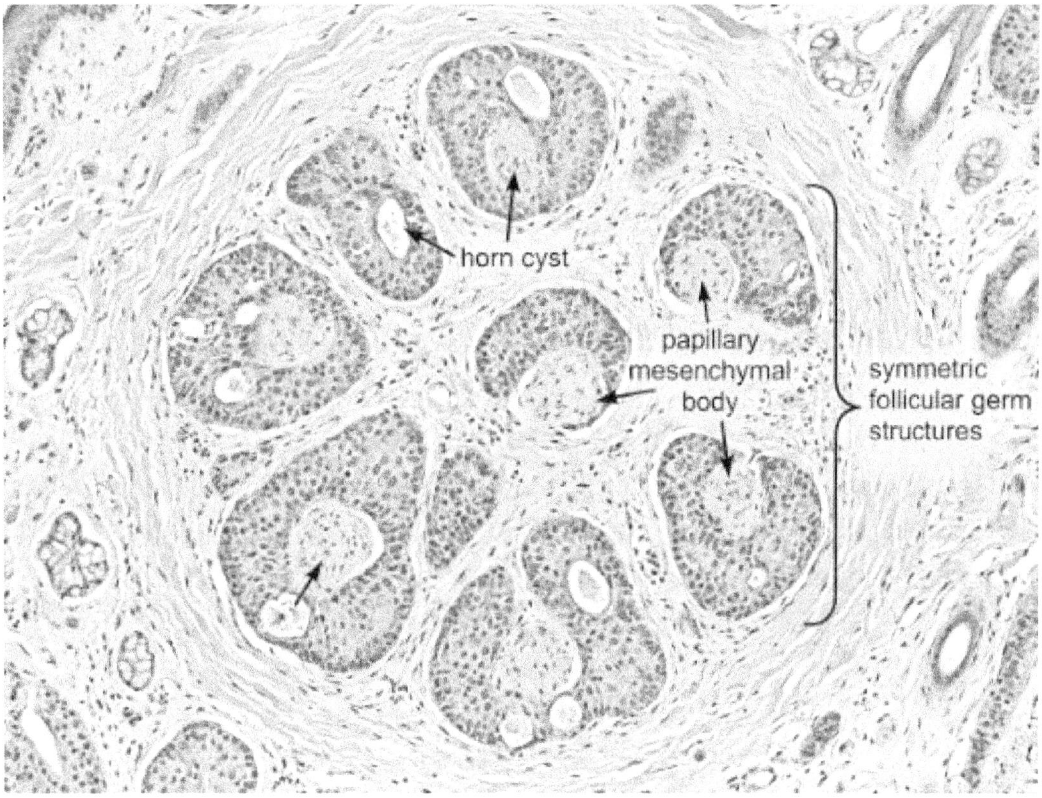

Etiology and Pathogenesis

CYLD Mutations and the Brooke-Spiegler Syndrome Spectrum

Trichoepithelioma, spiradenoma, and cylindroma share a common molecular pathway involving loss-of-function mutations in CYLD, a tumor suppressor gene encoding a deubiquitinating enzyme that normally restrains nuclear factor kappa B signaling, explaining why these three histologically distinct entities are grouped together as a related tumor family and why they co-occur, sometimes within a single composite lesion, in both sporadic and hereditary settings. Brooke-Spiegler syndrome, an autosomal dominant condition caused by germline CYLD mutations, produces numerous trichoepitheliomas, spiradenomas, and cylindromas, the latter classically producing multiple confluent scalp nodules historically termed a turban tumor given their cumulative appearance, a hereditary syndrome this chapter notes given its implications for genetic counseling and lifelong surveillance for the malignant transformation, while rare, that these tumors carry in the syndromic setting.

CTNNB1 Mutations Driving Pilomatricoma

Pilomatricoma is driven predominantly by activating mutations in CTNNB1 (beta-catenin), producing constitutive Wnt pathway activation that drives the characteristic transition from basaloid matrical cells to anucleate shadow (ghost) cells discussed in the histopathologic features section below, a molecular pathway shared with a subset of pilomatrical carcinoma, the rare malignant counterpart of this entity, though the great majority of CTNNB1-mutant pilomatricomas follow an entirely benign clinical course.

PTEN Mutations and Cowden Syndrome Recognition

Multiple tricholemmomas, particularly when numerous and presenting in a young patient, are a hallmark cutaneous finding of Cowden syndrome, caused by germline PTEN mutations and associated with a substantially elevated lifetime risk of breast, thyroid, and endometrial carcinoma, a hereditary association this chapter emphasizes because recognizing multiple tricholemmomas histologically can represent the first diagnostic clue leading to this syndrome's identification and, correspondingly, to the systemic malignancy screening and genetic counseling referral discussed in the management implications section below.

Mismatch Repair Deficiency and Muir-Torre Syndrome Identification

A subset of sebaceous neoplasms, sebaceous adenoma, sebaceoma, and sebaceous carcinoma, arise in the setting of Muir-Torre syndrome, a variant of Lynch syndrome caused by germline mutations in DNA mismatch repair genes, most commonly MSH2 and, less commonly, MLH1, MSH6, or PMS2, producing microsatellite instability within the tumor and an associated markedly elevated lifetime risk of colorectal, endometrial, and other Lynch syndrome-associated internal malignancies, an association this chapter develops further in the ancillary studies and management implications sections below given its direct, actionable implications for the patient and their family. The number of sebaceous neoplasms a given Muir-Torre syndrome patient develops over a lifetime is highly variable, ranging from a single lesion to numerous tumors, and sebaceous neoplasm development can precede, coincide with, or follow the internal Lynch syndrome-associated malignancy, meaning a cutaneous sebaceous neoplasm diagnosis should never be dismissed as syndromically insignificant simply because a patient has no known personal history of colorectal or endometrial cancer at the time of skin biopsy.

Sporadic Versus Syndromic Adnexal Presentation Patterns

Distinguishing a sporadic adnexal neoplasm from a syndromic presentation rests substantially on multiplicity, age at onset, and specific anatomic distribution: a single trichoepithelioma, tricholemmoma, cylindroma, or sebaceous neoplasm in an older adult is overwhelmingly likely to be sporadic, while multiple lesions of the same entity, particularly presenting at a younger age or in a characteristic distribution (centrofacial for multiple trichoepitheliomas, scalp-predominant for multiple cylindromas), should prompt the pathologist to explicitly note this pattern in the report and recommend clinical correlation for a possible underlying hereditary syndrome, a proactive reporting practice this chapter emphasizes given how often the diagnostic clue to a hereditary tumor predisposition syndrome first surfaces in a dermatopathology report rather than through primary clinical suspicion.

THE REACTION PATTERN RECOGNITION SYSTEM — Line of Differentiation as the Universal Adnexal Classification Anchor

---

The Pattern: Line of Differentiation, Follicular, Sebaceous, Eccrine, or Apocrine, as the Foundational Axis for Classifying Every Adnexal Neoplasm in This Chapter, from the Smallest Benign Papule to the Deepest Infiltrative Malignancy

Histologic Signature: Horn cysts and papillary mesenchymal bodies signal follicular differentiation; multivacuolated sebocytes with scalloped nuclei signal sebaceous differentiation; ductal or poroid cell structures signal eccrine differentiation; decapitation secretion signals apocrine differentiation; and deep, sclerotic, perineurally infiltrative small ducts signal microcystic adnexal carcinoma specifically.

The Decision: Identify the line of differentiation first using these signature structures, then assess architecture and cytology for organization, symmetry, and atypia to place the specific entity along its benign-to-malignant spectrum, escalating to the ancillary studies detailed below whenever a syndromic association is suspected, biopsy depth is inadequate to exclude deep infiltration, or the benign-versus-malignant distinction remains genuinely ambiguous.

Trap Logic: Trichoepithelioma is readily mistaken for basal cell carcinoma given shared basaloid cytomorphology; poroma can transform into porocarcinoma with subtle rather than dramatic histologic change; sebaceous carcinoma can closely mimic basal cell or squamous cell carcinoma, particularly outside the periocular region where clinical suspicion is often lower; and microcystic adnexal carcinoma's bland superficial component can mimic syringoma on a shallow biopsy, concealing its deep perineural invasion.

Pattern Anchor: Identify the line of differentiation first, follicular, sebaceous, eccrine, or apocrine, using its signature structure, then assess for organization versus destruction to determine benign versus malignant potential. Any sebaceous neoplasm outside the eyelid, any suspicion of a hereditary syndrome, or any facial plaque where microcystic adnexal carcinoma is a consideration triggers the specific ancillary workup and adequate-depth biopsy detailed below.

Histopathologic Features and Diagnostic Criteria

Diagnostic Histopathologic Features of the Follicular Tumor Family

Trichoepithelioma shows a symmetric dermal proliferation of basaloid keratinocytes forming horn cysts and follicular germinative structures, surrounded by characteristic papillary mesenchymal bodies, fibroblast-rich stromal condensations resembling the follicular papilla, without the retraction artifact, mucinous stroma, or significant mitotic activity typical of basal cell carcinoma, features developed further in the differential diagnosis section below given this specific distinction's clinical importance. Pilomatricoma shows a well-circumscribed dermal nodule composed of basaloid matrical cells at the periphery transitioning to eosinophilic, anucleate shadow (ghost) cells centrally, frequently with dystrophic calcification and, in longstanding lesions, ossification, a distinctive transition pattern that is essentially pathognomonic once recognized. Tricholemmoma shows a lobular proliferation of clear, glycogen-rich cells with peripheral palisading and a thickened, eosinophilic basement membrane resembling the outer root sheath of the normal hair follicle, features that, when multiple tricholemmomas are identified in a single patient, should prompt consideration of Cowden syndrome as discussed in the etiology section above. Trichofolliculoma, a less common but distinctive follicular entity, shows a central, dilated, keratin-filled cystic cavity from which numerous small, radiating secondary hair follicles emanate, a distinctive architecture resembling a miniature, disorganized hair follicle unit that, once recognized, is essentially diagnostic and rarely confused with the other follicular entities in this chapter.

Diagnostic Features of the Eccrine and Apocrine Tumor Family

Syringoma shows small, comma-shaped or tadpole-shaped ducts lined by two layers of cuboidal cells embedded within a fibrous stroma, confined to the superficial dermis. Eccrine poroma shows broad, anastomosing bands of small, uniform cuboidal (poroid) cells extending from the epidermis into the dermis, with ductal differentiation identifiable as small lumina within the tumor, a distinctive architecture with direct relevance to the poroma versus porocarcinoma differential developed below. Spiradenoma and cylindroma, closely related entities sharing the CYLD pathway discussed in the etiology section above, show basaloid cells arranged in a jigsaw-puzzle pattern of nests separated by thin fibrous septa, with cylindroma additionally showing characteristic thick, hyaline (basement membrane-like) material rimming and permeating the tumor nests, spiradenoma classically presenting as a single well-circumscribed dermal nodule and cylindroma more often as multiple coalescing nodules, particularly in the syndromic setting.

Diagnostic Features of the Sebaceous Neoplasm Spectrum

Sebaceous adenoma shows a well-circumscribed dermal lobular proliferation predominantly composed of mature sebocytes, cells with the characteristic multivacuolated, bubbly cytoplasm and central, scalloped nuclei that define sebaceous differentiation throughout this chapter, with only a thin peripheral rim of basaloid germinative cells, a proportion, mature sebocytes outnumbering basaloid cells, that distinguishes this entity from sebaceoma, discussed next, and provides a useful, reproducible quantitative anchor for this specific differential. Sebaceoma shows the inverse proportion, basaloid germinative cells predominating over a comparatively smaller population of mature, multivacuolated sebocytes, together with a more lobular, organoid architecture than sebaceous carcinoma, and, critically, an absence of the infiltrative growth, marked cytologic atypia, and pagetoid intraepidermal spread that define frank sebaceous carcinoma, discussed further in the differential diagnosis section below.

Diagnostic Features of Microcystic Adnexal Carcinoma

Microcystic adnexal carcinoma shows small, keratin-filled cysts and horn cysts in the superficial dermis transitioning, with increasing depth, to narrow, angulated cords and small ducts embedded within a densely sclerotic, desmoplastic stroma, a superficial-to-deep transition that means a shallow biopsy can show only the deceptively bland superficial component, mimicking a syringoma or desmoplastic trichoepithelioma, while missing the deeply infiltrative, perineural component entirely, a well-recognized and clinically consequential sampling pitfall this chapter emphasizes given its direct bearing on both diagnostic accuracy and the adequate biopsy depth needed to establish this diagnosis confidently. Perineural invasion is characteristic and frequently extensive in microcystic adnexal carcinoma, extending well beyond the tumor's visible margin along nerve twigs, a finding with direct and substantial implications for the surgical approach discussed in the management implications section below.

Diagnostic Features of Hidradenoma and Apocrine Tumors

Apocrine hidrocystoma, a further apocrine-derived entity relevant to the classification above, shows a simple, unilocular or multilocular cystic space lined by a bilayered epithelium with apparent apocrine decapitation secretion in the inner layer, most common on the eyelid margin and presenting clinically as a translucent, fluid-filled papule that can be mistaken for a simple epidermal inclusion cyst until the specific bilayered, secretory epithelial lining is appreciated on histologic examination. Nodular hidradenoma shows a well-circumscribed, often partially cystic dermal nodule composed of polygonal cells with eosinophilic cytoplasm admixed with clear, glycogen-rich cells, together with variably prominent ductal differentiation, features that overlap with poroma given both entities' eccrine lineage but that are distinguished by hidradenoma's typically deeper, more solid and cystic architecture against poroma's characteristic broad epidermal attachment described above. Hidradenoma papilliferum shows a well-circumscribed, encapsulated papillary and cystic proliferation lined by a bilayered epithelium, an inner columnar secretory layer showing apocrine (decapitation) secretion and an outer myoepithelial layer, without significant cytologic atypia, a pattern this chapter notes as visually striking but reliably benign once its close histologic resemblance to an intraductal papilloma of the breast, discussed in the definition and classification section above, is correctly recognized as an expected feature of this specific anogenital entity rather than a diagnostic concern.

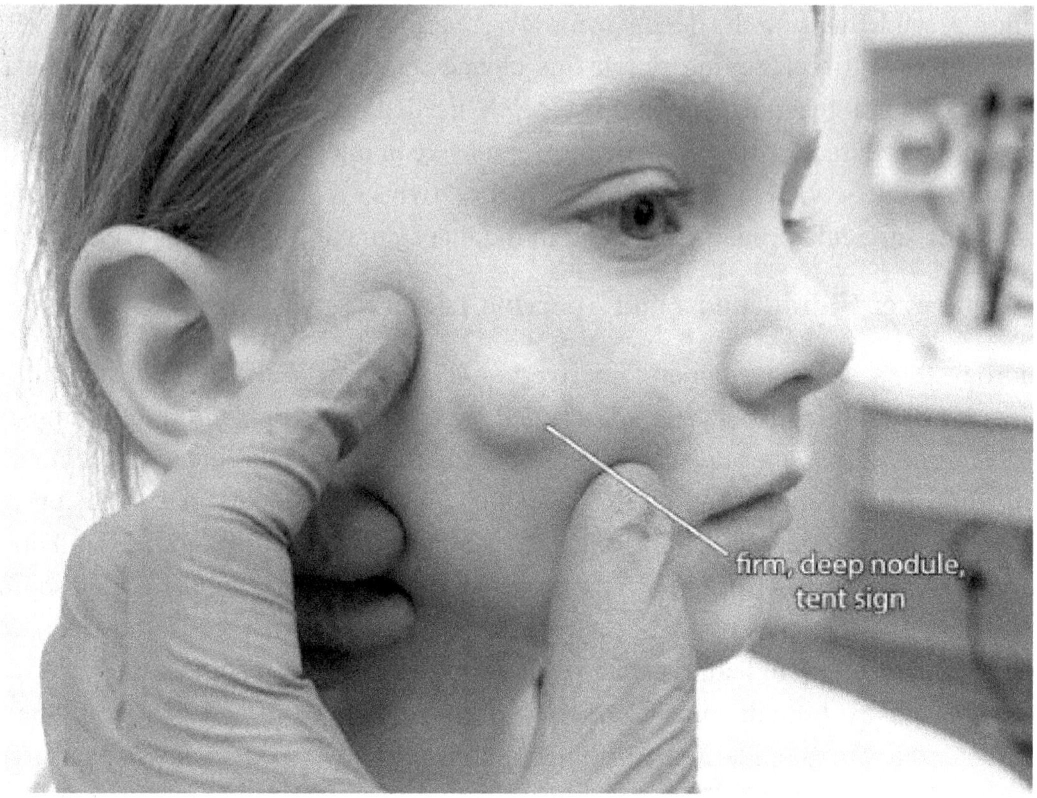

Clinical Presentation and Clinicopathologic Correlation

Clinical Morphology of Follicular Tumors

Trichoepitheliomas present as small, skin-colored, dome-shaped papules on the central face, most often solitary in sporadic cases but numerous, sometimes coalescing into a symmetric centrofacial distribution, in the syndromic setting of Brooke-Spiegler syndrome discussed above. Pilomatricoma presents classically as a firm, deep dermal or subcutaneous nodule, most common on the head, neck, and upper extremities of children and young adults, with a distinctive rock-hard consistency on palpation reflecting the calcification described in the histopathologic features section above, together with the tent sign, angulated, faceted skin surface changes elicited by stretching the overlying skin, a specific and useful clinical diagnostic sign for this entity. Tricholemmomas present as small, skin-colored, verrucous papules on the face, often clinically indistinguishable from a common wart or seborrheic keratosis when solitary, with multiplicity, as discussed above, warranting Cowden syndrome consideration.

Clinical Morphology of Eccrine and Apocrine Tumors

Apocrine hidrocystoma presents as a solitary, translucent, fluid-filled papule on the eyelid margin, often mistaken clinically for a simple sebaceous or epidermal inclusion cyst until histologic examination reveals its bilayered, secretory epithelial lining, while nodular hidradenoma presents as a solitary, slow-growing dermal or subcutaneous nodule at any body site without a distinctive site predilection, occasionally showing surface ulceration or serous discharge given its partially cystic architecture. Syringomas present as multiple small, skin-colored to slightly yellow papules, classically periorbital and most common in young to middle-aged women, a cosmetically motivated presentation in the great majority of cases. Eccrine poroma presents as a solitary, vascular-appearing papule or nodule, classically acral, on the palm or sole, sometimes with a peripheral collarette of scale, a presentation that can mimic a pyogenic granuloma or amelanotic melanoma clinically. Spiradenoma presents as a solitary, tender to spontaneously painful dermal nodule, a distinctive clinical feature among adnexal neoplasms that provides a useful diagnostic clue, while cylindroma presents as a firm, smooth, pink to red dermal nodule, most often on the scalp, that in the syndromic setting can progressively enlarge and coalesce into the turban tumor configuration discussed above.

Clinical Morphology of the Sebaceous Neoplasm Spectrum

Sebaceous adenoma and sebaceoma present as yellow to skin-colored papules or nodules, most common on the face and scalp of older patients, while sebaceous carcinoma presents most classically as a firm, yellow nodule of the eyelid, where it can mimic a chalazion or recurrent chronic blepharitis, a masquerade that is a well-documented contributor to delayed diagnosis of this specific, comparatively aggressive periocular malignancy discussed further in the management implications section below.

Special Populations: Congenital and Pediatric Presentations

Pilomatricoma, as discussed above, is disproportionately a pediatric and young adult diagnosis, and its firm, deep, sometimes rapidly enlarging clinical presentation can understandably raise concern for a soft tissue malignancy in this age group, underscoring the diagnostic value of the tent sign and rock-hard consistency discussed above as reassuring clinical features that, together with straightforward histologic confirmation once biopsied, typically resolve this concern definitively. Congenital and infantile presentations of certain adnexal neoplasms, including trichofolliculoma and, less commonly, syringoma, are recognized, generally following the same benign clinical course as their more typical later-onset counterparts, though any rapidly growing or atypical-appearing congenital nodule warrants the same biopsy threshold applied at any other age.

Clinical Presentation of Microcystic Adnexal Carcinoma

Microcystic adnexal carcinoma presents as a slowly enlarging, ill-defined, skin-colored to yellowish plaque or indurated nodule, most common on the central face, particularly the upper lip and periorbital region, of middle-aged and older patients, a subtle, slow-growing clinical presentation that, combined with the deceptively bland superficial histology discussed above, is a well-documented and specific contributor to substantial diagnostic delay for this tumor, frequently measured in years, underscoring why any longstanding, slowly enlarging, ill-defined facial plaque that fails to resolve or that shows any new sensory change, numbness or tingling suggesting perineural involvement, warrants biopsy with attention to obtaining adequate depth.

Hidradenoma Papilliferum and Anogenital Presentation

Hidradenoma papilliferum presents as a solitary, small, skin-colored to slightly erythematous nodule on the vulva or, less commonly, the perianal or perineal skin of adult women, occasionally with surface ulceration or bleeding that can raise clinical concern for a malignant anogenital neoplasm, a concern this chapter notes is reliably resolved by the characteristic bilayered papillary architecture described in the histopathologic features section above once biopsy is performed, given this entity's otherwise uniformly benign behavior.

Diagnostic Delay Considerations in Immunosuppressed and Elderly Patients

Immunosuppressed patients and elderly patients with multiple overlapping dermatologic diagnoses can experience compounded diagnostic delay for the malignant adnexal entities emphasized throughout this chapter, sebaceous carcinoma, porocarcinoma, and microcystic adnexal carcinoma, given both these populations' broader burden of concurrent skin findings that can obscure a single evolving lesion and, for immunosuppressed patients specifically, an elevated baseline burden of other cutaneous malignancies competing for clinical attention, a compounding effect this chapter notes because it reinforces the same practical lesson emphasized throughout this chapter: any adnexal-appearing lesion showing a change inconsistent with its presumed benign diagnosis, new growth, new pain, new sensory change, or bleeding, warrants biopsy or re-biopsy regardless of how many other, unrelated dermatologic findings a given patient happens to carry concurrently.

CLINICAL PEARL: A recurrent or treatment-resistant chalazion, particularly in an older patient, should prompt biopsy to exclude sebaceous carcinoma, given this tumor's well-documented tendency to masquerade as benign chronic eyelid inflammation and the meaningful diagnostic delay this masquerade has historically produced. The same low threshold applies to any slowly enlarging, ill-defined facial plaque, given microcystic adnexal carcinoma's parallel tendency toward delayed recognition.

Differential Diagnosis and Histologic Mimickers

Trichoepithelioma Versus Basal Cell Carcinoma

As introduced in Chapter 15, distinguishing trichoepithelioma from basal cell carcinoma rests on trichoepithelioma's organized, symmetric architecture with papillary mesenchymal bodies and horn cyst formation against basal cell carcinoma's peripheral palisading with retraction artifact, mucinous stroma, and infiltrative or destructive growth, criteria that, in a genuinely ambiguous small biopsy, are supported by the immunohistochemistry detailed in the ancillary studies section below, given the substantial management difference, observation or simple excision for trichoepithelioma against the more extensive surgical planning basal cell carcinoma warrants. This differential carries particular practical weight for the small, tangentially oriented shave biopsy commonly obtained for a facial papule, a specimen type that frequently fails to capture the deep architectural context, papillary mesenchymal bodies against retraction artifact and mucinous stroma, most useful for this distinction, underscoring why a genuinely ambiguous small facial biopsy in this specific differential often warrants either a deeper repeat biopsy or the supportive immunohistochemical panel detailed below rather than a forced categorical call on limited tissue.

Eccrine Poroma Versus Porocarcinoma

Porocarcinoma, the malignant counterpart of eccrine poroma, can arise de novo or, in a meaningful proportion of cases, within a pre-existing poroma, distinguished by cytologic atypia, an elevated mitotic rate including atypical forms, infiltrative rather than pushing deep margins, and, in more advanced lesions, lymphovascular invasion, features that can be subtle in early porocarcinoma and that warrant careful, deliberate examination of any poroma showing recent rapid growth, ulceration, or bleeding, clinical features that should lower the threshold for complete excision with histologic margin assessment rather than a more limited diagnostic biopsy alone.

A 64-year-old patient presents with a slowly enlarging, ill-defined, skin-colored plaque on the upper lip, present for approximately three years and previously biopsied elsewhere with a superficial shave biopsy read as syringoma, now referred given new mild perioral numbness. Repeat biopsy is performed as a deep incisional specimen extending into the subcutis. Pattern assignment identifies small keratin-filled cysts in the superficial dermis, as seen on the prior superficial biopsy, but now transitioning with depth to narrow, angulated cords and small ducts infiltrating a densely sclerotic stroma throughout the deep dermis and subcutis, with unequivocal perineural invasion identified around multiple nerve twigs at the deep margin. Differential narrowing confirms microcystic adnexal carcinoma, explaining both the prior superficial biopsy's misleadingly reassuring syringoma-like appearance and the patient's new sensory symptoms, directly attributable to the perineural invasion now identified at depth. Diagnosis of microcystic adnexal carcinoma is rendered, with the report explicitly noting the extensive perineural involvement and recommending Mohs micrographic surgery given this tumor's characteristic deep, infiltrative growth pattern and the well-documented risk of incomplete excision with conventional margins.

A 58-year-old patient with a history of Lynch syndrome-associated colorectal cancer presents with a 6-millimeter, yellow, waxy papule on the cheek, present for several months. Pattern assignment identifies a well-circumscribed dermal proliferation of basaloid and mature sebocytes, the latter showing the characteristic multivacuolated, scalloped nuclei of sebaceous differentiation, arranged in lobules without significant cytologic atypia, necrosis, or infiltrative growth. Differential narrowing favors sebaceoma over sebaceous carcinoma given the absence of significant atypia or infiltration, and given the patient's known Lynch syndrome history, immunohistochemistry for the mismatch repair proteins is pursued as an ancillary step. Immunohistochemistry shows loss of MSH2 and MSH6 nuclear staining within the tumor, consistent with mismatch repair deficiency. Diagnosis of sebaceoma with loss of MSH2/MSH6 expression, consistent with Muir-Torre syndrome in the setting of known Lynch syndrome, is rendered, with the report recommending correlation with the patient's known germline testing and continued adherence to Lynch syndrome-associated cancer surveillance given this histologic confirmation of syndrome-associated mismatch repair deficiency within the cutaneous tumor.

Pilomatricoma Versus Calcified Epidermal Cyst and Ossifying Panniculitis

A partially degenerated or calcified pilomatricoma can be mistaken for a calcified epidermal (infundibular) cyst or, when calcification is extensive, ossifying panniculitis, distinguished by identification of the characteristic basaloid-to-shadow cell transition described in the histopathologic features section above, which, even when focal within an otherwise degenerated and calcified lesion, remains the defining diagnostic feature, against the squamous lining and lamellar keratin of an epidermal cyst or the purely reactive, non-epithelial ossification of ossifying panniculitis, a distinction with limited management consequence given both entities' benign nature but genuine value for accurate diagnostic classification and patient counseling.

Cylindroma Versus Adenoid Cystic Basal Cell Carcinoma

Cylindroma's jigsaw-puzzle basaloid nests with prominent hyaline basement membrane material can be mistaken for the adenoid cystic variant of basal cell carcinoma, a distinction resting on cylindroma's characteristic two-cell population, small basaloid cells at the nest periphery and larger, paler cells centrally, together with its distinctive nested jigsaw-puzzle arrangement without the retraction artifact and infiltrative growth typical of basal cell carcinoma, criteria that, supported by the CD34 and CK15 immunohistochemistry discussed in the ancillary studies section below when needed, resolve this differential in the great majority of cases.

Microcystic Adnexal Carcinoma Versus Syringoma and Desmoplastic Trichoepithelioma

As introduced in the histopathologic features section above, microcystic adnexal carcinoma's superficial component can closely mimic syringoma or desmoplastic trichoepithelioma, a sclerosing trichoepithelioma variant showing narrow strands of basaloid cells within a fibrotic stroma; the distinguishing features are found specifically at depth and include microcystic adnexal carcinoma's extension into the deep dermis and subcutis with perineural invasion, findings absent in both syringoma, which remains confined to the superficial dermis, and desmoplastic trichoepithelioma, which, despite its infiltrative-appearing strands, retains horn cyst formation and lacks true perineural invasion, a differential this chapter emphasizes as the single most important reason adequate biopsy depth, ideally a deep punch or incisional biopsy extending into the subcutis, is essential whenever this specific entity is a clinical or histologic consideration.

Sebaceous Carcinoma Versus Basal Cell Carcinoma and Squamous Cell Carcinoma

Sebaceous carcinoma, particularly the less differentiated or extraocular variant, can closely mimic basal cell carcinoma or squamous cell carcinoma histologically, distinguished by identification of at least focal sebocytic differentiation, multivacuolated cells with scalloped, hyperchromatic nuclei and a foamy, lipid-containing cytoplasm best appreciated on frozen section or with oil red O staining given lipid dissolution during standard tissue processing, together with the pagetoid intraepidermal spread pattern this tumor characteristically shows, a spread pattern that, given its resemblance to Paget disease or melanoma in situ, is itself a recognized secondary diagnostic pitfall addressed further by the ancillary immunohistochemistry discussed below. Extraocular sebaceous carcinoma, arising on the trunk, extremities, or head and neck skin outside the periocular region, carries a comparatively worse baseline diagnostic recognition rate than the periocular subtype given the correspondingly lower routine clinical suspicion for sebaceous differentiation at these non-classic sites, reinforcing why an unexplained atypical basaloid or squamous-appearing tumor at any site benefits from deliberate, explicit consideration of sebaceous differentiation as part of the systematic differential this chapter has emphasized throughout, rather than sebaceous carcinoma being reserved as a diagnostic consideration for periocular lesions alone.

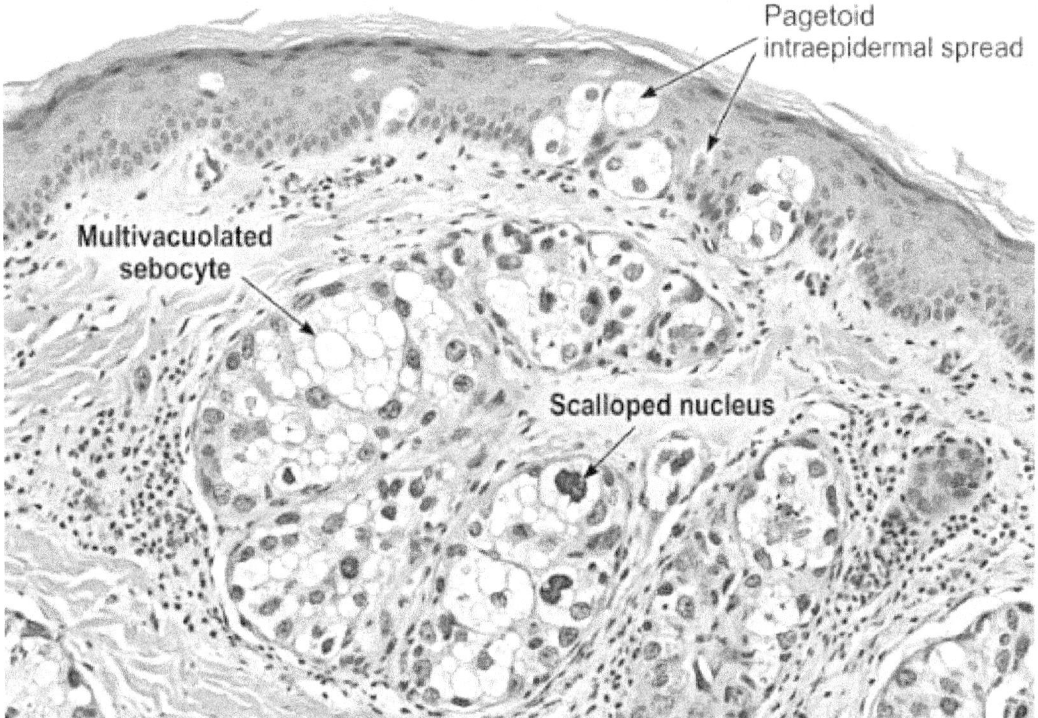

Ancillary Studies

Immunohistochemistry Distinguishing Trichoepithelioma From Basal Cell Carcinoma

CD34 immunohistochemistry highlights the fibroblast-rich stroma of trichoepithelioma's papillary mesenchymal bodies, a pattern absent in the mucinous, myxoid stroma of basal cell carcinoma, while CK15 and PHLDA1 show more consistent positivity in trichoepithelioma's follicular germinative cells relative to basal cell carcinoma, together with BerEP4, discussed in Chapter 15, which remains preferentially positive in basal cell carcinoma, this combined immunohistochemical panel providing meaningful supportive evidence in the genuinely ambiguous small biopsy scenario discussed in the differential diagnosis section above.

Mismatch Repair Immunohistochemistry for Muir-Torre Syndrome Screening

Immunohistochemistry for the mismatch repair proteins MSH2, MSH6, MLH1, and PMS2, performed as a screening tool on any sebaceous neoplasm, sebaceous adenoma, sebaceoma, or sebaceous carcinoma, particularly when arising outside the eyelid, when multiple, or when occurring in a patient younger than the typical age for sporadic sebaceous neoplasia, identifies loss of nuclear staining for one or more mismatch repair proteins as demonstrated in the worked case above, a finding that, together with clinical and family history, supports referral for germline genetic testing and Lynch syndrome-associated systemic malignancy surveillance, making this immunohistochemical panel a genuinely consequential, patient-altering ancillary study rather than a purely academic exercise.

Immunohistochemistry Supporting Sebaceous and Ductal Differentiation

Adipophilin immunohistochemistry highlights the lipid droplets characteristic of sebaceous differentiation with greater sensitivity than routine hematoxylin and eosin staining alone, providing valuable support in the sebaceous carcinoma versus basal or squamous cell carcinoma differential discussed above, while carcinoembryonic antigen and epithelial membrane antigen highlight true ductal luminal differentiation in eccrine and apocrine tumors, supporting the identification of poroma, syringoma, and their malignant counterparts when architectural ductal differentiation is subtle or focal.

Immunohistochemistry Supporting the Microcystic Adnexal Carcinoma Differential

Distinguishing microcystic adnexal carcinoma from desmoplastic trichoepithelioma, discussed in the differential diagnosis section above, can be supported by CD34 and androgen receptor immunohistochemistry, both more consistently positive in desmoplastic trichoepithelioma's fibroblast-rich stroma and germinative cells respectively, together with Ber-EP4 and p63, both more diffusely and strongly positive in microcystic adnexal carcinoma, an immunohistochemical panel that, while helpful, remains secondary to the single most important diagnostic maneuver for this specific differential, ensuring the biopsy specimen is deep enough to demonstrate or definitively exclude the perineural invasion and deep infiltrative growth that anchor this diagnosis, as emphasized throughout this chapter.

Molecular Testing: CYLD and CTNNB1 Confirmatory Testing

While the great majority of cases in this chapter are diagnosed confidently on histomorphology alone, targeted molecular testing for CYLD mutations, in a genuinely ambiguous cylindroma or spiradenoma, particularly when multiplicity or a suggestive family history raises Brooke-Spiegler syndrome concern, or for CTNNB1 mutations, in an atypical or incompletely differentiated pilomatricoma, can provide confirmatory support, though these molecular studies are reserved for genuinely diagnostically uncertain or syndromically significant cases rather than applied routinely, consistent with this book's overall emphasis on morphology and targeted, clinically indicated ancillary testing rather than reflexive, exhaustive molecular panels for every diagnosis.

KEY POINT: Mismatch repair protein immunohistochemistry on a sebaceous neoplasm is not merely a diagnostic refinement; a positive finding of protein loss directly triggers germline genetic testing referral and, when confirmed, lifelong Lynch syndrome-associated internal malignancy surveillance for the patient and screening discussions for their first-degree relatives, making this a genuinely high-yield ancillary test relative to its comparatively low cost and turnaround time.

Management Implications

Surgical Management by Entity and Risk

The great majority of benign adnexal neoplasms in this chapter, trichoepithelioma, pilomatricoma, tricholemmoma, syringoma, and eccrine poroma without atypical features, are managed with simple excision for symptomatic, cosmetically bothersome, or diagnostically uncertain lesions, while sebaceous carcinoma and porocarcinoma, given their malignant potential and, for sebaceous carcinoma specifically, propensity for pagetoid intraepidermal spread that can extend well beyond the apparent clinical tumor margin, are generally managed with wide local excision or Mohs micrographic surgery with careful margin assessment specifically accounting for this characteristic spread pattern. Microcystic adnexal carcinoma, given its characteristic deep, extensive, and perineural growth described above, is managed essentially exclusively with Mohs micrographic surgery or another complete circumferential margin assessment technique, given the well-documented high local recurrence rate that follows standard excision with conventional margins for this specific tumor, a management approach directly dictated by this tumor's histologic growth pattern rather than any single fixed margin distance.

For sebaceous carcinoma specifically, periocular tumors are frequently managed in close coordination with oculoplastic surgery given the anatomic complexity and functional preservation demands of this specific site, often incorporating conjunctival mapping biopsies to assess for the pagetoid intraepidermal spread discussed above extending into the palpebral conjunctiva, a site-specific evaluation not routinely required for the other malignant adnexal entities in this chapter and one that illustrates how closely this chapter's histopathologic findings translate into concrete, site-specific surgical planning decisions.

Syndrome Recognition and Coordinated Genetic Counseling

Recognition of Brooke-Spiegler syndrome, Cowden syndrome, or Muir-Torre syndrome based on the specific adnexal neoplasm pattern, multiplicity, and mismatch repair or other ancillary findings discussed throughout this chapter triggers referral for formal genetic counseling and germline testing, together with syndrome-specific surveillance protocols, periodic colonoscopy and endometrial surveillance for Muir-Torre syndrome, breast, thyroid, and endometrial surveillance for Cowden syndrome, and dermatologic surveillance for progressive cylindroma and spiradenoma development in Brooke-Spiegler syndrome, a coordinated, multidisciplinary management pathway this chapter emphasizes as extending well beyond the dermatopathologist's initial diagnostic role.

This coordinated pathway depends on timely, unambiguous communication from the dermatopathology report to the referring clinician, since a genetic counseling referral delayed by weeks or months carries genuine consequence when the underlying concern is an elevated risk of internal malignancy; accordingly, when a syndromic pattern is identified or strongly suspected, this chapter recommends direct, proactive communication with the ordering clinician beyond the written report alone, a practice this book has emphasized at several points for genuinely high-stakes ancillary findings and one that applies with particular force to the syndrome recognition scenarios addressed throughout this chapter.

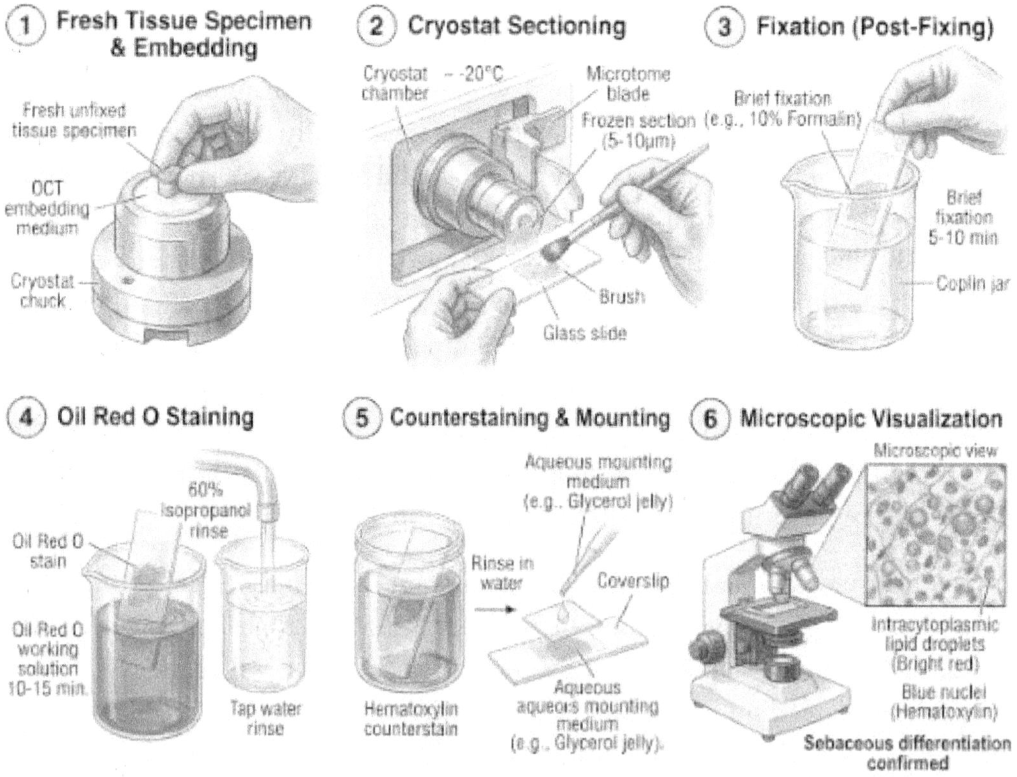

Documentation and Multidisciplinary Coordination

A dermatopathology report for an adnexal neoplasm should explicitly document the identified line of differentiation, the specific entity and its benign or malignant classification, and, whenever multiplicity, syndromic distribution, or a positive ancillary study result is present, an explicit statement recommending clinical correlation and genetic counseling referral, a documentation standard that ensures the syndrome recognition responsibility this chapter has emphasized throughout does not depend on the receiving clinician independently recognizing a pattern that the pathologist, reviewing the complete histologic and immunohistochemical picture, is frequently best positioned to identify first.

Complications and Prognosis

The great majority of entities in this chapter carry an excellent prognosis once appropriately excised, reflecting their fundamentally benign biological behavior, while malignant transformation, though uncommon, is a recognized risk for longstanding or syndromic cylindroma and spiradenoma, for pilomatricoma (pilomatrical carcinoma), and for eccrine poroma (porocarcinoma transformation), underscoring why any of these specific benign entities showing recent rapid growth, ulceration, or bleeding warrants a lower threshold for complete excision with histologic evaluation rather than continued clinical observation.

Microcystic adnexal carcinoma, sebaceous carcinoma, and porocarcinoma each carry a comparatively more guarded local prognosis than the benign entities in this chapter, though all three share a comparatively low metastatic rate relative to the local recurrence risk that dominates their overall clinical course, microcystic adnexal carcinoma given its deep, perineural growth pattern discussed throughout this chapter, sebaceous carcinoma given its pagetoid intraepidermal spread and periocular location's functional and cosmetic constraints on surgical margins, and porocarcinoma given its capacity for subtle, easily underrecognized malignant transformation within a pre-existing benign poroma. Regional lymph node metastasis, while uncommon for each of these three malignant entities, is more frequently reported for sebaceous carcinoma and advanced porocarcinoma than for microcystic adnexal carcinoma, a distinction that informs the more selective use of sentinel lymph node biopsy consideration for the former two entities in advanced or high-risk presentations.

Prevention and Screening

Unlike the ultraviolet-driven keratinocytic and melanocytic tumor families covered in Chapters 13 through 15, the great majority of entities in this chapter lack a well-established modifiable environmental risk factor, meaning prevention in this chapter is directed less at primary risk reduction and more at early recognition, structured surveillance for patients with an identified or suspected hereditary syndrome discussed throughout this chapter, and maintained clinical awareness of the specific deceptive presentations, the masquerading chalazion, the slowly enlarging facial plaque, the multiplying centrofacial papules, that this chapter has emphasized as the practical entry point to timely diagnosis for this comparatively rare but diagnostically consequential tumor family. Patients with a confirmed hereditary syndrome benefit from periodic full skin examination specifically oriented toward the syndrome-associated adnexal neoplasm pattern, in addition to, rather than instead of, the systemic surveillance protocols discussed in the syndrome recognition section above.

Patient Education and Counseling

Patients diagnosed with a syndromic adnexal neoplasm pattern benefit from clear, structured counseling regarding the identified or suspected hereditary syndrome, the rationale for genetic counseling referral, and the specific systemic surveillance recommendations that follow, delivered with attention to the anxiety a new hereditary cancer predisposition diagnosis can understandably provoke, together with reassurance that the great majority of the cutaneous tumors themselves, even in the syndromic setting, remain benign and effectively managed with excision alone. Patients diagnosed with microcystic adnexal carcinoma benefit from specific counseling regarding why Mohs micrographic surgery, rather than standard excision, is recommended, framed around this tumor's characteristic deep, subclinical extension rather than tumor aggressiveness alone, given that patients frequently equate the recommendation for a more extensive surgical technique with a worse overall prognosis when, for this specific tumor, the recommendation instead reflects the growth pattern's implications for achieving complete local excision.

Families of a patient newly diagnosed with a hereditary adnexal tumor syndrome benefit from coordinated counseling extending to at-risk relatives, since the identification of a specific pathogenic germline variant in the index patient allows targeted, predictive genetic testing for family members rather than the broader, less targeted surveillance protocols that would otherwise apply, a cascading family benefit this chapter notes as one of the most concrete, actionable outcomes that can follow from the accurate, pattern-aware adnexal neoplasm diagnosis this chapter has emphasized throughout.

THE REACTION PATTERN RECOGNITION SYSTEM — The Adnexal Neoplasm Differentiation Pattern Family

---

The Pattern: Adnexal neoplasms organized by line of differentiation, follicular, sebaceous, eccrine, and apocrine, spanning trichoepithelioma, pilomatricoma, tricholemmoma, syringoma, poroma, spiradenoma, cylindroma, and the sebaceous adenoma-to-carcinoma spectrum.

Histologic Signature: Horn cysts with papillary mesenchymal bodies define trichoepithelioma; shadow cells with calcification define pilomatricoma; jigsaw-puzzle basaloid nests with hyaline material define spiradenoma/cylindroma; multivacuolated scalloped sebocytes define the sebaceous spectrum.

The Decision: Identify line of differentiation first using signature structures, then assess organization versus destruction for malignant potential, escalating to CD34/CK15/BerEP4 for the trichoepithelioma-basal cell carcinoma differential and mismatch repair immunohistochemistry for any sebaceous neoplasm raising Muir-Torre concern.

Trap Logic: Trichoepithelioma mimics basal cell carcinoma; porocarcinoma can arise within a pre-existing poroma with subtle change; sebaceous carcinoma masquerades as chronic blepharitis or a recurrent chalazion; multiple tricholemmomas or a mismatch repair-deficient sebaceous neoplasm signal an underlying hereditary syndrome.

Pattern Anchor: Line of differentiation first, then organization versus destruction. A recurrent chalazion, a painful dermal nodule, or a sebaceous neoplasm outside the eyelid each warrant the specific ancillary workup and syndrome consideration detailed in this chapter.

Summary and Key Concepts

Cutaneous adnexal neoplasms are organized by line of differentiation, follicular, sebaceous, eccrine, and apocrine, each identified by a signature histologic structure recapitulating the corresponding normal adnexal component.

Trichoepithelioma, spiradenoma, and cylindroma share a CYLD mutation pathway and co-occur in Brooke-Spiegler syndrome, while pilomatricoma is driven by CTNNB1 mutations producing its characteristic shadow cell transition.

Multiple tricholemmomas signal possible Cowden syndrome (PTEN mutations), while sebaceous neoplasms with mismatch repair protein loss signal possible Muir-Torre syndrome, each triggering genetic counseling and systemic malignancy surveillance.

Trichoepithelioma is distinguished from basal cell carcinoma by symmetric architecture, papillary mesenchymal bodies, and supportive CD34/CK15 immunohistochemistry against basal cell carcinoma's retraction artifact and BerEP4 positivity.

Sebaceous carcinoma frequently masquerades as chronic blepharitis or a recurrent chalazion and shows characteristic pagetoid intraepidermal spread, requiring wide excision or Mohs surgery with attention to this specific spread pattern.

Microcystic adnexal carcinoma combines deceptively bland superficial cytology with deep, extensive perineural infiltration, meaning a shallow biopsy can mimic syringoma while a deep specimen is required to establish the diagnosis and guide Mohs micrographic surgery.

Eccrine poroma can undergo malignant transformation to porocarcinoma, sometimes with subtle rather than dramatic histologic change, warranting a lowered threshold for complete excision of any poroma showing recent growth, ulceration, or bleeding.

CHAPTER 17: CUTANEOUS MESENCHYMAL AND SOFT TISSUE TUMORS

Learning Objectives

1. Classify cutaneous mesenchymal tumors by line of differentiation: fibrohistiocytic, vascular, neural, adipocytic, and smooth muscle.
2. Identify the histopathologic features distinguishing dermatofibroma from dermatofibrosarcoma protuberans, and atypical fibroxanthoma from pleomorphic dermal sarcoma.
3. Recognize the diagnostic features of Kaposi sarcoma across its patch, plaque, and nodular stages, and its relationship to human herpesvirus 8.
4. Distinguish neurofibroma from schwannoma using architectural and immunohistochemical criteria.
5. Apply the immunohistochemical exclusion panel required to diagnose atypical fibroxanthoma and pleomorphic dermal sarcoma as diagnoses of exclusion.
6. Connect specific mesenchymal tumor diagnoses to their distinct surgical management pathways, including the role of Mohs micrographic surgery for infiltrative entities.

Definition and Classification

Mesenchymal Tumors Organized by Line of Differentiation

This chapter addresses the cutaneous mesenchymal and soft tissue tumors arising from the dermis and subcutis, organized, consistent with this book's approach to the adnexal tumors in Chapter 16, by line of differentiation, fibrohistiocytic, vascular, neural, adipocytic, and smooth muscle, a classification that provides the most reliable diagnostic scaffold for this genuinely heterogeneous tumor family. This chapter emphasizes throughout the specific differential diagnoses where benign and malignant entities sharing a common lineage overlap substantially in low-power appearance, dermatofibroma against dermatofibrosarcoma protuberans and atypical fibroxanthoma against pleomorphic dermal sarcoma foremost among them, given both differentials' outsized clinical consequence relative to their comparative diagnostic subtlety.

Entities Covered in This Chapter

Fibrohistiocytic entities include dermatofibroma, dermatofibrosarcoma protuberans, atypical fibroxanthoma, and pleomorphic dermal sarcoma. Vascular entities include pyogenic granuloma, angiosarcoma, and Kaposi sarcoma. Neural entities include neurofibroma and schwannoma. Adipocytic entities include lipoma and atypical lipomatous tumor, and smooth muscle entities include cutaneous leiomyoma and leiomyosarcoma, each developed in the sections that follow with particular emphasis on the specific pairs of entities most prone to diagnostic confusion.

Entity	Line of Differentiation	Key Distinguishing Feature	Malignant Potential
Dermatofibroma	Fibrohistiocytic	Storiform pattern, collagen trapping, overlying epidermal hyperplasia	None (benign)
Dermatofibrosarcoma protuberans	Fibrohistiocytic	Monotonous storiform spindle cells, honeycomb fat infiltration, CD34+	Low-grade malignant, locally aggressive
Atypical fibroxanthoma	Fibrohistiocytic	Pleomorphic spindle/epithelioid cells, superficial, exclusion diagnosis	Low-grade (superficial variant)
Pleomorphic dermal sarcoma	Fibrohistiocytic	Same cytology as AFX but deep/infiltrative with necrosis or perineural invasion	Higher-grade, metastatic potential
Kaposi sarcoma	Vascular	Spindle cells with slit-like vascular spaces, promontory sign, HHV-8+	Malignant (variable aggressiveness)
Neurofibroma	Neural	Wavy spindle cells, mast cells, myxoid stroma, unencapsulated	Low (plexiform variant in NF1)
Schwannoma	Neural	Encapsulated, Antoni A/B areas, Verocay bodies	None (benign)
Pyogenic granuloma	Vascular	Lobular capillary proliferation, collarette, ulceration	None (benign)
Angiosarcoma	Vascular	Anastomosing vascular channels dissecting collagen, multilayered atypical endothelium	High-grade malignant

Lipoma	Adipocytic	Mature adipocytes, thin fibrous capsule, uniform cell size	None (benign)
Atypical lipomatous tumor	Adipocytic	Adipocytic variation in size, atypical stromal cells, MDM2 amplification	Low-grade malignant, locally aggressive
Cutaneous leiomyoma	Smooth muscle	Interlacing eosinophilic spindle fascicles, blunt-ended nuclei, desmin+	None (benign)
Leiomyosarcoma	Smooth muscle	Cytologic atypia, elevated mitotic rate, necrosis, infiltrative margins	Malignant, metastatic potential

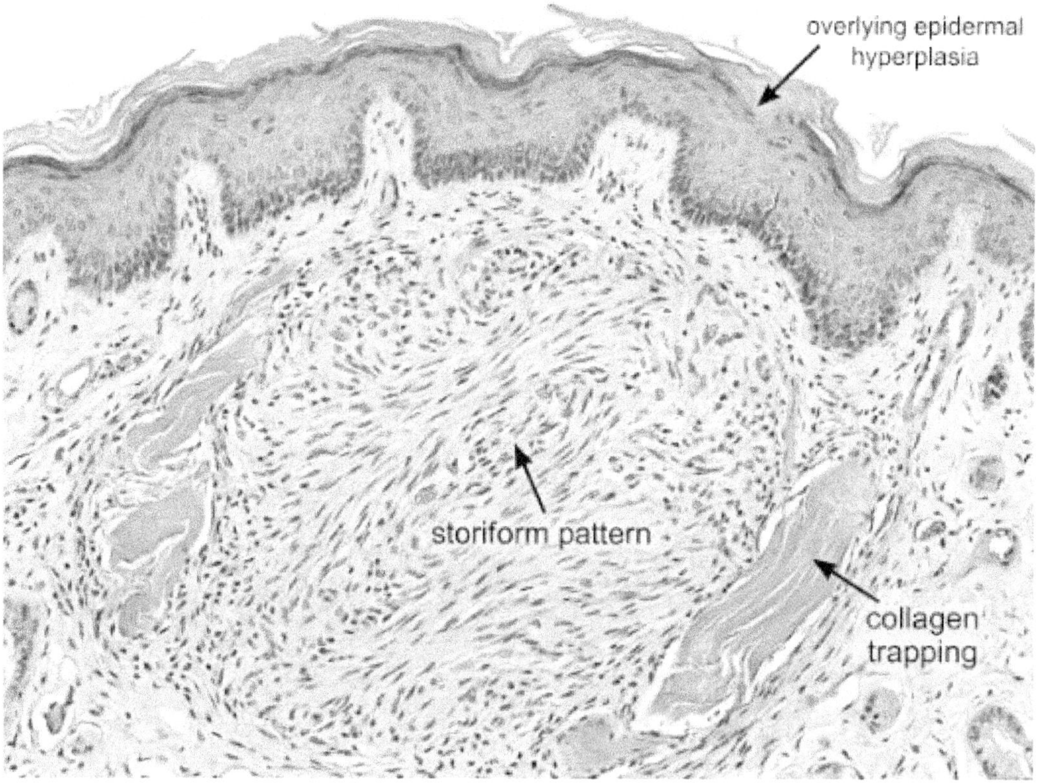

Epidemiology of Cutaneous Mesenchymal Tumors

Dermatofibroma is exceedingly common, encountered incidentally in routine dermatologic practice and disproportionately affecting women, most often on the lower extremities following minor antecedent trauma such as an insect bite or folliculitis, while dermatofibrosarcoma protuberans is comparatively rare, with an annual incidence on the order of four per million, most often diagnosed in the third to fifth decades of life and showing a recognized predilection for the trunk and proximal extremities. Atypical fibroxanthoma and pleomorphic dermal sarcoma both concentrate overwhelmingly in elderly patients with substantial cumulative ultraviolet exposure, the scalp, face, and ears of men in their seventh through ninth decades representing the classic demographic, a distribution this chapter notes mirrors the field cancerization pattern discussed for keratinocytic malignancies in Chapter 15. Lipoma is the single most common soft tissue tumor encountered in general practice, while atypical lipomatous tumor, though far less common, shows a strong predilection for the deep soft tissue of the proximal extremities and, less commonly, the trunk, with a comparatively even distribution across the fifth through seventh decades. Cutaneous leiomyoma is uncommon but not rare, arising from arrector pili smooth muscle (piloleiomyoma), from vascular smooth muscle (angioleiomyoma), or from dartos or mammary areolar smooth muscle (genital leiomyoma), while cutaneous leiomyosarcoma is rare, and angiosarcoma, though rare overall, shows three recognized clinical contexts developed further below: idiopathic scalp and face angiosarcoma of elderly patients, radiation-associated angiosarcoma arising in a prior radiation field, and lymphedema-associated angiosarcoma (Stewart-Treves syndrome) arising in a chronically lymphedematous limb, most classically following axillary lymph node dissection for breast carcinoma.

Etiology and Pathogenesis

COL1A1-PDGFB Fusion in Dermatofibrosarcoma Protuberans

Dermatofibrosarcoma protuberans is driven by a characteristic t(17;22) chromosomal translocation producing a COL1A1-PDGFB fusion gene, resulting in constitutive, ligand-independent activation of the platelet-derived growth factor receptor beta signaling pathway, a molecular alteration that directly drives this tumor's characteristic monotonous spindle cell proliferation and that, importantly, represents a therapeutically actionable target, imatinib and other tyrosine kinase inhibitors directed against platelet-derived growth factor receptor beta providing an effective systemic therapy option for unresectable, recurrent, or metastatic disease discussed further in the management implications section below. This fusion is identifiable by fluorescence in situ hybridization or reverse transcriptase polymerase chain reaction, ancillary studies developed in the ancillary studies section below that provide confirmatory molecular support in genuinely ambiguous cases.

Human Herpesvirus 8 and Kaposi Sarcoma

Kaposi sarcoma is causally driven by human herpesvirus 8 (HHV-8, also termed Kaposi sarcoma-associated herpesvirus) infection of endothelial and spindle cell precursors, with the virus's latency-associated nuclear antigen driving proliferative and angiogenic signaling that produces this tumor's characteristic vascular proliferation, discussed further in the histopathologic features section below. Four recognized clinical-epidemiologic subtypes share this common viral etiology but differ substantially in host immune context: classic Kaposi sarcoma, occurring in older patients of Mediterranean and Eastern European ancestry independent of HIV infection; endemic (African) Kaposi sarcoma; iatrogenic (immunosuppression-associated) Kaposi sarcoma, occurring in solid organ transplant recipients and other chronically immunosuppressed patients; and epidemic (AIDS-associated) Kaposi sarcoma, occurring in the setting of HIV infection and historically the most aggressive of the four subtypes prior to the advent of effective antiretroviral therapy, each subtype developed further in the clinical presentation section below.

NF1 Mutations and Neurofibromatosis Type 1

Sporadic neurofibromas arise from Schwann cell and perineurial cell proliferation without an identifiable germline mutation in the great majority of cases, while multiple neurofibromas, and particularly the plexiform neurofibroma variant, a distinctive, diffusely infiltrative growth pattern extending along a nerve and its branches, are hallmark findings of neurofibromatosis type 1, caused by germline NF1 mutations, a hereditary tumor predisposition syndrome this chapter notes given the plexiform variant's recognized, though uncommon, risk of malignant transformation to malignant peripheral nerve sheath tumor, discussed further in the differential diagnosis and management implications sections below.

MDM2 Amplification in Atypical Lipomatous Tumor

Atypical lipomatous tumor (well-differentiated liposarcoma when arising in deep soft tissue) is characterized by MDM2 gene amplification, typically on a supernumerary ring or giant marker chromosome, a molecular alteration absent in simple lipoma and one that provides the definitive ancillary distinction between these two entities when morphology alone leaves genuine uncertainty, developed further in the ancillary studies section below. This amplification is frequently accompanied by co-amplification of the neighboring CDK4 gene, and both markers are exploited diagnostically, discussed further below, given their shared amplicon on chromosome 12q13-15.

MYC Amplification and the Three Clinical Contexts of Angiosarcoma

Angiosarcoma arises through at least three distinct etiologic pathways that converge on a shared malignant endothelial phenotype. Idiopathic angiosarcoma of the scalp and face in elderly patients arises without a clear inciting factor, though chronic ultraviolet exposure has been proposed as a contributing influence given this variant's site predilection. Radiation-associated angiosarcoma arises within a prior radiation field, most classically the breast or chest wall following radiotherapy for breast carcinoma, typically after a latency of five to ten years, and is characterized molecularly by MYC gene amplification, a genetic alteration that both drives this tumor's aggressive behavior and, discussed further in the ancillary studies section below, provides a diagnostically useful immunohistochemical surrogate distinguishing radiation-associated angiosarcoma from benign radiation-associated atypical vascular lesions, a differential this chapter emphasizes given its substantial clinical consequence. Lymphedema-associated angiosarcoma (Stewart-Treves syndrome) arises within a chronically lymphedematous limb, classically following axillary lymph node dissection and radiotherapy for breast carcinoma, and is thought to reflect malignant transformation within a chronically stimulated, lymphatically congested vascular bed, though it does not characteristically show the same MYC amplification pattern as radiation-associated angiosarcoma.

Etiology of Cutaneous Leiomyoma and Leiomyosarcoma

Piloleiomyoma arises from the arrector pili muscle and can occur sporadically or, when multiple, as a manifestation of hereditary leiomyomatosis and renal cell cancer syndrome, caused by germline mutations in the fumarate hydratase gene, a hereditary tumor predisposition syndrome this chapter notes given its associated risk of an aggressive, early-onset variant of papillary renal cell carcinoma, making recognition of multiple piloleiomyomas a genuinely important clinical trigger for genetic counseling and renal imaging referral. Angioleiomyoma arises from vascular smooth muscle and is not associated with this syndrome. Cutaneous leiomyosarcoma, in contrast, arises sporadically without a well-characterized hereditary predisposition syndrome, and is generally considered a low-grade, dermal-based malignancy with a substantially more favorable prognosis than deep soft tissue or retroperitoneal leiomyosarcoma, a site-based prognostic distinction developed further in the complications and prognosis discussion below.

THE REACTION PATTERN RECOGNITION SYSTEM — Line of Differentiation and Depth as the Universal Mesenchymal Classification Anchor

---

The Pattern: Line of Differentiation Combined with Depth, Circumscription, and Cytologic Monotony Versus Pleomorphism as the Framework for Classifying Every Mesenchymal Tumor in This Chapter

Histologic Signature: Storiform spindle cells with collagen trapping signal fibrohistiocytic differentiation; slit-like vascular spaces and a promontory sign signal vascular differentiation; wavy spindle cells with mast cells signal neural differentiation; and pleomorphic spindle/epithelioid cells with high mitotic activity signal the atypical fibroxanthoma/pleomorphic dermal sarcoma spectrum.

The Decision: Identify the line of differentiation first, then assess depth of extension, circumscription versus infiltration, and cytologic monotony versus pleomorphism to place the entity along its benign-to-malignant spectrum, escalating to CD34, immunohistochemical exclusion panels, or molecular testing whenever the benign-versus-malignant or line-of-differentiation distinction remains genuinely ambiguous.

Trap Logic: Dermatofibrosarcoma protuberans can be mistaken for dermatofibroma given shared fibrohistiocytic lineage; atypical fibroxanthoma and pleomorphic dermal sarcoma share identical cytology and are distinguished only by depth and invasion; and Kaposi sarcoma's early patch stage can closely mimic a benign vascular or inflammatory process.

Pattern Anchor: Line of differentiation first, then depth and circumscription versus infiltration. Atypical fibroxanthoma and pleomorphic dermal sarcoma are diagnoses of exclusion requiring a negative immunohistochemical panel before either diagnosis is rendered.

Histopathologic Features and Diagnostic Criteria

Diagnostic Features of Dermatofibroma and Dermatofibrosarcoma Protuberans

Dermatofibroma shows a dermal proliferation of bland spindled fibroblasts and histiocytes arranged in a storiform (cartwheel) pattern, characteristically trapping thickened, hyalinized collagen bundles at the lesion's periphery, together with overlying epidermal hyperplasia and basal layer hyperpigmentation, features developed further in the ancillary studies section below given their direct relevance to the CD34 immunohistochemical distinction from dermatofibrosarcoma protuberans. Dermatofibrosarcoma protuberans shows a monotonous proliferation of bland spindle cells arranged in a more uniform, diffuse storiform pattern than dermatofibroma, infiltrating the subcutaneous fat in a characteristic honeycomb (lace-like) pattern, individual tumor cells surrounding and infiltrating between fat lobules rather than displacing them, a distinctive infiltrative growth pattern that extends well beyond the tumor's clinically apparent margin and that, together with the immunohistochemical distinction discussed below, anchors this tumor's diagnosis and directly informs the surgical approach detailed in the management implications section.

Diagnostic Features of Atypical Fibroxanthoma and Pleomorphic Dermal Sarcoma

Atypical fibroxanthoma and pleomorphic dermal sarcoma share identical cytologic features, markedly pleomorphic spindled and epithelioid cells with bizarre, hyperchromatic nuclei, frequent atypical mitotic figures, and admixed multinucleated giant cells, arising on chronically sun-damaged skin, most often the scalp, face, and ears of elderly patients, distinguished from one another not by cytology, which is indistinguishable between the two, but by depth and invasiveness: atypical fibroxanthoma is confined to the dermis without invasion into the subcutis, without perineural or lymphovascular invasion, and without necrosis, while pleomorphic dermal sarcoma shows extension into the subcutis, perineural or lymphovascular invasion, or tumor necrosis, features that upgrade the diagnosis and its associated metastatic risk substantially, a depth- and invasion-based distinction this chapter emphasizes as the single most consequential decision point in this specific tumor pair.

Diagnostic Features of Lipoma and Atypical Lipomatous Tumor

Lipoma shows a well-circumscribed lobule of mature adipocytes indistinguishable from normal subcutaneous fat other than its encapsulation by a thin fibrous rim, with uniform cell size, absent cytologic atypia, and no significant fibrous septation, a bland, monotonous appearance that this chapter emphasizes is the essential negative feature separating lipoma from atypical lipomatous tumor. Atypical lipomatous tumor shows adipocytic variation in cell size, thickened, hyalinized fibrous septa containing scattered atypical, hyperchromatic stromal cells, sometimes with bizarre, floret-like multinucleated forms, and, in a subset of cases, admixed lipoblasts, univacuolated or multivacuolated cells with hyperchromatic, scalloped nuclei indented by cytoplasmic fat vacuoles, features that individually can be subtle but that collectively, and particularly when supported by the MDM2/CDK4 ancillary confirmation discussed below, distinguish this entity from its far more common benign mimic.

Diagnostic Features of Cutaneous Leiomyoma and Leiomyosarcoma

Cutaneous leiomyoma shows interlacing fascicles of bland, eosinophilic spindle cells with abundant fibrillary cytoplasm and elongated, blunt-ended (cigar-shaped) nuclei, the defining cytologic feature of smooth muscle differentiation, arranged in a well-circumscribed, unencapsulated dermal nodule without significant mitotic activity or necrosis. Leiomyosarcoma shows the same fundamental smooth muscle cytology, interlacing fascicles of spindle cells with cigar-shaped nuclei, but with superimposed cytologic atypia, an elevated mitotic rate, and, in more advanced examples, tumor necrosis and infiltrative, poorly circumscribed margins extending into the subcutis, a combination of atypia, mitotic activity, and infiltrative growth that this chapter emphasizes as the diagnostic triad separating this malignant entity from its bland benign counterpart.

Diagnostic Features of Angiosarcoma

Angiosarcoma shows an infiltrative proliferation of anastomosing, irregular vascular channels dissecting between dermal collagen bundles, lined by atypical, hyperchromatic endothelial cells that characteristically pile up into multiple layers rather than the single, flattened endothelial layer of a benign vascular lesion, with the most poorly differentiated examples showing solid sheets of epithelioid or spindled cells in which the vasoformative architecture is only focally apparent, a diagnostically treacherous pattern this chapter notes can closely mimic a poorly differentiated carcinoma or melanoma on hematoxylin and eosin staining alone, developed further in the differential diagnosis section below. The characteristically ill-defined, infiltrative growth pattern, extending well beyond the tumor's clinically apparent margin in a manner reminiscent of dermatofibrosarcoma protuberans, directly informs this tumor's notoriously high rate of incomplete excision and local recurrence, discussed further in the management implications section below.

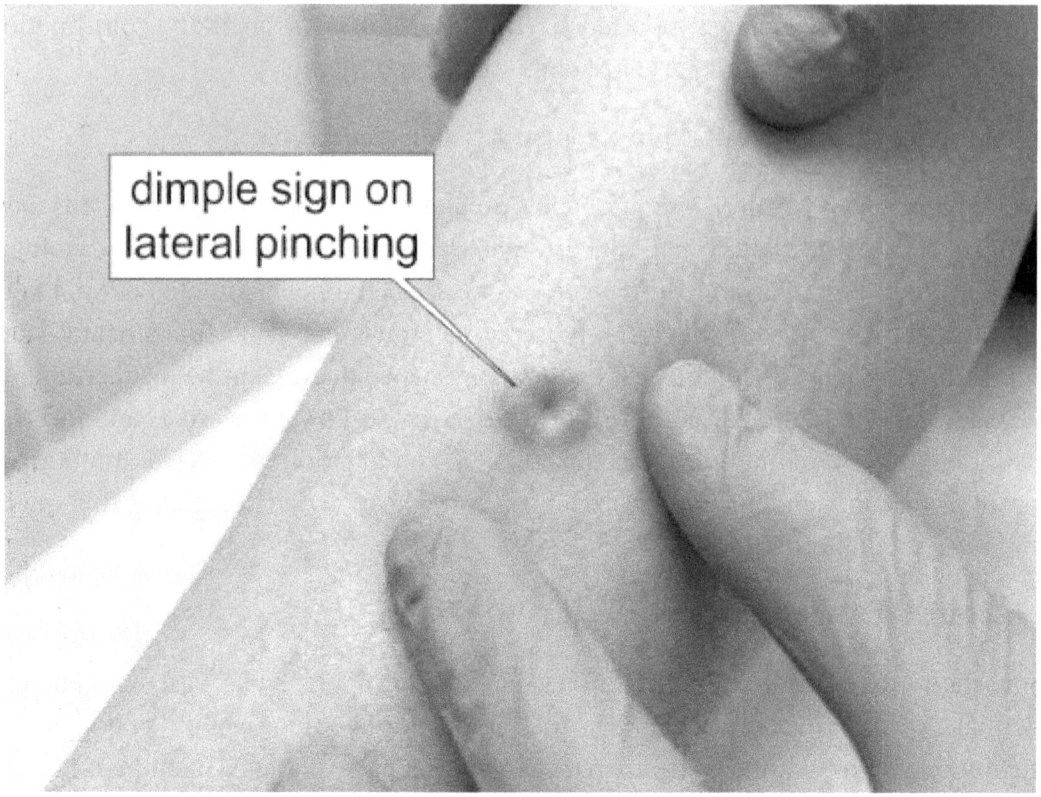

Clinical Presentation and Clinicopathologic Correlation

Clinical Morphology of Fibrohistiocytic Tumors

Dermatofibroma presents as a firm, tan-to-brown dermal papule or nodule, most common on the lower extremities, characteristically showing the dimple sign, central depression on lateral pinching of the lesion, a specific and useful bedside clinical diagnostic maneuver reflecting the tumor's dermal, rather than purely epidermal or subcutaneous, location and its tethering to the overlying skin. Dermatofibrosarcoma protuberans presents as a slowly enlarging, indurated plaque or nodule, most common on the trunk of young to middle-aged adults, that can be present for years before developing the protuberant, multinodular surface change that gives this entity its name, a comparatively subtle early presentation that, combined with this tumor's deceptively bland cytology described above, is a well-documented contributor to diagnostic delay and, correspondingly, to the more extensive surgical excision required once the tumor's true infiltrative extent is finally appreciated.

Clinical Morphology of Vascular Tumors

Pyogenic granuloma (lobular capillary hemangioma) presents as a rapidly growing, friable, easily bleeding red papule or nodule, often following minor trauma and frequently occurring during pregnancy given hormonally mediated vascular proliferation, a rapid growth and bleeding tendency that can raise clinical concern for amelanotic melanoma, developed further in the differential diagnosis section below. Kaposi sarcoma presents across a spectrum of clinical stages correlating with histologic progression: violaceous patches in the early patch stage, infiltrated violaceous plaques in the plaque stage, and violaceous to dark brown nodules, sometimes ulcerated, in the nodular stage, most common on the lower extremities in classic Kaposi sarcoma but with a broader distribution, including oral mucosa and visceral involvement, in epidemic (AIDS-associated) Kaposi sarcoma.

Clinical Morphology of Neural and Adipocytic Tumors

Neurofibroma presents as a soft, skin-colored papule or nodule showing the buttonhole sign, invagination of the lesion into the underlying subcutis on gentle pressure, reflecting this tumor's characteristic soft, myxoid consistency, while lipoma presents as a soft, mobile, subcutaneous nodule without overlying skin changes, the most common benign soft tissue tumor overall and generally requiring no ancillary workup beyond straightforward clinical and, when excised, routine histologic confirmation. Atypical lipomatous tumor, in contrast, typically presents as a deep-seated, slowly enlarging mass exceeding five centimeters in the proximal extremity or trunk, a size and depth threshold this chapter emphasizes as a genuine clinical red flag that should prompt cross-sectional imaging and, where feasible, MDM2/CDK4 ancillary confirmation before a presumptive diagnosis of simple lipoma is accepted.

Clinical Morphology of Smooth Muscle Tumors and Angiosarcoma

Piloleiomyoma presents as one or multiple firm, pink-to-brown dermal papules or nodules, most common on the trunk and extensor extremities, with a distinctive and clinically useful feature: paroxysmal pain on palpation, cold exposure, or emotional stress, reflecting arrector pili muscle contraction, a symptom this chapter notes is sufficiently characteristic that its presence should prompt specific inquiry into a family history of similar lesions and uterine fibroids given the hereditary leiomyomatosis and renal cell cancer syndrome association discussed in the etiology section above. Angioleiomyoma presents as a solitary, tender subcutaneous nodule, most common on the lower extremity of middle-aged women. Cutaneous leiomyosarcoma presents as a slowly enlarging, firm dermal or subcutaneous nodule, most common on the extremities, generally without the pain that characterizes piloleiomyoma, a presentation that, given the substantial cytologic overlap discussed above, underscores why histologic rather than clinical criteria drive this specific differential. Angiosarcoma of the scalp and face classically presents as an ill-defined, bruise-like violaceous patch or plaque that is easily mistaken for a resolving contusion or a benign vascular lesion, a deceptively innocuous early appearance that this chapter identifies as a major contributor to diagnostic delay, frequently progressing to nodular, ulcerated, and hemorrhagic lesions with satellite nodules as the disease advances; Stewart-Treves syndrome presents as violaceous nodules or plaques arising within a chronically lymphedematous limb, typically years after axillary dissection, a temporal and anatomic context that should immediately raise concern for this diagnosis in any new or changing lesion within a lymphedematous field.

CLINICAL PEARL: The dimple sign for dermatofibroma and the buttonhole sign for neurofibroma are both simple, reliable bedside clinical maneuvers that, while never a substitute for histologic confirmation when a lesion is excised, can meaningfully guide pretest clinical suspicion and patient counseling before biopsy results return. A new or changing bruise-like patch on the scalp or face of an elderly patient that fails to resolve over an expected timeframe should never be dismissed as ordinary trauma without at least considering angiosarcoma.

Differential Diagnosis and Histologic Mimickers

Dermatofibroma Versus Dermatofibrosarcoma Protuberans

As introduced in the histopathologic features section above, distinguishing dermatofibroma from dermatofibrosarcoma protuberans rests on the latter's more uniform, diffuse storiform architecture, honeycomb fat infiltration, and lack of significant collagen trapping or overlying epidermal hyperplasia, criteria supported decisively by CD34 immunohistochemistry, discussed in the ancillary studies section below, given this differential's outsized clinical consequence: dermatofibroma requires no further treatment beyond simple excision or observation, while dermatofibrosarcoma protuberans requires wide local excision or Mohs micrographic surgery given its characteristic subclinical extension, making an inaccurate call in either direction a genuinely consequential diagnostic error.

Atypical Fibroxanthoma and Pleomorphic Dermal Sarcoma Versus Spindle Cell Squamous Cell Carcinoma and Melanoma

Given atypical fibroxanthoma and pleomorphic dermal sarcoma's markedly pleomorphic cytology described above, both entities must be distinguished from spindle cell (sarcomatoid) squamous cell carcinoma and desmoplastic or spindle cell melanoma, each of which can show a similarly pleomorphic spindle cell morphology on hematoxylin and eosin staining alone; this distinction is made definitively, not by morphology, but by a negative immunohistochemical exclusion panel, pancytokeratin, S100/SOX10, and desmin at minimum, discussed further in the ancillary studies section below, meaning atypical fibroxanthoma and pleomorphic dermal sarcoma are, by definition, diagnoses of exclusion that cannot be rendered on morphology alone.

A 78-year-old patient presents with a 1.2-centimeter, rapidly growing, ulcerated nodule on the scalp, present for approximately six weeks, in a background of extensive actinic damage. Pattern assignment identifies a markedly pleomorphic dermal spindle and epithelioid cell proliferation with frequent atypical mitotic figures and multinucleated giant cells, confined to the dermis without extension into the subcutaneous fat, without perineural or lymphovascular invasion, and without necrosis. Differential narrowing requires exclusion of spindle cell squamous cell carcinoma and desmoplastic melanoma given the pleomorphic cytology, and an immunohistochemical panel is pursued: pancytokeratin, S100, SOX10, and desmin are all negative within the tumor cells, excluding squamous, melanocytic, and myogenic lineage respectively. Given the negative exclusion panel and the tumor's confinement to the dermis without invasive or necrotic features, diagnosis of atypical fibroxanthoma is rendered, with the report explicitly documenting the negative immunohistochemical panel supporting this diagnosis of exclusion and confirming the absence of the deep or invasive features that would upgrade this diagnosis to pleomorphic dermal sarcoma.

Pyogenic Granuloma Versus Amelanotic Melanoma and Bacillary Angiomatosis

As introduced in the clinical presentation section above, pyogenic granuloma's rapid growth and friable bleeding tendency can raise genuine clinical concern for amelanotic melanoma, discussed in Chapter 14, a differential resolved histologically by pyogenic granuloma's characteristic lobular architecture, discrete lobules of proliferating capillaries separated by fibromyxoid stroma, typically with a collarette of adjacent epidermis and a background of ulceration, against amelanotic melanoma's atypical melanocytic proliferation confirmable by SOX10 and Melan-A immunohistochemistry when morphology alone is ambiguous. A second important mimic, particularly in immunosuppressed or HIV-positive patients, is bacillary angiomatosis, a Bartonella-driven reactive vascular proliferation that can closely resemble pyogenic granuloma both clinically and, at low power, histologically, distinguished by bacillary angiomatosis's characteristic neutrophilic infiltrate with admixed granular, purplish bacillary clusters on Warthin-Starry staining, a distinction this chapter emphasizes carries direct therapeutic consequence, bacillary angiomatosis responding to antimicrobial therapy rather than surgical excision alone.

Lipoma Versus Atypical Lipomatous Tumor

As introduced in the clinical presentation section above, the distinction between lipoma and atypical lipomatous tumor rests on a combination of clinical red flags, size exceeding five centimeters, deep location, and progressive growth, and histologic findings, adipocytic size variation, thickened fibrous septa with atypical stromal cells, and, when present, lipoblasts, criteria that this chapter notes can be genuinely subtle on a small or superficial biopsy, making ancillary MDM2/CDK4 confirmation, discussed in the ancillary studies section below, an appropriately liberal practice whenever a fatty tumor shows any of these clinical or histologic red flags.

A 55-year-old patient presents with a slowly enlarging, deep-seated mass on the medial thigh, now measuring 6.5 centimeters, present for approximately eighteen months. Pattern assignment identifies a lobulated adipocytic proliferation with mild but definite variation in adipocyte size and scattered thickened fibrous septa containing rare hyperchromatic, atypical stromal cells, without definite lipoblasts identified. Differential narrowing weighs simple lipoma against atypical lipomatous tumor given the lesion's size, depth, and subtle septal atypia, and MDM2 and CDK4 immunohistochemistry are pursued as the deciding ancillary study: both markers show diffuse nuclear positivity within the atypical stromal cells, and fluorescence in situ hybridization confirms MDM2 amplification. Given the positive MDM2 amplification, a diagnosis of atypical lipomatous tumor is rendered, with the report explicitly noting the tumor's size and depth and recommending wide local excision with attention to margin status given this entity's locally aggressive behavior and recognized potential for local recurrence if incompletely excised.

Angiosarcoma Versus Benign Vascular Proliferations and Bruising

Given angiosarcoma's deceptively innocuous, bruise-like early clinical appearance described in the clinical presentation section above, this diagnosis must be distinguished from a resolving contusion, a benign vascular proliferation, and, in a radiation field specifically, an atypical vascular lesion, a benign, MYC-negative reactive vascular proliferation that can show architectural overlap with well-differentiated angiosarcoma on limited sampling; this distinction is supported decisively by MYC immunohistochemistry, discussed further in the ancillary studies section below, positive in radiation-associated angiosarcoma and negative in atypical vascular lesion, making any violaceous or bruise-like lesion within a prior radiation field that fails to resolve over an expected timeframe an appropriate trigger for biopsy rather than continued observation.

An 82-year-old patient presents with an ill-defined, violaceous, bruise-like patch on the scalp, present for approximately three months and initially attributed to minor trauma, now with a new area of nodularity at its margin. Pattern assignment identifies an infiltrative proliferation of anastomosing, irregular vascular channels dissecting between collagen bundles, lined by hyperchromatic endothelial cells showing multilayering and focal papillary tufting, with the nodular component showing more solid, epithelioid areas in which vasoformation is only focally discernible. Differential narrowing weighs a benign vascular proliferation against angiosarcoma given the patient's age, the lesion's ill-defined clinical margin, and the multilayered, atypical endothelial cytology, and CD31, ERG, and Ki-67 immunohistochemistry are pursued: CD31 and ERG confirm endothelial lineage within both the vasoformative and solid epithelioid areas, while Ki-67 shows a markedly elevated proliferative index. Given the infiltrative growth, multilayered atypical endothelium, and elevated proliferative index, a diagnosis of angiosarcoma is rendered, with the report recommending wide-margin re-excision and prompt multidisciplinary oncologic referral given this tumor's well-documented propensity for subclinical extension well beyond its apparent clinical margin and its comparatively poor overall prognosis relative to the other entities in this chapter.

Cutaneous Leiomyoma Versus Leiomyosarcoma

Distinguishing piloleiomyoma or angioleiomyoma from cutaneous leiomyosarcoma rests on the histologic triad introduced in the histopathologic features section above, cytologic atypia, elevated mitotic rate, and infiltrative margins with or without necrosis, criteria supported by desmin and smooth muscle actin immunohistochemistry, which confirm smooth muscle lineage in both benign and malignant entities but do not by themselves distinguish one from the other, making Ki-67 proliferative index and careful assessment of mitotic count per high-power field, discussed further in the ancillary studies section below, the practically decisive ancillary studies whenever cytologic assessment alone leaves genuine uncertainty.

A 61-year-old patient presents with a firm, slowly enlarging subcutaneous nodule on the posterior thigh, present for approximately one year, without the paroxysmal pain on palpation that would suggest piloleiomyoma. Pattern assignment identifies interlacing fascicles of eosinophilic spindle cells with cigar-shaped nuclei, definite cytologic atypia, and a mitotic count exceeding the threshold expected for a benign smooth muscle tumor, together with an infiltrative margin extending focally into the immediately adjacent subcutaneous fat, without frank necrosis. Differential narrowing weighs cutaneous leiomyoma against leiomyosarcoma given the combination of atypia, elevated mitotic activity, and infiltrative margin, and desmin, smooth muscle actin, and Ki-67 immunohistochemistry are pursued: desmin and smooth muscle actin confirm smooth muscle lineage, while Ki-67 shows a proliferative index substantially higher than expected for piloleiomyoma. Given the cytologic atypia, elevated mitotic rate, and infiltrative margin, a diagnosis of cutaneous leiomyosarcoma is rendered, with the report recommending wide local excision and noting the generally favorable prognosis associated with dermal-based, as opposed to deep soft tissue, leiomyosarcoma.

Neurofibroma Versus Schwannoma

Neurofibroma shows an unencapsulated, dermal proliferation of wavy, spindled Schwann cells and fibroblasts admixed with mast cells within a loose, myxoid to collagenous stroma, while schwannoma shows a well-encapsulated tumor composed of alternating Antoni A areas (compact, spindled cells) and Antoni B areas (looser, myxoid, hypocellular regions), with characteristic Verocay bodies, palisaded nuclear arrangements flanking anuclear zones, a distinguishing feature not seen in neurofibroma, together with diffuse, strong S100 immunoreactivity in both entities, discussed further in the ancillary studies section below, given the shared Schwann cell lineage these two entities share despite their distinct architectural presentations.

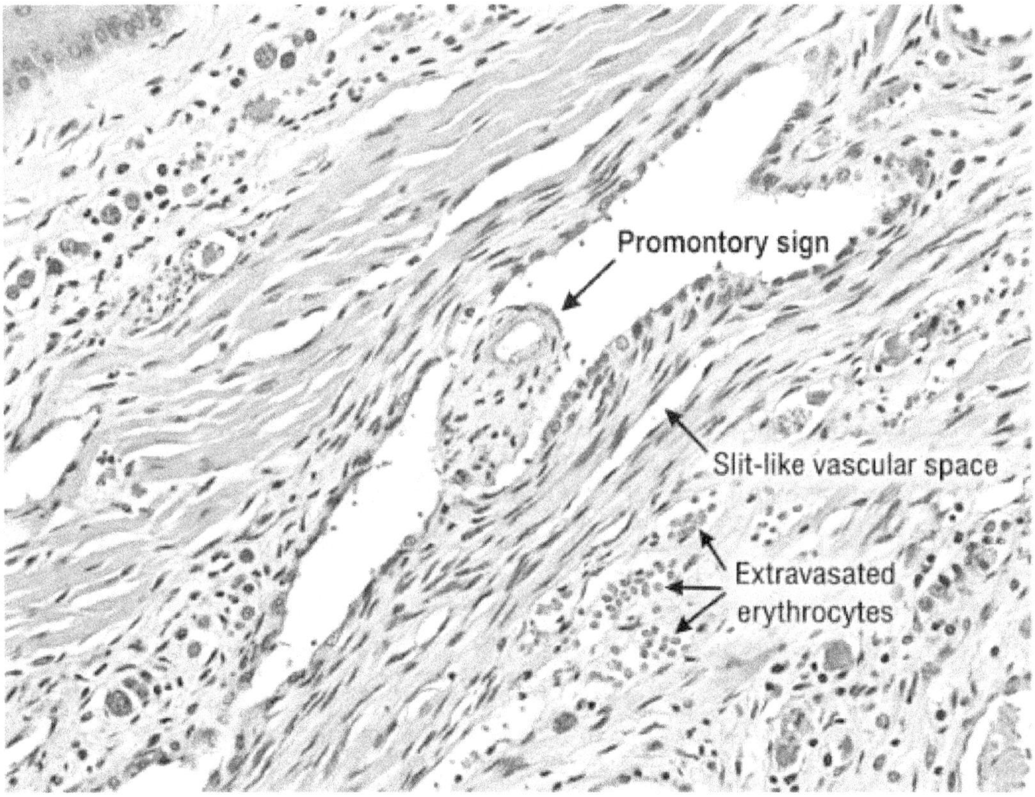

Ancillary Studies

CD34 and Factor XIIIa Immunohistochemistry

CD34 immunohistochemistry shows strong, diffuse positivity in dermatofibrosarcoma protuberans and characteristic negativity or only focal, weak staining in dermatofibroma, while Factor XIIIa shows the inverse pattern, positive in dermatofibroma's histiocytic component and negative in dermatofibrosarcoma protuberans, together forming a reciprocal immunohistochemical panel that resolves this chapter's most clinically consequential differential decisively in the great majority of cases, reserving molecular fluorescence in situ hybridization testing for the COL1A1-PDGFB fusion discussed in the etiology section above for the comparatively rare cases where the immunohistochemical panel remains genuinely ambiguous.

The Immunohistochemical Exclusion Panel for Atypical Fibroxanthoma and Pleomorphic Dermal Sarcoma

As demonstrated in the worked case above, diagnosing atypical fibroxanthoma or pleomorphic dermal sarcoma requires a negative immunohistochemical panel excluding the mimickers discussed in the differential diagnosis section: pancytokeratin (excluding spindle cell squamous cell carcinoma), S100 and SOX10 (excluding desmoplastic and spindle cell melanoma), and desmin or smooth muscle actin (excluding leiomyosarcoma), a panel that must be negative across all markers before either diagnosis is appropriately rendered, making this one of the few entities in this book where the diagnosis is defined as much by what the tumor is not as by any single positive, defining marker of its own.

HHV-8 Immunohistochemistry for Kaposi Sarcoma

Immunohistochemistry for HHV-8 latency-associated nuclear antigen shows strong, diffuse nuclear positivity within the spindle cell component of Kaposi sarcoma across all clinical stages, including the subtle, easily overlooked patch stage, providing a highly sensitive and specific confirmatory marker for this diagnosis and one that this chapter recommends applying liberally to any biopsy from a patient with HIV infection, transplant immunosuppression, or a violaceous lesion of uncertain etiology given the clinical importance of an accurate, timely Kaposi sarcoma diagnosis in these specific populations.

MDM2 and CDK4 Immunohistochemistry and Fluorescence In Situ Hybridization for Atypical Lipomatous Tumor

As demonstrated in the worked case above, MDM2 and CDK4 immunohistochemistry, showing diffuse nuclear positivity within the atypical stromal cells, provide a sensitive initial screen for atypical lipomatous tumor, with fluorescence in situ hybridization confirmation of MDM2 amplification, discussed in the etiology section above, reserved for cases where immunohistochemical staining is equivocal or where a definitive molecular confirmation is clinically warranted given the management implications that follow a positive result, wide excision rather than the simple excision appropriate for conventional lipoma.

Desmin, Smooth Muscle Actin, and Ki-67 for Smooth Muscle Tumors

Desmin and smooth muscle actin immunohistochemistry confirm smooth muscle lineage in both cutaneous leiomyoma and leiomyosarcoma, showing diffuse, strong cytoplasmic positivity in both entities and therefore functioning primarily to confirm the fundamental smooth muscle differentiation of a spindle cell lesion rather than to distinguish benign from malignant, a distinction that instead relies substantially on Ki-67 proliferative index, elevated in leiomyosarcoma relative to leiomyoma, together with the mitotic count, cytologic atypia, and infiltrative margin assessment performed on hematoxylin and eosin staining discussed in the differential diagnosis section above.

CD31, ERG, and MYC for Angiosarcoma

CD31 and ERG immunohistochemistry confirm endothelial lineage in angiosarcoma, including in the poorly differentiated, solid epithelioid areas where vasoformative architecture is not readily apparent on hematoxylin and eosin staining alone, functioning analogously to the pancytokeratin and S100/SOX10 exclusion panel discussed above for atypical fibroxanthoma in confirming lineage when morphology alone is genuinely ambiguous. MYC immunohistochemistry, reflecting the MYC gene amplification discussed in the etiology section above, shows diffuse nuclear positivity in radiation-associated angiosarcoma and characteristic negativity in benign atypical vascular lesion, providing the practically decisive ancillary distinction between these two entities whenever a vascular proliferation arises within a prior radiation field.

KEY POINT: CD34 and Factor XIIIa immunohistochemistry resolve the dermatofibroma versus dermatofibrosarcoma protuberans differential in the great majority of cases; a negative pancytokeratin, S100/SOX10, and desmin panel is required before diagnosing atypical fibroxanthoma or pleomorphic dermal sarcoma; HHV-8 immunohistochemistry confirms Kaposi sarcoma even at its subtle patch stage; MDM2/CDK4 confirm atypical lipomatous tumor; and MYC positivity distinguishes radiation-associated angiosarcoma from benign atypical vascular lesion.

Management Implications

Surgical Management by Entity

Dermatofibroma requires no further treatment beyond the diagnostic biopsy or excision itself, while dermatofibrosarcoma protuberans, given its characteristic subclinical infiltrative extension described throughout this chapter, is managed with Mohs micrographic surgery or wide local excision with wide margins and careful pathologic margin assessment, given the well-documented high local recurrence rate that follows conventional excision with standard margins for this specific tumor. Atypical fibroxanthoma is generally managed with complete excision given its low but present local recurrence risk, while pleomorphic dermal sarcoma, given its deeper invasion and metastatic potential, warrants wider excision and closer clinical follow-up, with the depth- and invasion-based distinction discussed in the histopathologic features section above directly determining which management pathway a given tumor receives.

Systemic and Site-Specific Management of Kaposi Sarcoma and Neural Tumors

Management of Kaposi sarcoma is directed substantially at the underlying immune context: initiation or optimization of antiretroviral therapy for epidemic (AIDS-associated) Kaposi sarcoma, and reduction of immunosuppression when feasible for iatrogenic Kaposi sarcoma, frequently produces meaningful regression given this tumor's fundamentally virus- and immune-context-driven pathogenesis, with localized therapy, excision, radiation, or intralesional therapy, and systemic chemotherapy reserved for extensive, rapidly progressive, or visceral disease. Neurofibroma and schwannoma are managed with simple excision for symptomatic or diagnostically uncertain lesions, while the plexiform neurofibroma variant associated with neurofibromatosis type 1, given its diffuse, often unresectable extent and recognized risk of malignant transformation discussed in the etiology section above, warrants longitudinal surveillance and prompt biopsy of any area showing new pain, rapid growth, or a change in consistency.

Management of Adipocytic and Smooth Muscle Tumors

Lipoma is managed with simple excision when symptomatic or of cosmetic concern, or with observation when small and asymptomatic, requiring no further workup once the diagnosis is clinically or histologically confirmed, while atypical lipomatous tumor, given its locally aggressive behavior and recognized recurrence risk following incomplete excision, is managed with wide local excision and, given its deep-seated location, appropriate cross-sectional imaging for surgical planning, together with longitudinal clinical follow-up given this tumor's potential, albeit rare, for dedifferentiation to a higher-grade sarcoma. Piloleiomyoma and angioleiomyoma are managed conservatively, excision reserved for symptomatic lesions given the paroxysmal pain that piloleiomyoma characteristically produces, while cutaneous leiomyosarcoma is managed with wide local excision, with Mohs micrographic surgery increasingly employed for anatomically sensitive sites given this tumor's generally more favorable prognosis relative to deep soft tissue leiomyosarcoma discussed further below.

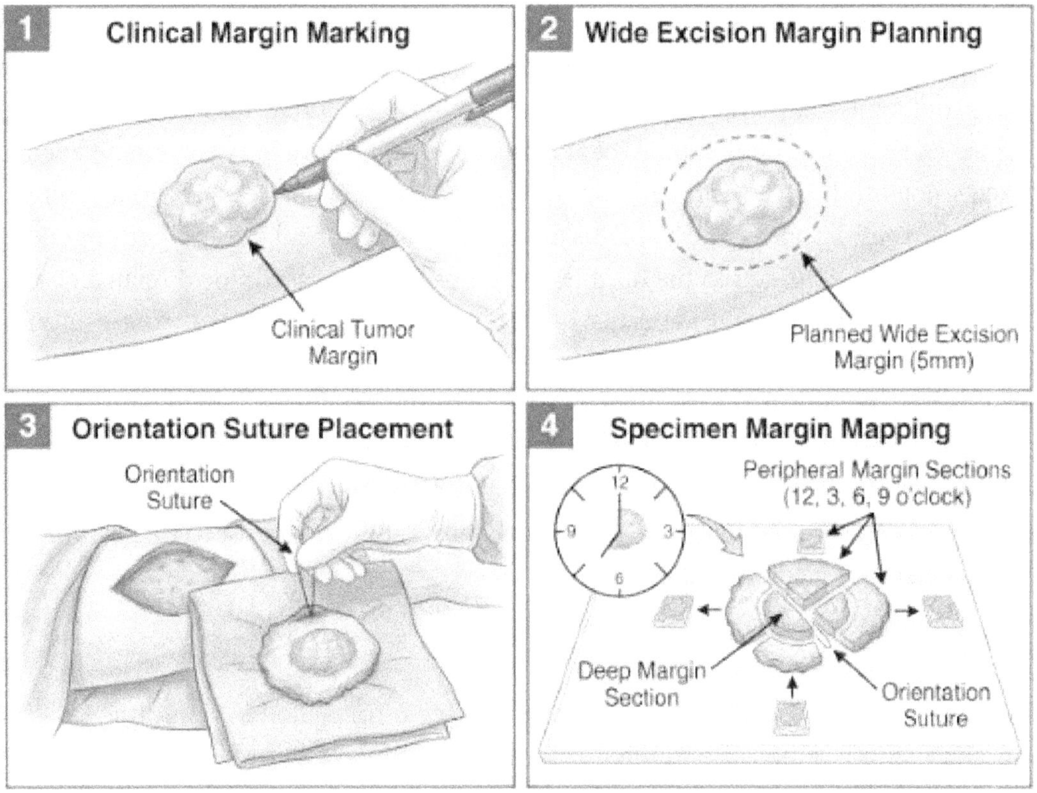

Multidisciplinary Management of Angiosarcoma

Angiosarcoma, given its characteristic subclinical extension well beyond the apparent clinical margin, high local recurrence rate, and substantial metastatic potential, warrants prompt multidisciplinary oncologic referral rather than dermatologic management in isolation, with wide local excision, frequently requiring staged or Mohs-assisted margin control given the difficulty of clinically defining this tumor's true extent, combined with adjuvant radiation therapy to the surgical field, and systemic therapy, paclitaxel-based chemotherapy or antiangiogenic agents among the regimens employed, reserved for extensive, multifocal, or metastatic disease. Stewart-Treves syndrome carries a particularly poor prognosis and is managed similarly, though the affected limb's chronic lymphedema can complicate both surgical planning and wound healing, a management complexity this chapter notes underscores the importance of preventing chronic lymphedema in the first instance through careful surgical and radiotherapy planning for the primary breast malignancy.

Complications and Prognosis

Dermatofibrosarcoma protuberans carries a low but genuine metastatic potential, concentrated in tumors showing fibrosarcomatous transformation, an area of higher-grade, more mitotically active tumor arising within an otherwise conventional dermatofibrosarcoma protuberans, a transformation this chapter notes warrants explicit reporting given its independent prognostic significance. Pleomorphic dermal sarcoma carries a meaningfully higher local recurrence and metastatic rate than atypical fibroxanthoma, directly reflecting the deeper invasion, perineural or lymphovascular involvement, or necrosis that defines this upgraded diagnosis, while Kaposi sarcoma's prognosis varies substantially by clinical subtype, generally indolent for classic Kaposi sarcoma and historically more aggressive for untreated epidemic Kaposi sarcoma, though outcomes have improved substantially with effective antiretroviral therapy. Atypical lipomatous tumor carries a low but genuine local recurrence risk following incomplete excision and a rare but recognized potential for dedifferentiation to a higher-grade sarcoma, while cutaneous leiomyosarcoma, in contrast to its deep soft tissue and retroperitoneal counterparts, generally carries a favorable prognosis when confined to the dermis and completely excised, local recurrence representing a greater practical concern than distant metastasis for this site-restricted variant. Angiosarcoma carries the least favorable prognosis of any entity in this chapter, with five-year survival historically reported in the range of approximately ten to fifty percent depending on tumor size, depth, and completeness of excision, reflecting this tumor's combination of subclinical local extension, high local recurrence rate, and substantial metastatic potential, a sobering prognosis this chapter attributes directly to the diagnostic delay that this tumor's deceptively innocuous bruise-like early presentation, discussed in the clinical presentation section above, so often produces.

Special Populations

Multiple piloleiomyomas in a young patient warrant referral for genetic counseling and renal imaging given the hereditary leiomyomatosis and renal cell cancer syndrome association discussed in the etiology section above, a special-population consideration this chapter emphasizes given the syndrome's associated aggressive, early-onset renal cell carcinoma phenotype. Kaposi sarcoma in a pediatric or young adult patient should prompt evaluation for underlying HIV infection or another immunosuppressed state given this tumor's fundamentally immune-context-driven pathogenesis discussed in the etiology section above, while plexiform neurofibroma identified in a child warrants comprehensive neurofibromatosis type 1 evaluation and longitudinal dermatologic and neuro-oncologic surveillance given this population's lifelong exposure to the malignant transformation risk discussed above. Solid organ transplant recipients and other chronically immunosuppressed patients warrant a lower threshold for biopsy of any new or enlarging violaceous lesion given their elevated risk of iatrogenic Kaposi sarcoma, and any patient with longstanding lymphedema of a limb, whether following axillary, inguinal, or pelvic lymph node dissection, warrants prompt biopsy of any new nodule or plaque arising within the affected field given the Stewart-Treves syndrome risk discussed above, a surveillance point this chapter emphasizes given the substantial survival benefit associated with earlier detection of this otherwise poor-prognosis malignancy.

Documentation and Reporting Standards

The pathology report for any dermal spindle cell or fibrohistiocytic tumor should explicitly document depth of invasion, presence or absence of subcutaneous, perineural, or lymphovascular extension, and mitotic activity given these features' direct role in distinguishing benign from malignant entities throughout this chapter, together with the specific immunohistochemical panel performed and its results, particularly for atypical fibroxanthoma and pleomorphic dermal sarcoma given their status as diagnoses of exclusion. For dermatofibrosarcoma protuberans, the report should note whether fibrosarcomatous transformation is present given its independent prognostic significance discussed above, and for atypical lipomatous tumor and angiosarcoma, the report should explicitly state MDM2/CDK4 or MYC ancillary results respectively, given these markers' direct bearing on the surgical margin and adjuvant therapy decisions that follow. Margin status should be reported using standardized distance measurements wherever feasible rather than a binary positive or negative designation alone, providing the surgeon with the quantitative information needed to plan re-excision when margins are close but technically clear.

Patient Education and Counseling

Patients diagnosed with dermatofibrosarcoma protuberans benefit from clear counseling regarding why Mohs micrographic surgery or wide excision is recommended despite this tumor's low-grade histologic appearance, framed around its characteristic subclinical extension rather than aggressive short-term behavior, while patients diagnosed with atypical fibroxanthoma or pleomorphic dermal sarcoma benefit from counseling regarding the specific depth- and invasion-based distinction that determined their diagnosis and the corresponding surveillance recommendation that follows. Patients diagnosed with angiosarcoma benefit from clear, compassionate counseling regarding the multidisciplinary management pathway and the prognosis discussed above, framed around the concrete surgical, radiotherapeutic, and systemic options available rather than prognosis alone, while patients with hereditary leiomyomatosis and renal cell cancer syndrome benefit from counseling regarding the lifelong renal surveillance this diagnosis warrants for themselves and at-risk family members.

THE REACTION PATTERN RECOGNITION SYSTEM — The Mesenchymal Tumor Differentiation and Depth Pattern Family

The Pattern: Mesenchymal tumors organized by line of differentiation, fibrohistiocytic, vascular, neural, adipocytic, and smooth muscle, with benign-versus-malignant status determined by depth, circumscription, and cytologic monotony versus pleomorphism.

Histologic Signature: Storiform pattern with collagen trapping defines dermatofibroma; honeycomb fat infiltration with CD34 positivity defines dermatofibrosarcoma protuberans; slit-like vascular spaces with a promontory sign define Kaposi sarcoma; Verocay bodies define schwannoma.

The Decision: Identify line of differentiation, then assess depth and circumscription versus infiltration, escalating to CD34/Factor XIIIa for the dermatofibroma differential, HHV-8 for suspected Kaposi sarcoma, and the full exclusion panel before diagnosing atypical fibroxanthoma or pleomorphic dermal sarcoma.

Trap Logic: Dermatofibrosarcoma protuberans mimics dermatofibroma; atypical fibroxanthoma and pleomorphic dermal sarcoma share identical cytology distinguished only by depth and invasion; Kaposi sarcoma's patch stage is subtle and easily overlooked without HHV-8 confirmation.

Pattern Anchor: Line of differentiation first, then depth and circumscription versus infiltration. Atypical fibroxanthoma and pleomorphic dermal sarcoma are exclusion diagnoses; a negative pancytokeratin, S100/SOX10, and desmin panel is mandatory before either diagnosis is rendered.

Summary and Key Concepts

Mesenchymal tumors are organized by line of differentiation, fibrohistiocytic, vascular, neural, adipocytic, and smooth muscle, with benign versus malignant status determined by depth, circumscription, and cytologic pleomorphism.

Dermatofibroma is distinguished from dermatofibrosarcoma protuberans by storiform architecture and collagen trapping against honeycomb fat infiltration, resolved definitively by reciprocal CD34 and Factor XIIIa immunohistochemistry.

Atypical fibroxanthoma and pleomorphic dermal sarcoma share identical pleomorphic cytology and are distinguished only by depth of invasion, requiring a negative pancytokeratin, S100/SOX10, and desmin exclusion panel before diagnosis.

Kaposi sarcoma, driven by HHV-8 infection, presents across patch, plaque, and nodular stages with slit-like vascular spaces and a promontory sign, confirmed by HHV-8 latency-associated nuclear antigen immunohistochemistry.

Neurofibroma and schwannoma share Schwann cell lineage but differ architecturally, unencapsulated wavy spindle cells with mast cells against encapsulated Antoni A/B areas with Verocay bodies, with plexiform neurofibroma carrying malignant transformation risk in neurofibromatosis type 1.

CHAPTER 18: CUTANEOUS LYMPHOPROLIFERATIVE DISORDERS AND LYMPHOMA

Learning Objectives

1. Classify primary cutaneous lymphomas by T-cell versus B-cell lineage and recognize the major entities within each category.
2. Identify the histopathologic features distinguishing mycosis fungoides from its benign inflammatory mimickers at the patch stage.
3. Distinguish lymphomatoid papulosis from primary cutaneous anaplastic large cell lymphoma and from systemic anaplastic large cell lymphoma with secondary skin involvement.
4. Recognize the diagnostic criteria for Sézary syndrome and its relationship to mycosis fungoides.
5. Apply T-cell receptor and immunoglobulin heavy chain gene rearrangement studies appropriately to support, rather than independently establish, a diagnosis of cutaneous lymphoma.
6. Connect clinical stage in mycosis fungoides to prognosis and to the corresponding skin-directed versus systemic management pathway.

Definition and Classification

Primary Cutaneous Lymphomas and the WHO-EORTC Classification

Primary cutaneous lymphomas are a heterogeneous group of non-Hodgkin lymphomas that present in the skin without evidence of extracutaneous disease at the time of diagnosis, a definitional distinction this chapter emphasizes as clinically fundamental given that a histologically identical lymphoma presenting primarily in the skin carries a substantially different prognosis and management pathway than the same lymphoma subtype presenting as secondary cutaneous involvement of a systemic nodal process. The World Health Organization-European Organisation for Research and Treatment of Cancer classification, the framework this chapter follows throughout, organizes primary cutaneous lymphomas first by T-cell versus B-cell lineage and then by specific clinicopathologic entity, a two-tier organizational structure that mirrors this chapter's approach to mesenchymal tumors in Chapter 17 and to melanocytic lesions in Chapters 13 and 14: identify the fundamental lineage first, then apply entity-specific criteria to arrive at a precise diagnosis.

T-Cell Versus B-Cell Lineage as the Foundational Distinction

Cutaneous T-cell lymphomas are substantially more common than cutaneous B-cell lymphomas, with mycosis fungoides representing the single most common subtype overall, accounting for the majority of all primary cutaneous lymphomas encountered in routine dermatopathologic practice. The CD30-positive lymphoproliferative disorders, lymphomatoid papulosis and primary cutaneous anaplastic large cell lymphoma, form a distinct clinicopathologic spectrum within the T-cell category, sharing a common CD30-positive immunophenotype but differing substantially in clinical course, a spectrum developed in detail throughout this chapter given its outsized diagnostic importance. Cutaneous B-cell lymphomas are less common and are further divided into indolent entities, primary cutaneous marginal zone lymphoma and primary cutaneous follicle center lymphoma, and the more aggressive primary cutaneous diffuse large B-cell lymphoma, leg type, a site-specific designation reflecting this entity's characteristic, though not exclusive, predilection for the lower extremity. Two additional, comparatively rare entities, subcutaneous panniculitis-like T-cell lymphoma and extranodal NK/T-cell lymphoma, nasal type, are developed later in this chapter given their distinct clinical presentations and the specific, high-stakes differential diagnoses each raises against a benign panniculitis or a destructive infectious process respectively.

Entity	Lineage	Key Distinguishing Feature	Clinical Behavior
Mycosis fungoides	T-cell	Epidermotropism, Pautrier microabscesses, cerebriform lymphocytes	Indolent, stage-dependent
Sézary syndrome	T-cell	Erythroderma, lymphadenopathy, circulating Sézary cells	Aggressive leukemic variant
Lymphomatoid papulosis	T-cell (CD30+)	Waxing and waning papulonodules, self-resolving	Indolent, recurrent
Primary cutaneous anaplastic large cell lymphoma	T-cell (CD30+)	Solitary or localized nodule, sheets of anaplastic cells	Indolent to intermediate
Subcutaneous panniculitis-like T-cell lymphoma	T-cell (alpha-beta)	Rimming of adipocytes by atypical lymphocytes	Indolent (alpha-beta type)
Primary cutaneous marginal zone lymphoma	B-cell	Nodular marginal zone cells, plasmacytic differentiation	Indolent

Primary cutaneous follicle center lymphoma	B-cell	Follicular or diffuse centrocyte/centroblast proliferation	Indolent
Primary cutaneous diffuse large B-cell lymphoma, leg type	B-cell	Sheets of centroblasts/immunoblasts, MYD88 mutation common	More aggressive

Epidemiology of Cutaneous Lymphoma

This section situates each entity discussed in this chapter within its expected demographic and clinical context, information this chapter emphasizes is directly relevant to pretest diagnostic suspicion. Mycosis fungoides shows a male predominance and a peak incidence in the fifth through seventh decades, though it can arise, less commonly, in children and young adults, particularly the hypopigmented variant discussed in the special populations section below, with an overall incidence that, while representing the most common cutaneous lymphoma, remains substantially lower than nodal non-Hodgkin lymphoma overall. Sézary syndrome is comparatively rare, representing a small minority of cutaneous T-cell lymphoma presentations, while the CD30-positive lymphoproliferative disorder spectrum, taken together, represents the second most common category of cutaneous T-cell lymphoma after mycosis fungoides, lymphomatoid papulosis in particular showing a chronic, often decades-long natural history that this chapter notes contributes to its comparatively high point prevalence relative to its annual incidence. Cutaneous B-cell lymphomas are collectively less common than cutaneous T-cell lymphomas, primary cutaneous marginal zone lymphoma and primary cutaneous follicle center lymphoma both showing a comparatively even age distribution across middle-aged and older adults, while primary cutaneous diffuse large B-cell lymphoma, leg type, shows a strong predilection for elderly women, a demographic pattern this chapter notes remains incompletely explained.

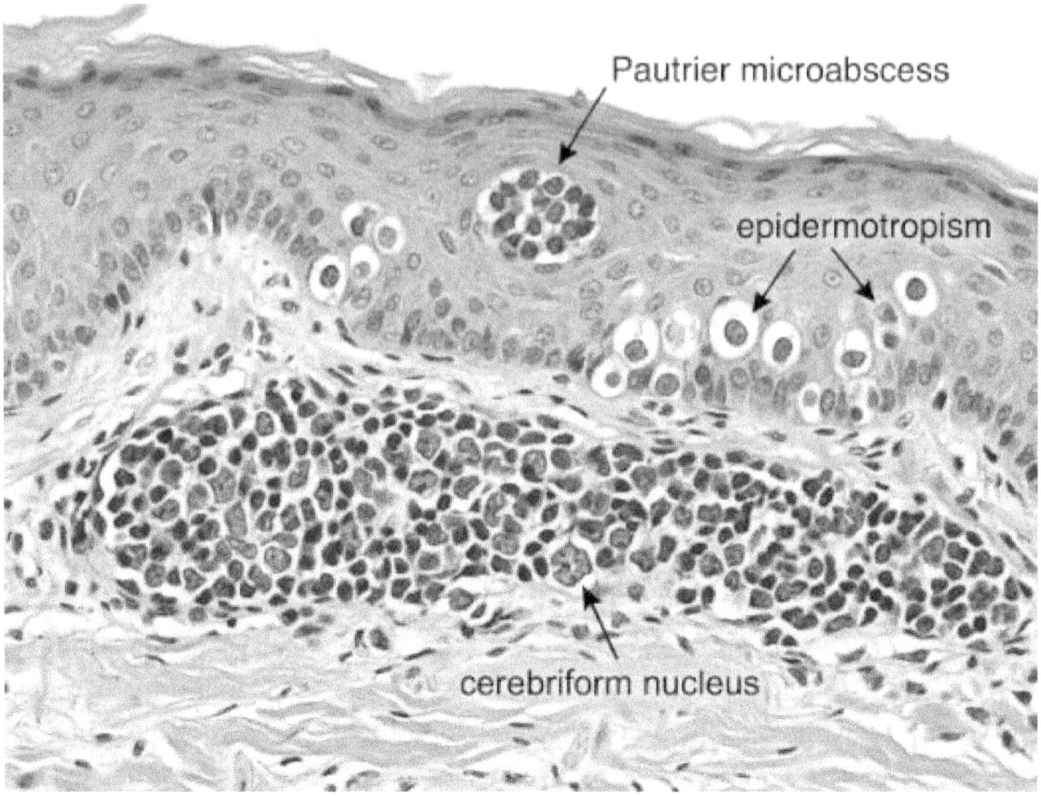

Etiology and Pathogenesis

Clonal T-Cell Expansion and the Chronic Antigen Stimulation Hypothesis

Mycosis fungoides arises from the clonal proliferation of a skin-homing CD4-positive memory T-cell, though the inciting molecular events driving this clonal expansion remain incompletely defined; the leading pathogenetic hypothesis holds that chronic antigenic stimulation, whether from a persistent environmental exposure, an occult infectious agent, or an unidentified autoantigen, drives sustained proliferation of a T-cell clone that progressively accumulates additional genetic alterations, including loss-of-function mutations in tumor suppressor genes and activating mutations in T-cell receptor signaling pathway components, over the course of disease progression from patch through plaque to tumor stage, a stepwise molecular evolution that parallels this disease's characteristic stepwise clinical progression developed further in the clinical presentation section below.

CD30 Biology in Lymphomatoid Papulosis and Primary Cutaneous Anaplastic Large Cell Lymphoma

CD30 is a member of the tumor necrosis factor receptor superfamily whose expression on activated lymphocytes drives proliferative and anti-apoptotic signaling; its aberrant, sustained expression is the defining immunophenotypic feature shared across the CD30-positive lymphoproliferative disorder spectrum discussed in the definition and classification section above. A subset of primary cutaneous anaplastic large cell lymphoma and, less commonly, lymphomatoid papulosis harbors a DUSP22-IRF4 gene rearrangement on chromosome 6p25.3, a molecular alteration this chapter notes is generally associated with a favorable prognosis, in contrast to the ALK gene rearrangement characteristic of systemic anaplastic large cell lymphoma, a molecular distinction developed further in the differential diagnosis section below given its direct bearing on distinguishing primary cutaneous from secondary cutaneous anaplastic large cell lymphoma.

MYD88 and Other Molecular Alterations in Cutaneous B-Cell Lymphoma

Primary cutaneous diffuse large B-cell lymphoma, leg type, frequently harbors an activating MYD88 L265P mutation, a molecular alteration that drives constitutive nuclear factor kappa B signaling and that is shared with several other extranodal large B-cell lymphomas, while primary cutaneous marginal zone lymphoma has been associated in some cases with chronic antigenic stimulation from Borrelia burgdorferi infection in geographic regions where this organism is endemic, an association substantially weaker and more geographically restricted than the well-established Helicobacter pylori association with gastric marginal zone lymphoma but one this chapter notes as relevant to the differential consideration of antibiotic therapy in appropriately selected, localized cases.

Alpha-Beta T-Cell Receptor Phenotype in Subcutaneous Panniculitis-like T-Cell Lymphoma

Subcutaneous panniculitis-like T-cell lymphoma arises from a cytotoxic T-cell expressing the alpha-beta T-cell receptor phenotype, a lineage distinction this chapter emphasizes as clinically pivotal, since the histologically overlapping but immunophenotypically distinct gamma-delta T-cell receptor-expressing primary cutaneous gamma-delta T-cell lymphoma carries a substantially more aggressive clinical course, developed further in the differential diagnosis section below. A subset of alpha-beta subcutaneous panniculitis-like T-cell lymphoma has been associated with somatic or, less commonly, germline HAVCR2 mutations affecting the TIM-3 immune checkpoint pathway, an alteration proposed to contribute to this entity's occasionally accompanying hemophagocytic lymphohistiocytosis, discussed further in the complications and prognosis section below.

Epstein-Barr Virus and Extranodal NK/T-Cell Lymphoma, Nasal Type

Extranodal NK/T-cell lymphoma, nasal type, though most classically a mucosal and nasal cavity malignancy, can present with primary or secondary cutaneous involvement and is driven causally by Epstein-Barr virus infection of natural killer or, less commonly, T-cells, with the virus detectable within the neoplastic cells in essentially all cases, a near-universal association that, discussed further in the ancillary studies section below, provides both a defining etiologic link and a highly sensitive diagnostic marker for this comparatively rare but clinically aggressive entity.

THE REACTION PATTERN RECOGNITION SYSTEM — Epidermotropism and Clonality as the Universal Cutaneous Lymphoma Anchor

---

The Pattern: Lineage (T-cell versus B-cell) Combined with Epidermotropism, Cytologic Atypia, and Depth of Dermal Involvement as the Framework for Classifying Every Cutaneous Lymphoproliferative Disorder in This Chapter

Histologic Signature: Disproportionate epidermotropism with Pautrier microabscess formation signals mycosis fungoides; sheets of large anaplastic CD30-positive cells signal the CD30-positive lymphoproliferative disorder spectrum; nodular or diffuse small-to-medium B-cell infiltrates with reactive germinal centers signal indolent B-cell lymphoma or pseudolymphoma; and sheets of centroblasts or immunoblasts without epidermotropism signal aggressive B-cell lymphoma.

The Decision: Determine lineage by morphology and confirm with immunohistochemistry, then assess epidermotropism, cytologic atypia, and growth pattern, escalating to T-cell receptor or immunoglobulin heavy chain gene rearrangement studies whenever a clonal lymphoid process is suspected but morphology and immunophenotype alone leave genuine diagnostic uncertainty.

Trap Logic: Patch-stage mycosis fungoides can closely mimic benign inflammatory dermatoses including eczema and psoriasis; lymphomatoid papulosis can mimic primary cutaneous or systemic anaplastic large cell lymphoma given shared CD30 positivity; and cutaneous pseudolymphoma can mimic marginal zone lymphoma given overlapping nodular lymphoid architecture.

Pattern Anchor: Lineage first, then epidermotropism, cytologic atypia, and depth. Clonality studies support but never independently establish a lymphoma diagnosis; correlation with morphology, immunophenotype, and clinical course is mandatory in every case.

Histopathologic Features and Diagnostic Criteria

Mycosis Fungoides Across Patch, Plaque, and Tumor Stage

Patch-stage mycosis fungoides shows a band-like or lichenoid superficial dermal infiltrate of small-to-medium lymphocytes with hyperchromatic, cerebriform (irregularly convoluted) nuclear contours, together with disproportionate epidermotropism, individual atypical lymphocytes within the epidermis unaccompanied by the spongiosis that would be expected in a comparably cellular benign inflammatory infiltrate, a specific and diagnostically pivotal discordance this chapter emphasizes as the single most useful low-power clue distinguishing early mycosis fungoides from its inflammatory mimickers, developed further in the differential diagnosis section below. Plaque-stage disease shows a denser dermal infiltrate with more pronounced epidermotropism, often forming Pautrier microabscesses, discrete intraepidermal collections of atypical lymphocytes, a finding that, when present, is highly specific for mycosis fungoides. Tumor-stage disease shows a dense, diffuse dermal and often subcutaneous infiltrate of atypical lymphocytes with reduced or absent epidermotropism, a paradoxical loss of the very feature that anchors earlier-stage diagnosis, together with an increasing proportion of large, transformed cells, a transformation this chapter notes carries independent prognostic significance discussed further in the complications and prognosis section below.

Histologic Variants of Mycosis Fungoides

Folliculotropic mycosis fungoides shows atypical lymphocytic infiltration concentrated around and within hair follicle epithelium, often with associated mucinous degeneration of the follicular epithelium (follicular mucinosis), rather than the epidermotropism of classic mycosis fungoides, a distinct histologic pattern that correlates clinically with a comparatively less favorable prognosis given this variant's characteristic involvement of the deeper, follicular-based skin compartment, developed further in the management implications section below given its relative resistance to skin-directed therapy that depends on epidermal penetration. Pagetoid reticulosis shows marked, florid epidermotropism with relative sparing of the dermis, individual atypical lymphocytes percolating throughout the full thickness of a markedly hyperplastic epidermis, a localized, indolent variant confined to a solitary plaque, most often on an acral site. Granulomatous slack skin, a rare variant, shows a granulomatous infiltrate with scattered multinucleated giant cells engulfing (emperipolesis) elastic fibers, resulting in progressive loss of dermal elastic tissue and the characteristic pendulous, lax skin folds that give this variant its name, most often affecting the axillae and groin.

Sézary Syndrome

Sézary syndrome shows histologic features overlapping with mycosis fungoides, though epidermotropism is frequently less pronounced than in classic plaque-stage mycosis fungoides, and the diagnosis in practice rests substantially on the combined clinical triad and peripheral blood findings developed in the clinical presentation section below rather than on skin histology in isolation, skin biopsy in a genuinely erythrodermic patient sometimes showing only a nonspecific perivascular lymphocytic infiltrate.

Histopathology of the CD30-Positive Lymphoproliferative Disorder Spectrum

Lymphomatoid papulosis shows a wedge-shaped dermal infiltrate that varies histologically across recognized subtypes: type A, the most common, shows scattered large, CD30-positive anaplastic cells admixed with numerous inflammatory cells, neutrophils, eosinophils, and small lymphocytes; type B shows a band-like infiltrate of small, atypical, cerebriform lymphocytes closely resembling mycosis fungoides; and type C shows sheets of large, CD30-positive anaplastic cells with comparatively sparse admixed inflammation, closely resembling primary cutaneous anaplastic large cell lymphoma on histology alone. Primary cutaneous anaplastic large cell lymphoma shows a dense, diffuse infiltrate of large, cohesive, CD30-positive anaplastic cells with abundant cytoplasm and pleomorphic, sometimes horseshoe-shaped (hallmark cell) nuclei, a histologic overlap with lymphomatoid papulosis type C that this chapter emphasizes is resolved substantially by clinical presentation and course rather than histology alone, developed further in the differential diagnosis section below.

Histopathology of Subcutaneous Panniculitis-like T-Cell Lymphoma and Extranodal NK/T-Cell Lymphoma

Subcutaneous panniculitis-like T-cell lymphoma shows a lobular panniculitis pattern with atypical lymphocytes characteristically rimming individual adipocytes, a distinctive architectural feature, together with karyorrhectic debris and, frequently, a background of reactive histiocytes, including foamy macrophages that can show hemophagocytosis, a finding that correlates with this entity's occasionally accompanying hemophagocytic lymphohistiocytosis discussed in the etiology section above. Extranodal NK/T-cell lymphoma, nasal type, shows an angiocentric and angiodestructive infiltrate of atypical lymphocytes with frequent, often extensive, coagulative necrosis, a combination of vascular destruction and necrosis this chapter notes reflects the tumor's characteristic biological aggressiveness and directly produces the deep, midline destructive ulceration developed in the clinical presentation section below.

Clinical Presentation and Clinicopathologic Correlation

Staging of Mycosis Fungoides

Mycosis fungoides progresses, in the classic though not universal disease course, through three clinical stages that correlate with the histologic progression described above: patch stage, presenting as scaly, erythematous to violaceous patches in a characteristic "bathing trunk" distribution favoring sun-protected sites including the buttocks, groin, and breasts; plaque stage, presenting as infiltrated, well-demarcated plaques that can arise de novo or evolve from pre-existing patches; and tumor stage, presenting as dome-shaped or ulcerated nodules that can arise within existing plaques or, less commonly, on previously uninvolved skin, an occurrence this chapter notes should prompt consideration of large cell transformation given its documented association with tumor-stage disease arising outside the expected progression sequence.

Sézary Syndrome Diagnostic Triad

Sézary syndrome is defined by a clinical and laboratory triad: erythroderma involving the great majority of the body surface area, generalized lymphadenopathy, and the presence of clonally related, circulating atypical lymphocytes with cerebriform nuclei (Sézary cells) meeting specific quantitative or immunophenotypic thresholds on peripheral blood flow cytometry, developed further in the ancillary studies section below, a triad this chapter emphasizes must be assessed together given that erythroderma alone has a broad differential extending well beyond Sézary syndrome, discussed further in the differential diagnosis section below.

Clinical Presentation of the CD30-Positive Spectrum and Cutaneous B-Cell Lymphomas

Lymphomatoid papulosis presents as recurrent crops of papules and small nodules that characteristically wax and wane, individual lesions spontaneously resolving over weeks even as new lesions continue to appear, a self-limited natural history that stands in useful clinical contrast to primary cutaneous anaplastic large cell lymphoma, which presents as a solitary or localized nodule or tumor that does not spontaneously resolve, though it can show partial regression, a distinction developed further in the differential diagnosis section below. Primary cutaneous marginal zone lymphoma and primary cutaneous follicle center lymphoma both present as slowly growing, asymptomatic papules, plaques, or nodules, most common on the trunk and extremities for marginal zone lymphoma and on the scalp, forehead, and trunk for follicle center lymphoma, while primary cutaneous diffuse large B-cell lymphoma, leg type, presents as a more rapidly growing, often ulcerated nodule or tumor, most common, as its name indicates, on the lower extremity of elderly patients.

Clinical Presentation of Subcutaneous Panniculitis-like T-Cell Lymphoma and Extranodal NK/T-Cell Lymphoma

Subcutaneous panniculitis-like T-cell lymphoma presents as deep, firm, erythematous to violaceous subcutaneous nodules or plaques, most common on the extremities and trunk, a presentation that closely mimics erythema nodosum or lupus panniculitis and is frequently accompanied by systemic symptoms, fever, fatigue, and cytopenias, particularly when hemophagocytic lymphohistiocytosis complicates the disease course, discussed in the etiology section above. Extranodal NK/T-cell lymphoma, nasal type, presents with progressive, deep, midline facial destruction, most classically involving the nasal cavity, palate, and surrounding midfacial soft tissue, an aggressive, ulcerative, and destructive presentation historically termed lethal midline granuloma before this entity's neoplastic, Epstein-Barr virus-driven nature was established.

CLINICAL PEARL: The waxing and waning natural history of lymphomatoid papulosis, individual lesions resolving spontaneously over a period of weeks even as the overall process persists, is itself a diagnostically useful clinical feature that should prompt this diagnosis whenever a biopsy shows a CD30-positive infiltrate in a patient describing this specific recurrent, self-resolving pattern. Deep, tender subcutaneous nodules accompanied by unexplained fever or cytopenias warrant early consideration of subcutaneous panniculitis-like T-cell lymphoma rather than a routine panniculitis workup alone.

Differential Diagnosis and Histologic Mimickers

Patch-Stage Mycosis Fungoides Versus Benign Inflammatory Dermatoses

As introduced in the histopathologic features section above, patch-stage mycosis fungoides must be distinguished from chronic eczematous dermatitis, psoriasis, and other chronic inflammatory dermatoses, a differential this chapter identifies as among the most genuinely difficult in dermatopathology given the marked histologic overlap and the well-documented reality that a single biopsy can be non-diagnostic even in a patient with established mycosis fungoides. The key discriminating features favor mycosis fungoides: disproportionate epidermotropism relative to the degree of spongiosis, lymphocytes with cerebriform nuclear atypia, lymphocytes haloed by clear spaces within the epidermis, alignment of lymphocytes along the dermoepidermal junction, and Pautrier microabscess formation when present, while a benign inflammatory dermatosis more typically shows lymphocytes and spongiosis occurring in proportion to one another, without significant cytologic atypia. Given this differential's genuine difficulty, correlation with clinical presentation, T-cell receptor gene rearrangement studies discussed in the ancillary studies section below, and, when the diagnosis remains uncertain, repeat biopsy after an interval or comparison of multiple simultaneous biopsies from different sites, are appropriately liberal practices rather than exceptions.

A 52-year-old patient presents with several years of scaly, mildly pruritic, erythematous patches confined to the buttocks and inner thighs, previously treated as chronic eczema without sustained improvement. Pattern assignment identifies a superficial, band-like lymphocytic infiltrate with mild epidermotropism, lymphocytes present within the epidermis at a density disproportionate to the comparatively mild spongiosis, several lymphocytes showing haloed clearing and subtle cerebriform nuclear contours, without a well-formed Pautrier microabscess. Differential narrowing weighs chronic eczematous dermatitis against early mycosis fungoides given the disproportionate epidermotropism and subtle cytologic atypia, and T-cell receptor gene rearrangement studies are pursued: a dominant clonal T-cell receptor gamma gene rearrangement is identified, concordant with the clinical distribution and chronicity. Given the disproportionate epidermotropism, cytologic atypia, and confirmed T-cell clonality in the appropriate clinical context, a diagnosis of patch-stage mycosis fungoides is rendered, with the report explicitly noting that the histologic findings alone were suggestive but not definitive, and that the diagnosis was established through integration with the confirmed clonal rearrangement and the multi-year clinical course.

Lymphomatoid Papulosis Versus Primary Cutaneous and Systemic Anaplastic Large Cell Lymphoma

Given lymphomatoid papulosis type C's histologic overlap with primary cutaneous anaplastic large cell lymphoma described in the histopathologic features section above, this differential is resolved substantially by clinical course, lymphomatoid papulosis showing the characteristic recurrent, self-resolving papulonodular eruption described above against primary cutaneous anaplastic large cell lymphoma's solitary or localized, non-spontaneously-resolving nodule or tumor. Both entities must additionally be distinguished from systemic anaplastic large cell lymphoma with secondary cutaneous involvement, a distinction with substantial prognostic and management consequence given systemic disease's less favorable prognosis, supported by ALK immunohistochemistry, positive in a meaningful subset of systemic anaplastic large cell lymphoma and characteristically negative in primary cutaneous disease, together with clinical staging to exclude nodal or visceral involvement, discussed further in the management implications section below.

A 45-year-old patient presents with a solitary, rapidly enlarging 2.5-centimeter nodule on the forearm, present for approximately four weeks without a preceding history of recurrent, self-resolving papules. Pattern assignment identifies a dense, diffuse dermal infiltrate of large, cohesive anaplastic cells with abundant cytoplasm and pleomorphic hallmark cell nuclei, extending focally into the subcutis, with comparatively sparse admixed inflammatory cells. Differential narrowing weighs lymphomatoid papulosis type C, primary cutaneous anaplastic large cell lymphoma, and systemic anaplastic large cell lymphoma with secondary skin involvement given the solitary, non-waxing-and-waning presentation and anaplastic cytology, and CD30, ALK, and DUSP22-IRF4 rearrangement studies are pursued alongside complete nodal and visceral staging imaging: CD30 is diffusely positive, ALK is negative, and staging imaging shows no nodal or visceral disease. Given the solitary presentation, negative ALK, absent systemic disease, and lack of a preceding recurrent papular history, a diagnosis of primary cutaneous anaplastic large cell lymphoma is rendered, with the report noting the favorable prognosis generally associated with this diagnosis and recommending localized excision or radiation therapy over systemic chemotherapy.

Sézary Syndrome and Erythroderma Versus Other Causes of Generalized Erythroderma

Given that erythroderma has a broad differential extending well beyond Sézary syndrome, atopic dermatitis, psoriasis, drug reaction, and, in select cases, other causes of erythrodermic exfoliative dermatitis must each be considered, a differential this chapter emphasizes is resolved not by skin biopsy alone, which, as noted in the histopathologic features section above, can show only a nonspecific infiltrate in genuine Sézary syndrome, but by the combined clinical triad and peripheral blood flow cytometric findings discussed in the clinical presentation and ancillary studies sections. A history of pre-existing, longstanding patch or plaque-stage mycosis fungoides preceding the onset of erythroderma favors a diagnosis of erythrodermic mycosis fungoides evolving toward Sézary syndrome, while acute-onset erythroderma without such a preceding history, particularly in temporal association with a new medication, should prompt primary consideration of a drug reaction before an extensive lymphoma workup is pursued, though this chapter notes the two are not mutually exclusive and biopsy with clonality assessment remains appropriate whenever diagnostic uncertainty persists.

Cutaneous Pseudolymphoma Versus Primary Cutaneous Marginal Zone Lymphoma

Cutaneous lymphoid hyperplasia (pseudolymphoma), a reactive, polyclonal lymphoid proliferation that can arise in response to an arthropod bite, tattoo pigment, medication, or another identifiable antigenic stimulus, can closely mimic primary cutaneous marginal zone lymphoma given shared nodular lymphoid architecture with reactive-appearing germinal centers; this differential is resolved by a combination of architectural features, pseudolymphoma typically showing a top-heavy, superficial and mid-dermal nodular infiltrate with preserved germinal center polarization and a mixed population of B-cells, T-cells, and histiocytes, against marginal zone lymphoma's more monotonous marginal zone cell population with light chain restriction on immunohistochemistry or in situ hybridization and, when present, clonal immunoglobulin heavy chain gene rearrangement, discussed further in the ancillary studies section below.

Subcutaneous Panniculitis-like T-Cell Lymphoma Versus Lupus Panniculitis and Primary Cutaneous Gamma-Delta T-Cell Lymphoma

As introduced in the clinical presentation section above, subcutaneous panniculitis-like T-cell lymphoma's overlap with lupus panniculitis (lupus profundus) is a well-documented and genuinely difficult differential, both entities showing a lobular panniculitis with lymphocytic infiltration, the distinction resting on adipocyte rimming, cytologic atypia, and karyorrhectic debris favoring lymphoma, against lupus panniculitis's characteristic overlying interface dermatitis, dermal mucin deposition, and lymphoid follicles with reactive germinal centers, together with clinical and serologic correlation for systemic or cutaneous lupus erythematosus, given that some patients can show overlapping or sequential features of both processes. Subcutaneous panniculitis-like T-cell lymphoma must additionally be distinguished from the histologically similar but clinically more aggressive primary cutaneous gamma-delta T-cell lymphoma, a distinction resolved definitively by T-cell receptor immunophenotyping, discussed further in the ancillary studies section below, given this differential's substantial prognostic and management consequence.

A 34-year-old patient presents with several firm, tender subcutaneous nodules on the thighs, accompanied by low-grade fever and mild pancytopenia, initially treated empirically as erythema nodosum without improvement. Pattern assignment identifies a lobular panniculitis with atypical lymphocytes rimming individual adipocytes, karyorrhectic debris, and scattered hemophagocytic macrophages, without a significant overlying interface dermatitis or dermal mucin deposition. Differential narrowing weighs lupus panniculitis against subcutaneous panniculitis-like T-cell lymphoma given the adipocyte rimming and hemophagocytosis, and T-cell receptor immunophenotyping and gene rearrangement studies are pursued: the atypical lymphocytes express an alpha-beta T-cell receptor phenotype with a dominant clonal T-cell receptor gamma gene rearrangement, and antinuclear antibody testing is negative. Given the adipocyte rimming, confirmed alpha-beta phenotype and clonality, and absence of serologic or histologic support for lupus, a diagnosis of subcutaneous panniculitis-like T-cell lymphoma is rendered, with the report recommending close hematologic monitoring given the patient's cytopenias and the recognized association with hemophagocytic lymphohistiocytosis.

Folliculotropic Mycosis Fungoides Versus Alopecia Mucinosa

Folliculotropic mycosis fungoides, given its characteristic follicular mucinosis described in the histopathologic features section above, must be distinguished from primary (idiopathic) alopecia mucinosa, a benign, self-limited condition most common in children and young adults that shows histologically identical follicular mucin deposition without the atypical, clonal lymphocytic infiltrate that defines the neoplastic variant, a distinction resting substantially on the density and cytologic atypia of the associated lymphocytic infiltrate, supported by T-cell receptor gene rearrangement studies and, importantly, by longitudinal clinical follow-up, given that idiopathic alopecia mucinosa in an older patient or with an atypical clinical course should prompt reconsideration of the folliculotropic mycosis fungoides diagnosis.

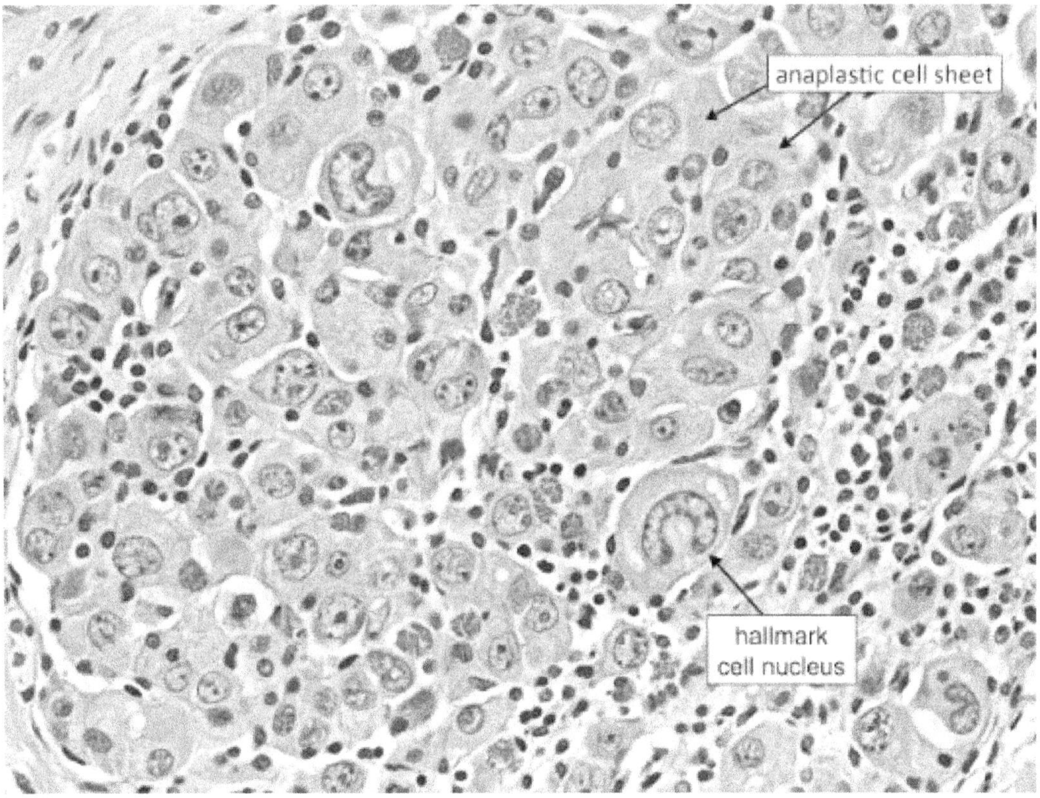

Ancillary Studies

Immunohistochemical Panels by Entity

A comprehensive immunohistochemical panel, rather than a single marker in isolation, is the appropriate practice throughout this chapter given the substantial morphologic overlap among the entities discussed, with panel composition tailored to the leading clinical and histologic differential in a given case rather than applied uniformly, mirroring this book's general approach to immunohistochemical exclusion panels established for atypical fibroxanthoma in Chapter 17.

Mycosis fungoides typically shows a CD3-positive, CD4-positive, CD8-negative T-cell immunophenotype with characteristic loss of one or more pan-T-cell antigens, CD2, CD5, or CD7, an aberrant antigen loss that, while not entity-specific, supports a neoplastic rather than reactive process when identified in conjunction with the morphologic findings described above. The CD30-positive lymphoproliferative disorder spectrum is defined immunophenotypically by CD30 positivity in the large atypical cell population, with ALK immunohistochemistry applied specifically to exclude systemic anaplastic large cell lymphoma as discussed in the differential diagnosis section above. Cutaneous B-cell lymphomas are evaluated with a CD20, CD79a, and CD3 panel to confirm B-cell lineage and exclude T-cell lymphoma, together with kappa and lambda light chain immunohistochemistry or in situ hybridization to assess for light chain restriction, and BCL2 and BCL6 immunohistochemistry, useful in supporting a diagnosis of follicle center lymphoma when follicular architecture is present.

T-Cell Receptor and Immunoglobulin Heavy Chain Gene Rearrangement Studies

T-cell receptor gene rearrangement studies, most often performed by polymerase chain reaction targeting the T-cell receptor gamma gene, identify a dominant clonal peak supporting a diagnosis of cutaneous T-cell lymphoma, as demonstrated in the worked case above, though this chapter emphasizes that clonality alone is not diagnostic of malignancy, since a subset of benign inflammatory dermatoses can show a detectable clonal or oligoclonal population, and, conversely, early or partially treated mycosis fungoides can occasionally show a polyclonal result, making integration with morphology and clinical course, rather than reliance on gene rearrangement results in isolation, the mandatory practice in every case. Immunoglobulin heavy chain gene rearrangement studies play an analogous supportive role in distinguishing primary cutaneous marginal zone or follicle center lymphoma from cutaneous pseudolymphoma, discussed in the differential diagnosis section above, again functioning as one component of an integrated diagnosis rather than a standalone determinant.

High-Throughput Sequencing for Molecular Staging and Minimal Residual Disease

High-throughput sequencing of the T-cell receptor beta or gamma gene provides substantially greater sensitivity and specificity than conventional polymerase chain reaction-based clonality assessment, allowing not only more confident identification of a dominant clone in genuinely ambiguous early-stage cases but also, when the specific clonal sequence is known, sensitive tracking of minimal residual disease in the peripheral blood, a capability this chapter notes is of particular value in Sézary syndrome and advanced mycosis fungoides, where confirming the same clone across skin and blood compartments provides definitive evidence of blood involvement, directly informing staging and reinforcing the flow cytometric findings discussed below.

Peripheral Blood Flow Cytometry for Sézary Syndrome

Peripheral blood flow cytometry in suspected Sézary syndrome assesses for an expanded population of CD4-positive T-cells with an abnormal CD4-to-CD8 ratio and loss of pan-T-cell antigens, most often CD7 or CD26, together with quantification of circulating Sézary cells, findings that, combined with the clinical triad described in the clinical presentation section above and, where available, confirmation of T-cell clonality in the peripheral blood, establish this diagnosis and additionally serve as the primary staging and treatment-response monitoring tool for this specific entity.

T-Cell Receptor Beta F1 and Epstein-Barr Virus-Encoded RNA In Situ Hybridization

As demonstrated in the worked case above, T-cell receptor beta F1 immunohistochemistry, positive in alpha-beta lineage subcutaneous panniculitis-like T-cell lymphoma and negative in the gamma-delta lineage primary cutaneous gamma-delta T-cell lymphoma, together with CD4, CD8, and CD56 immunophenotyping, resolves this chapter's most consequential panniculitic differential decisively, given the substantially more aggressive course associated with the gamma-delta phenotype. Epstein-Barr virus-encoded RNA in situ hybridization shows diffuse positivity within the neoplastic cells of extranodal NK/T-cell lymphoma, nasal type, a near-universal finding, discussed in the etiology section above, that functions as this entity's defining and essentially mandatory confirmatory ancillary study, together with a CD2, CD56, and cytotoxic marker (granzyme B, TIA-1) immunophenotype supporting natural killer or cytotoxic T-cell lineage.

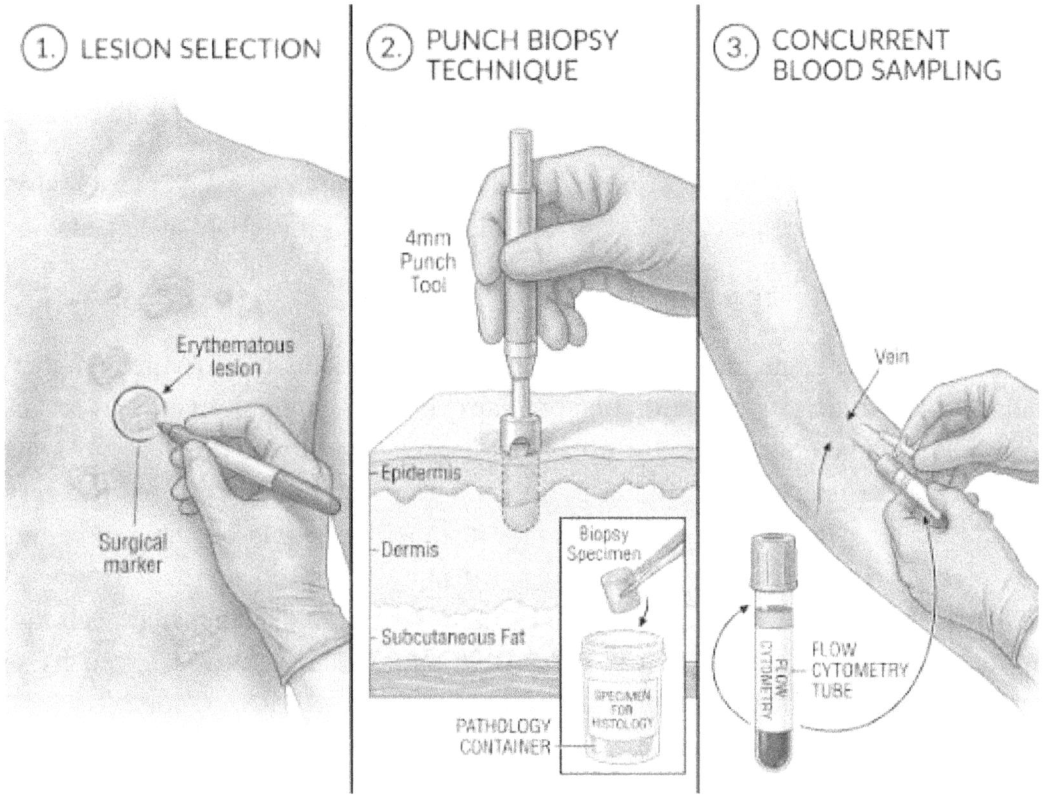

Management Implications

Staging Workup

Mycosis fungoides and Sézary syndrome are staged using the TNMB (tumor, node, metastasis, blood) system, incorporating the extent and morphology of skin involvement, lymph node status, visceral involvement, and peripheral blood involvement, a staging system this chapter notes directly governs prognosis and treatment selection, discussed further below, making complete staging evaluation, including physical examination for lymphadenopathy, appropriate imaging, and peripheral blood assessment, standard practice at diagnosis for any patient beyond limited patch-stage disease.

Clinical Stage	Skin Involvement	Approximate Prognosis
IA	Patches/plaques, less than 10% body surface area	Near-normal life expectancy
IB	Patches/plaques, 10% or more body surface area	Favorable, majority long-term survival
IIB	One or more tumors present	Intermediate, stage-dependent

III	Erythroderma, 80% or more body surface area	Variable, blood involvement worsens prognosis
IV	Nodal, visceral, or significant blood involvement	Less favorable

KEY POINT: TNMB staging in mycosis fungoides and Sézary syndrome directly determines the treatment pathway, skin-directed therapy for limited patch and plaque-stage disease against systemic therapy for tumor-stage, erythrodermic, or blood-involved disease, making accurate staging at diagnosis, rather than histologic diagnosis alone, the practical determinant of appropriate management.

Skin-Directed and Systemic Therapy

Limited patch and plaque-stage mycosis fungoides is managed with skin-directed therapy, topical corticosteroids, topical nitrogen mustard, phototherapy (narrowband ultraviolet B or psoralen plus ultraviolet A), or localized radiation therapy, given this stage's generally favorable, often chronic-indolent course. More extensive plaque-stage, tumor-stage, or erythrodermic disease, and Sézary syndrome, warrant systemic therapy, retinoids, interferon, histone deacetylase inhibitors, extracorporeal photopheresis particularly for Sézary syndrome, or, for more advanced or refractory disease, targeted monoclonal antibody therapy or systemic chemotherapy, with allogeneic stem cell transplantation reserved for selected advanced or refractory cases. Lymphomatoid papulosis, given its self-resolving natural history, is frequently managed with observation alone or low-dose methotrexate for symptomatic or frequently recurring disease, while primary cutaneous anaplastic large cell lymphoma is managed with excision or localized radiation for solitary lesions, given this entity's generally favorable prognosis discussed further below.

Management of Folliculotropic Mycosis Fungoides, Subcutaneous Panniculitis-like T-Cell Lymphoma, and Extranodal NK/T-Cell Lymphoma

Folliculotropic mycosis fungoides, given its follicular-based, deeper involvement discussed in the histopathologic features section above, is comparatively resistant to standard skin-directed therapy and frequently requires phototherapy combined with topical or systemic retinoids, localized radiation, or systemic therapy earlier in its course than classic mycosis fungoides at an equivalent clinical stage. Subcutaneous panniculitis-like T-cell lymphoma of the alpha-beta phenotype is generally managed with systemic corticosteroids or other immunosuppressive or immunomodulatory therapy given its relatively indolent course, reserving multiagent chemotherapy for refractory disease or cases complicated by hemophagocytic lymphohistiocytosis, while the gamma-delta phenotype, given its markedly more aggressive behavior, is managed with multiagent chemotherapy analogous to peripheral T-cell lymphoma from the outset. Extranodal NK/T-cell lymphoma, nasal type, is managed with combined radiation and asparaginase-based chemotherapy regimens, reflecting this tumor's relative resistance to anthracycline-based regimens used in other peripheral T-cell lymphomas, with prompt multidisciplinary oncologic referral warranted given this entity's aggressive natural history.

Documentation and Reporting Standards

The pathology report for a suspected cutaneous lymphoma should explicitly document the pattern and degree of epidermotropism or, for panniculitic and deeper processes, the pattern of subcutaneous involvement, the immunophenotype obtained, and the result and interpretation of any gene rearrangement or in situ hybridization study performed, together with an explicit statement regarding whether the histologic findings are considered diagnostic in isolation or require clinical correlation, given the genuine diagnostic difficulty of early-stage mycosis fungoides and the panniculitic lymphomas discussed throughout this chapter. For Sézary syndrome, the report should reference the peripheral blood flow cytometry findings when available, and for extranodal NK/T-cell lymphoma, the report should explicitly document the Epstein-Barr virus-encoded RNA in situ hybridization result given its near-mandatory role in this entity's diagnosis. Multidisciplinary correlation with the treating oncologist or dermatologist at the time of reporting, rather than a report issued in isolation, is good practice for any diagnosis in this chapter given the degree of clinical, laboratory, and histologic integration each requires.

Management of Cutaneous B-Cell Lymphomas

Primary cutaneous marginal zone lymphoma and primary cutaneous follicle center lymphoma, given their indolent course, are managed with localized radiation therapy or excision for solitary or limited lesions, with observation an appropriate option for asymptomatic marginal zone lymphoma, particularly where an identifiable antigenic driver can be addressed. Where Borrelia burgdorferi infection is identified or clinically suspected in an appropriately endemic geographic setting, discussed in the etiology section above, a trial of antibiotic therapy is a reasonable initial approach for localized marginal zone lymphoma before proceeding to radiation or excision, reflecting this subset's documented potential for regression with infection eradication. Primary cutaneous diffuse large B-cell lymphoma, leg type, given its more aggressive behavior, is managed with systemic rituximab-based chemoimmunotherapy analogous to nodal diffuse large B-cell lymphoma, reflecting this entity's comparatively higher risk of extracutaneous dissemination relative to the other cutaneous B-cell lymphomas discussed in this chapter. Multifocal cutaneous B-cell lymphoma of any subtype warrants staging evaluation to exclude systemic or nodal involvement before a primary cutaneous designation, and the corresponding indolent management pathway, is finalized.

Large Cell Transformation

Large cell transformation, defined as the presence of large atypical cells, generally accepted as exceeding four times the size of a small lymphocyte, comprising more than twenty-five percent of the infiltrate or forming discrete microscopic nodules, can arise in mycosis fungoides at any stage but is most frequently encountered in tumor-stage disease, discussed in the histopathologic features section above, and carries independent prognostic significance beyond clinical stage alone, generally portending a less favorable course and often prompting escalation to more aggressive systemic therapy. CD30 immunohistochemistry should be performed whenever large cell transformation is identified or suspected, since a subset of transformed mycosis fungoides expresses CD30, a finding that, while not equivalent to a diagnosis of primary cutaneous anaplastic large cell lymphoma given the pre-existing mycosis fungoides context, can carry therapeutic relevance given the availability of CD30-targeted therapy for appropriately selected patients.

Complications and Prognosis

Prognosis in mycosis fungoides correlates directly with clinical stage at diagnosis, patch and plaque-stage disease confined to the skin carrying a favorable, near-normal life expectancy in many patients, while tumor-stage disease, particularly with large cell transformation discussed in the histopathologic features and complications sections above, and disease with nodal or visceral involvement, carries a substantially less favorable prognosis, underscoring why the staging evaluation discussed above, rather than histologic subtype alone, is the practical determinant of prognostic counseling for an individual patient. Sézary syndrome carries a less favorable prognosis than early-stage mycosis fungoides given its inherently more advanced, leukemic presentation. Lymphomatoid papulosis and primary cutaneous anaplastic large cell lymphoma both carry excellent long-term prognosis despite their sometimes locally destructive or recurrent course, though patients with lymphomatoid papulosis carry a small but well-documented increased lifetime risk of developing a second lymphoma, most often mycosis fungoides or systemic anaplastic large cell lymphoma, warranting longitudinal dermatologic surveillance. Primary cutaneous diffuse large B-cell lymphoma, leg type, carries a less favorable prognosis than the indolent cutaneous B-cell lymphomas, reflecting its greater propensity for extracutaneous spread. Folliculotropic mycosis fungoides carries a less favorable prognosis than classic mycosis fungoides at an equivalent clinical stage, reflecting its deeper, treatment-resistant follicular involvement, while subcutaneous panniculitis-like T-cell lymphoma of the alpha-beta phenotype carries a generally favorable prognosis except when complicated by hemophagocytic lymphohistiocytosis, a complication that meaningfully worsens outcome, in contrast to the gamma-delta phenotype, which carries a poor prognosis regardless. Extranodal NK/T-cell lymphoma, nasal type, carries a variable but generally guarded prognosis correlating with disease extent and response to the combined radiation and chemotherapy approach discussed above.

Special Populations

Mycosis fungoides in patients with darker skin phototypes can present with hypopigmented, rather than the classically described erythematous to violaceous, patches, a presentation this chapter emphasizes is disproportionately encountered in children and young adults and can be mistaken for a benign hypopigmented dermatosis without a sufficiently high index of suspicion, making biopsy of a persistent, treatment-resistant hypopigmented patch an appropriately liberal practice in this population. Multiple lesions of lymphomatoid papulosis in a child should prompt the same diagnostic consideration and monitoring approach applied in adults, this entity's favorable natural history holding across age groups. Immunosuppressed and solid organ transplant recipients warrant a lower threshold for biopsy and ancillary clonality testing of a persistent or atypical dermatosis given both a documented elevated risk of cutaneous lymphoproliferative disease in this population and the potential for iatrogenic immunosuppression to mask or alter the typical clinical appearance of an underlying lymphoma, a special-population consideration this chapter notes parallels the elevated skin cancer risk discussed for this same population in Chapter 15.

Patient Education and Counseling

Patients diagnosed with early-stage mycosis fungoides benefit from clear counseling regarding this disease's characteristically chronic, often indolent course and the corresponding expectation of skin-directed rather than systemic therapy, framed around long-term disease control rather than cure, while patients diagnosed with lymphomatoid papulosis benefit from counseling regarding this entity's expected waxing and waning course and the small but genuine long-term risk of a second lymphoma warranting continued surveillance. Patients with Sézary syndrome or advanced-stage mycosis fungoides benefit from counseling regarding the systemic nature of the treatment pathway ahead and realistic expectations regarding disease control given this stage's less favorable natural history. Patients diagnosed with subcutaneous panniculitis-like T-cell lymphoma of the alpha-beta phenotype benefit from reassurance regarding the generally favorable prognosis associated with this diagnosis, tempered by clear counseling regarding the warning signs of hemophagocytic lymphohistiocytosis, persistent fever, worsening cytopenias, and fatigue, that should prompt urgent reevaluation, while patients diagnosed with extranodal NK/T-cell lymphoma benefit from early, direct counseling regarding the combined-modality treatment pathway and the importance of prompt initiation of therapy given this entity's aggressive natural history. Across all cutaneous lymphoma diagnoses, patients benefit from an explicit explanation of why the diagnosis required correlation of histology, immunophenotype, and molecular clonality studies rather than histology in isolation, a point of genuine diagnostic nuance this chapter has emphasized throughout and one that helps patients understand both the diagnostic process and the rationale for any repeat biopsies performed along the way.

THE REACTION PATTERN RECOGNITION SYSTEM — The Cutaneous Lymphoma Clonality and Stage Pattern Family

The Pattern: Cutaneous lymphoproliferative disorders organized first by T-cell versus B-cell lineage, then by epidermotropism, cytologic atypia, and depth, with clinical stage and course determining prognosis and management within each lineage.

Histologic Signature: Disproportionate epidermotropism with Pautrier microabscesses defines mycosis fungoides; sheets of CD30-positive anaplastic cells with hallmark nuclei define the CD30-positive lymphoproliferative disorder spectrum; nodular marginal zone or follicle center proliferations define indolent cutaneous B-cell lymphoma.

The Decision: Determine lineage, then assess epidermotropism, atypia, and architecture, escalating to T-cell receptor or immunoglobulin heavy chain gene rearrangement studies and, for suspected Sézary syndrome, peripheral blood flow cytometry, whenever morphology and immunophenotype alone leave genuine uncertainty.

Trap Logic: Patch-stage mycosis fungoides mimics benign inflammatory dermatoses; lymphomatoid papulosis mimics primary cutaneous and systemic anaplastic large cell lymphoma; cutaneous pseudolymphoma mimics marginal zone lymphoma.

Pattern Anchor: Lineage first, then epidermotropism, atypia, and depth. Clonality studies support but never independently establish a lymphoma diagnosis; integration with morphology and clinical course is mandatory in every case.

Summary and Key Concepts

Primary cutaneous lymphomas are classified by T-cell versus B-cell lineage, with mycosis fungoides the most common overall subtype and the CD30-positive lymphoproliferative disorder spectrum, lymphomatoid papulosis and primary cutaneous anaplastic large cell lymphoma, forming a distinct clinicopathologic continuum.

Mycosis fungoides is distinguished from benign inflammatory dermatoses by disproportionate epidermotropism, cerebriform nuclear atypia, and Pautrier microabscess formation, with T-cell receptor gene rearrangement studies supporting, but never independently establishing, the diagnosis.

Sézary syndrome is defined by the triad of erythroderma, lymphadenopathy, and circulating clonal Sézary cells confirmed by peripheral blood flow cytometry.

Lymphomatoid papulosis shows a characteristic waxing and waning natural history distinguishing it clinically from primary cutaneous anaplastic large cell lymphoma, with ALK immunohistochemistry excluding systemic anaplastic large cell lymphoma when the differential arises.

Cutaneous B-cell lymphomas range from indolent marginal zone and follicle center lymphoma to the more aggressive diffuse large B-cell lymphoma, leg type, with cutaneous pseudolymphoma remaining an important reactive mimicker throughout this differential.

CHAPTER 19: GENODERMATOSES, PEDIATRIC, AND METABOLIC/DEPOSITION DISORDERS OF THE SKIN

Learning Objectives

1. Classify the major subtypes of epidermolysis bullosa by the level of the dermoepidermal junction at which blistering occurs and the corresponding defective structural protein.
2. Distinguish ichthyosis vulgaris, X-linked ichthyosis, and epidermolytic ichthyosis by their underlying genetic defect, histopathology, and clinical presentation.
3. Recognize the histopathologic and clinical features of cutaneous mastocytosis and apply Darier's sign appropriately in clinical evaluation.
4. Distinguish primary cutaneous amyloidosis from systemic amyloidosis with cutaneous involvement, and explain why this distinction carries major clinical consequence.
5. Identify the histopathologic features of scleromyxedema and lichen myxedematosus and their associated paraproteinemia.
6. Apply immunofluorescence antigen mapping and electron microscopy appropriately in the diagnostic workup of epidermolysis bullosa.

Definition and Classification

Genodermatoses and Metabolic/Deposition Disorders as a Shared Framework

The entities addressed in this chapter span a wide range of inheritance patterns, ages of onset, and clinical stakes, from the entirely benign and self-limited to the potentially life-threatening, a genuine heterogeneity that this chapter organizes not by clinical severity but by the shared diagnostic logic, defective protein or deposited substance combined with its precise anatomic level, developed throughout below. This chapter addresses two related but distinct categories of skin disease: genodermatoses, inherited disorders arising from a defined single-gene defect affecting a specific structural or functional skin protein, and metabolic and deposition disorders, conditions defined by the abnormal accumulation of an endogenous substance, amyloid, mucin, or lipid, within the skin, whether as a primary cutaneous process or as a cutaneous manifestation of systemic disease. Despite their distinct etiologies, both categories share a common diagnostic architecture that organizes this chapter throughout: identify the specific defective protein or deposited substance first, then localize its level within the skin, epidermal, junctional, or dermal, to arrive at a precise diagnosis, a framework directly analogous to this book's approach to the immunobullous and mesenchymal chapters.

Level of the Dermoepidermal Junction as the Organizing Principle for Epidermolysis Bullosa

Epidermolysis bullosa, the genodermatosis this chapter develops in greatest depth given its diagnostic complexity and clinical consequence, is classified into four major types based on the precise ultrastructural level at which blistering occurs: epidermolysis bullosa simplex, intraepidermal, at the level of the basal keratinocyte; junctional epidermolysis bullosa, within the lamina lucida; dystrophic epidermolysis bullosa, below the lamina densa; and the more recently characterized Kindler epidermolysis bullosa, showing blistering at mixed and multiple levels, a level-based classification that directly determines both the specific defective protein involved and the disease's overall severity and prognosis.

Entity	Defective Protein/Gene	Level of Blistering	Severity
Epidermolysis bullosa simplex	Keratin 5/14	Intraepidermal (basal keratinocyte)	Generally mild
Junctional epidermolysis bullosa	Laminin 332, collagen XVII	Lamina lucida	Variable, severe in generalized subtype
Dystrophic epidermolysis bullosa	Collagen VII (COL7A1)	Sub-lamina densa	Variable, severe in recessive subtype
Ichthyosis vulgaris	Filaggrin (FLG)	Stratum corneum/granulosum	Mild
X-linked ichthyosis	Steroid sulfatase (STS)	Stratum corneum	Mild-moderate
Epidermolytic ichthyosis	Keratin 1/10	Stratum spinosum/granulosum	Moderate-severe
Cutaneous mastocytosis	KIT (somatic, lesional)	Dermis	Variable
Primary cutaneous amyloidosis	N/A (keratin-derived amyloid)	Papillary dermis	Benign, localized
Systemic (AL) amyloidosis	Immunoglobulin light chain	Dermis, vessel walls	Life-threatening if untreated
Scleromyxedema	N/A (paraprotein-associated)	Reticular dermis	Chronic, systemic associations
Neurofibromatosis type 1	NF1	Dermis (neurofibroma), melanocyte (café-au-lait macule)	Variable, tumor predisposition
Tuberous sclerosis complex	TSC1/TSC2	Dermis, adnexal structures	Variable, multi-organ hamartomas

Incontinentia pigmenti	IKBKG/NEMO	Epidermis, dermis (stage-dependent)	X-linked, variable extracutaneous
Juvenile xanthogranuloma	N/A (reactive histiocytic)	Dermis	Benign, self-limited
Xanthoma	N/A (lipid-driven)	Dermis	Benign, marker of lipid disorder
Porphyria cutanea tarda	Uroporphyrinogen decarboxylase (UROD)	Subepidermal, dermal vessel walls	Chronic, photosensitive
Calcinosis cutis	N/A (dystrophic/metastatic/idiopathic)	Dermis/subcutis	Variable, underlying-cause dependent

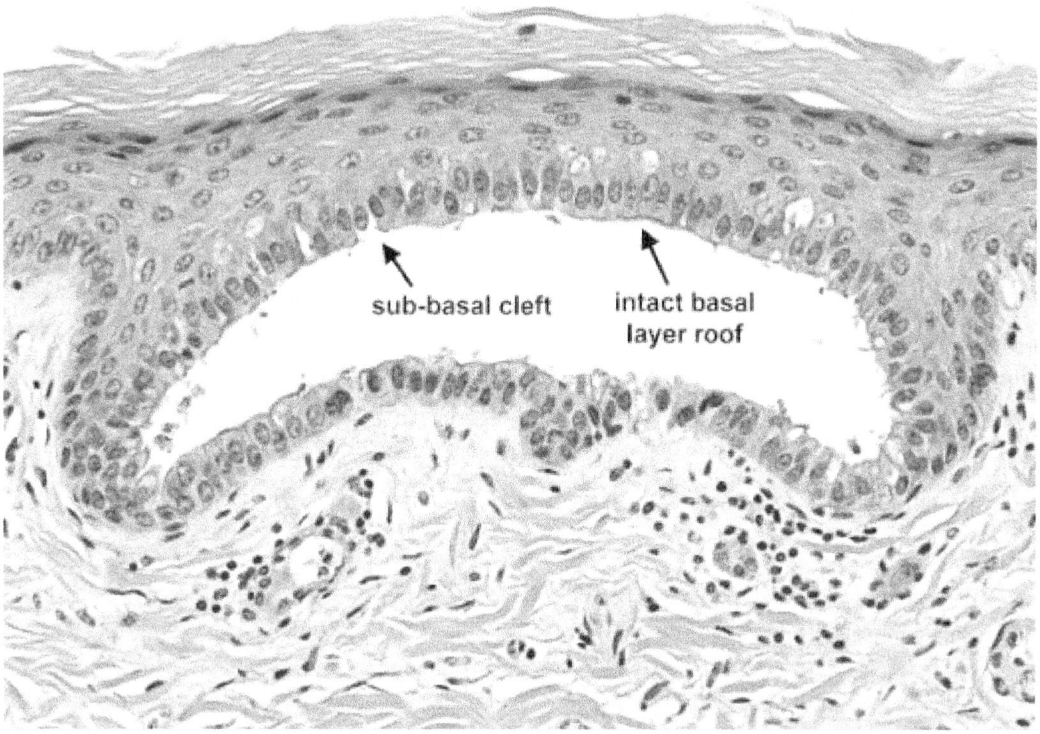

Etiology and Pathogenesis

Keratin, Laminin, and Collagen VII Mutations in Epidermolysis Bullosa

Epidermolysis bullosa simplex arises from mutations in the keratin 5 or keratin 14 genes, encoding the intermediate filament proteins that provide basal keratinocytes with their mechanical resilience, such that even minor mechanical trauma produces cytolysis and intraepidermal blister formation. Junctional epidermolysis bullosa arises from mutations in genes encoding laminin 332 or, in a milder subtype, collagen XVII, both components of the hemidesmosomal-anchoring filament complex that adheres the basal keratinocyte to the underlying basement membrane, with severe generalized junctional epidermolysis bullosa, historically termed the Herlitz subtype, arising from complete absence of functional laminin 332 and carrying a substantially worse prognosis than the milder, non-Herlitz subtypes. Dystrophic epidermolysis bullosa arises from mutations in COL7A1, encoding type VII collagen, the principal structural component of the anchoring fibrils that secure the basement membrane to the underlying papillary dermis, with both dominant and recessive inheritance patterns recognized, recessive dystrophic epidermolysis bullosa generally producing more severe, mutilating scarring given more complete loss of functional collagen VII.

Filaggrin, Steroid Sulfatase, and Keratin Mutations in Ichthyosis

Ichthyosis vulgaris, the most common inherited ichthyosis, arises from loss-of-function mutations in the filaggrin gene, encoding a protein essential to terminal keratinocyte differentiation and stratum corneum barrier formation, with heterozygous carriers showing a milder phenotype than homozygous or compound heterozygous individuals, a dose-dependent genotype-phenotype relationship this chapter notes is additionally relevant given filaggrin mutations' well-established association with atopic dermatitis risk, discussed elsewhere in this book. X-linked ichthyosis arises from deletion or mutation of the steroid sulfatase gene on the X chromosome, resulting in accumulation of cholesterol sulfate within the stratum corneum that impairs normal corneocyte desquamation, an X-linked recessive inheritance pattern that, unlike ichthyosis vulgaris, essentially exclusively affects males. Epidermolytic ichthyosis arises from mutations in keratin 1 or keratin 10, producing structural fragility within the suprabasal epidermis that manifests as both the erosive, blistering neonatal presentation and the progressive hyperkeratosis that characterizes this disorder's later clinical course, developed further below.

KIT Mutations in Mastocytosis

Cutaneous mastocytosis arises from activating mutations in the KIT gene, encoding the stem cell factor receptor that drives mast cell proliferation and survival, with the specific D816V mutation most commonly identified in adult-onset and systemic disease, while pediatric-onset mastocytosis, generally confined to the skin and often showing spontaneous regression around puberty, less consistently harbors this specific mutation, a childhood-versus-adult distinction this chapter emphasizes carries direct prognostic and management relevance discussed further in the management implications section below.

Immunoglobulin Light Chain Deposition and Paraproteinemia in Deposition Disorders

Systemic AL amyloidosis arises from clonal plasma cell production of an amyloidogenic immunoglobulin light chain that misfolds into insoluble beta-pleated sheet fibrils deposited within the skin and multiple visceral organs, in contrast to primary cutaneous amyloidosis, which arises instead from degenerated keratin filaments released by apoptotic keratinocytes that aggregate locally within the papillary dermis without any underlying plasma cell dyscrasia, a fundamentally different pathogenesis this chapter emphasizes as the biological basis for these two entities' dramatically different prognoses despite a superficially similar histologic appearance of dermal amyloid deposition, developed further in the differential diagnosis section below. Scleromyxedema is associated in the great majority of cases with an underlying monoclonal gammopathy, most often IgG-lambda, though the precise mechanism by which the paraprotein drives the characteristic dermal mucin deposition and fibroblast proliferation described in the histopathologic features section below remains incompletely understood.

NF1 and TSC1/TSC2 Mutations in Neurofibromatosis Type 1 and Tuberous Sclerosis Complex

Neurofibromatosis type 1, whose plexiform and dermal neurofibroma manifestations were introduced in Chapter 17, arises from germline mutations in the NF1 tumor suppressor gene, encoding neurofibromin, a negative regulator of RAS signaling, such that loss of functional neurofibromin drives unchecked proliferative signaling within Schwann cells and, distinctly, within epidermal melanocytes, producing this disorder's characteristic café-au-lait macules developed further in the histopathologic features section below. Tuberous sclerosis complex arises from germline mutations in TSC1 or TSC2, encoding hamartin and tuberin respectively, both components of a complex that normally inhibits mTOR signaling, such that loss of function drives constitutive mTOR pathway activation and the multi-organ hamartomatous growths, angiofibroma, shagreen patch, and ash-leaf macule among the cutaneous manifestations developed further below, that define this disorder.

IKBKG/NEMO Mutations in Incontinentia Pigmenti

Incontinentia pigmenti arises from mutations in IKBKG (NEMO), an X-linked gene encoding a regulatory component of the nuclear factor kappa B signaling pathway essential for cellular protection against tumor necrosis factor-alpha-induced apoptosis; because this X-linked pattern is generally lethal in hemizygous males, incontinentia pigmenti overwhelmingly affects females, surviving male cases generally reflecting either a postzygotic somatic mutation or an associated Klinefelter karyotype, a genetic mechanism this chapter notes directly explains this disorder's characteristic X-linked, female-predominant inheritance pattern.

Lipid Metabolism, Porphyrin Metabolism, and Calcium Deposition in Metabolic Disorders

Xanthomas arise from dermal deposition of lipid-laden macrophages (foam cells) driven by an underlying disturbance in lipid metabolism, whether a primary genetic dyslipidemia, familial hypercholesterolemia foremost among them, or a secondary cause including diabetes mellitus, nephrotic syndrome, or cholestatic liver disease, with the specific xanthoma subtype, developed further in the clinical presentation section below, often providing a useful clue to the underlying lipid abnormality. Porphyria cutanea tarda, the most common porphyria overall, arises from acquired or, less commonly, inherited deficiency of uroporphyrinogen decarboxylase, an enzyme in the heme biosynthetic pathway, resulting in accumulation of photoreactive porphyrin intermediates that, upon ultraviolet light exposure, generate reactive oxygen species producing the characteristic photodistributed blistering and skin fragility developed below; hepatitis C infection, excess alcohol use, estrogen therapy, and hepatic iron overload are recognized and clinically important precipitating or exacerbating factors. Calcinosis cutis arises through three distinct mechanisms: dystrophic calcification, deposition within previously damaged or inflamed tissue with normal serum calcium and phosphate, the most common mechanism and one frequently encountered in the connective tissue disease chapter's dermatomyositis and systemic sclerosis discussions elsewhere in this book; metastatic calcification, deposition driven by abnormal serum calcium or phosphate homeostasis, as in chronic kidney disease; and idiopathic calcification, arising without an identifiable underlying tissue damage or metabolic derangement.

THE REACTION PATTERN RECOGNITION SYSTEM — Protein Defect and Level of Involvement as the Universal Genodermatosis and Deposition Disorder Anchor

The Pattern: Defective Structural Protein or Deposited Substance Combined with Its Precise Anatomic Level as the Framework for Classifying Every Genodermatosis and Deposition Disorder in This Chapter

Histologic Signature: Intraepidermal cleft signals epidermolysis bullosa simplex; sub-basal cleft with intact basal roof signals junctional epidermolysis bullosa; sub-lamina densa cleft signals dystrophic epidermolysis bullosa; dermal mast cell infiltrate signals mastocytosis; Congo red-positive, apple-green birefringent papillary dermal deposits signal amyloidosis; and diffuse dermal mucin with fibroblast proliferation signals scleromyxedema.

The Decision: Identify the level of involvement or the deposited substance first, then apply the specific ancillary study, immunofluorescence antigen mapping or electron microscopy for epidermolysis bullosa, Congo red polarization for amyloid, or serum protein electrophoresis for suspected paraproteinemia, required to reach a definitive, prognostically accurate diagnosis.

Trap Logic: The distinct epidermolysis bullosa subtypes can appear similar on routine hematoxylin and eosin staining alone without antigen mapping; primary cutaneous and systemic amyloidosis show histologically similar dermal deposits despite dramatically different prognosis; and scleromyxedema can be mistaken for scleroderma or scleredema given overlapping sclerodermoid clinical features.

Pattern Anchor: Level of involvement or deposited substance first, then the specific confirmatory ancillary study. Primary cutaneous and systemic amyloidosis are never distinguished by dermal histology alone; systemic workup is mandatory whenever this distinction is clinically uncertain.

Histopathologic Features and Diagnostic Criteria

Histopathology of Epidermolysis Bullosa Subtypes

Epidermolysis bullosa simplex shows an intraepidermal blister cavity forming within or immediately above the basal keratinocyte layer, with cytolysis of basal keratinocytes evident at the blister base, a level of cleavage that, while suggestive, is not by itself sufficient to confirm this specific subtype without the ancillary confirmation discussed below given overlapping low-power appearance with other superficial blistering processes. Junctional epidermolysis bullosa shows a clean, sub-basal cleft with an intact, non-cytolyzed basal keratinocyte layer forming the roof of the blister cavity, a comparatively bland, minimally inflammatory blister that this chapter notes can be a useful low-power distinguishing clue from the more inflammatory blisters typical of the immunobullous disorders. Dystrophic epidermolysis bullosa shows a sub-lamina densa cleft, similarly bland and minimally inflammatory on routine hematoxylin and eosin staining, such that all three major epidermolysis bullosa subtypes, despite their genuinely distinct levels of involvement, can appear deceptively similar without the ancillary confirmation developed in the ancillary studies section below.

Histopathology of Ichthyosis

Ichthyosis vulgaris shows compact orthokeratotic hyperkeratosis with a diminished or absent granular layer, a specific and useful histologic clue given that most other ichthyoses and simple xerosis show a normal or thickened granular layer, reflecting filaggrin's specific role in granular layer keratohyalin granule formation. X-linked ichthyosis shows compact orthokeratotic hyperkeratosis with a normal or mildly thickened granular layer, distinguishing it from ichthyosis vulgaris on this specific feature. Epidermolytic ichthyosis shows the distinctive histologic finding of epidermolytic hyperkeratosis, perinuclear vacuolization of keratinocytes within the upper spinous and granular layers together with coarse, irregular keratohyalin granules and compact hyperkeratosis, a specific and diagnostic pattern that this chapter notes can also be encountered as an incidental finding within an otherwise unrelated lesion, discussed further in the differential diagnosis section below.

Histopathology of Mastocytosis

Cutaneous mastocytosis shows an increased number of mast cells within the papillary and superficial reticular dermis, ranging from a subtle perivascular increase in adult-onset maculopapular cutaneous mastocytosis to a dense, monomorphic dermal infiltrate in solitary mastocytoma, mast cells identifiable on routine hematoxylin and eosin staining by their round-to-oval nuclei and finely granular cytoplasm but more reliably and sensitively highlighted by the special stains and immunohistochemistry discussed in the ancillary studies section below given how subtle the infiltrate can be in adult-onset disease.

Histopathology of NF1 Café-Au-Lait Macules and Incontinentia Pigmenti

The café-au-lait macule of neurofibromatosis type 1 shows increased melanin within basal keratinocytes without an increase in melanocyte number, together with characteristic giant melanosomes visible ultrastructurally, a subtle histologic finding that this chapter notes is rarely biopsied in practice given the diagnosis's overwhelmingly clinical basis, discussed further in the clinical presentation section below. Incontinentia pigmenti shows a distinct histologic appearance at each of its four clinical stages: the vesicular stage shows eosinophilic spongiosis with intraepidermal vesicles containing numerous eosinophils; the verrucous stage shows epidermal hyperplasia with dyskeratosis; the hyperpigmented stage shows pigment incontinence, melanin-laden macrophages within the papillary dermis, without a significant overlying inflammatory infiltrate; and the atrophic/hypopigmented stage shows epidermal thinning with diminished adnexal structures, a stage-dependent histologic progression that, discussed further in the clinical presentation section below, mirrors this disorder's characteristic evolving clinical appearance over infancy and childhood.

Histopathology of Juvenile Xanthogranuloma, Xanthoma, Porphyria Cutanea Tarda, and Calcinosis Cutis

Juvenile xanthogranuloma shows a dense dermal infiltrate of foamy histiocytes admixed with characteristic Touton giant cells, multinucleated giant cells with a wreath-like ring of nuclei surrounding a central, non-foamy eosinophilic zone and a peripheral foamy cytoplasmic rim, a specific and diagnostic morphology this chapter emphasizes as the single most useful low-power clue to this diagnosis. Xanthoma shows sheets of lipid-laden foamy histiocytes within the dermis, generally without the Touton giant cells or admixed inflammatory cells characteristic of juvenile xanthogranuloma, a comparatively monotonous foam cell population that, developed further in the differential diagnosis section below, is the principal histologic feature distinguishing these two foam cell-rich entities. Porphyria cutanea tarda shows a subepidermal blister with minimal inflammatory infiltrate and characteristic festooning of the dermal papillae protruding upward into the blister cavity, together with thickened, hyalinized ("caterpillar body"-containing) superficial dermal vessel walls reflecting periodic acid-Schiff-positive basement membrane reduplication, findings that, combined with the clinical photodistribution and precipitating factors discussed above, anchor this diagnosis. Calcinosis cutis shows deposits of basophilic, granular calcium salts within the dermis or subcutis, at times provoking a surrounding foreign body giant cell reaction, with the precise clinical and histologic context, discussed in the etiology section above, determining whether the underlying mechanism is dystrophic, metastatic, or idiopathic.

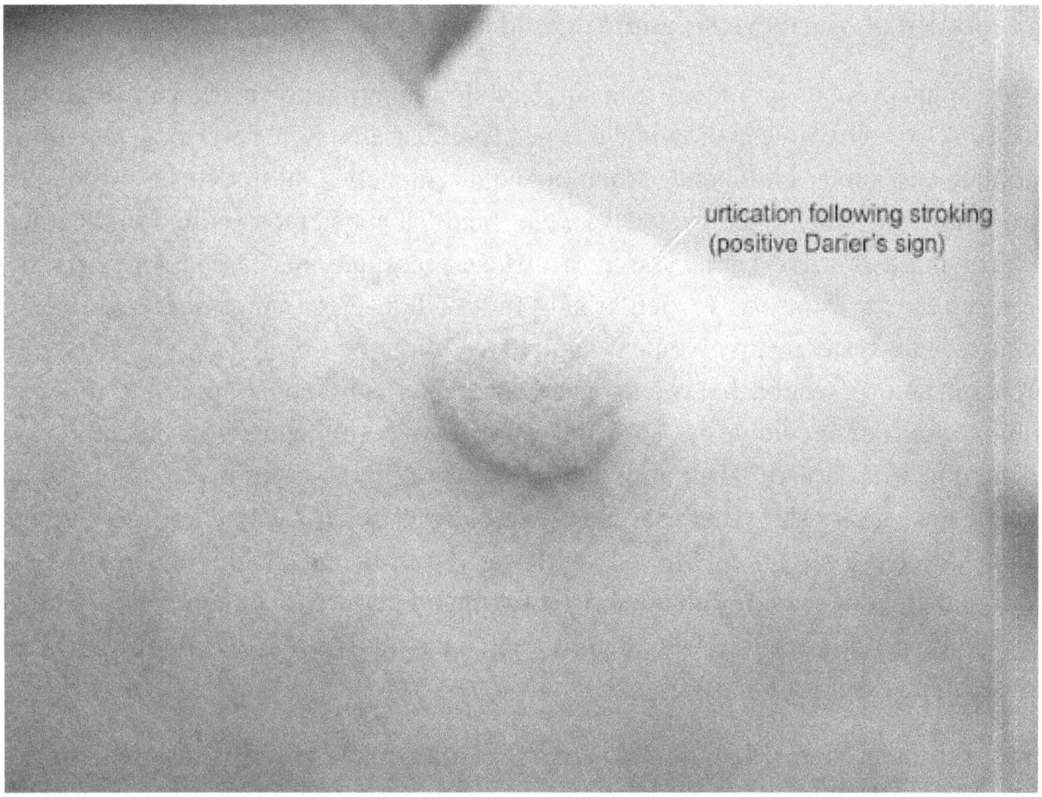

Clinical Presentation and Clinicopathologic Correlation

Clinical Presentation of Epidermolysis Bullosa and Ichthyosis

Epidermolysis bullosa simplex presents in the localized (Weber-Cockayne) subtype with blistering confined to the palms and soles, precipitated by friction and heat, generally sparing internal mucosa and healing without significant scarring, while the generalized subtypes show more widespread blistering from birth or early infancy. Junctional and dystrophic epidermolysis bullosa present with more widespread blistering evident from birth, frequently involving oral and other mucosal surfaces, with severe generalized junctional epidermolysis bullosa carrying a poor early infancy prognosis and recessive dystrophic epidermolysis bullosa producing progressive scarring, milia formation, and characteristic digital fusion (pseudosyndactyly, "mitten deformity") over the course of childhood. Ichthyosis vulgaris presents as fine, white to gray scale concentrated on the extensor extremities with characteristic sparing of the flexural creases, generally appearing in early childhood and improving somewhat with age and in warmer, more humid climates, while X-linked ichthyosis presents with larger, darker, adherent scale, notably involving the flexural creases that ichthyosis vulgaris characteristically spares, a distinguishing clinical distribution this chapter emphasizes as a useful bedside distinguishing feature. Epidermolytic ichthyosis presents at birth with widespread erythema and superficial blistering, evolving over infancy and childhood into the characteristic thick, verrucous, dark hyperkeratosis with an increased risk of superimposed bacterial infection given the underlying epidermal barrier defect.

Clinical Presentation of Mastocytosis and Amyloidosis

Solitary mastocytoma presents in infancy as a single yellow-tan to reddish-brown plaque or nodule, most often on the trunk or extremities, showing the positive Darier's sign described above, and generally resolving spontaneously over childhood. Maculopapular cutaneous mastocytosis (urticaria pigmentosa) presents with numerous small, red-brown macules and papules, most common on the trunk, each individually showing a positive Darier's sign, a diffuse presentation this chapter notes should prompt evaluation for systemic mastocytosis when arising in an adult, given adult-onset disease's substantially higher association with systemic involvement relative to childhood-onset disease, discussed further in the management implications section below. Primary cutaneous amyloidosis presents in its two principal clinical variants, macular amyloidosis, showing rippled, hyperpigmented macules and patches, most common on the upper back, and lichen amyloidosis, showing intensely pruritic, hyperkeratotic papules, most common on the anterior shins, both variants classically associated with chronic friction or scratching. Systemic AL amyloidosis presents cutaneously with waxy, translucent papules and plaques, most common periorbitally, together with the highly characteristic finding of periorbital or generalized purpura occurring spontaneously or after minor trauma ("pinch purpura"), a distinctive vascular fragility reflecting amyloid infiltration of dermal vessel walls.

Clinical Presentation of Neurofibromatosis Type 1, Tuberous Sclerosis Complex, and Incontinentia Pigmenti

Neurofibromatosis type 1 presents cutaneously with multiple café-au-lait macules, well-demarcated, uniformly tan-brown patches, together with axillary or inguinal freckling (Crowe's sign) and, as developed in Chapter 17, cutaneous and plexiform neurofibromas, with the diagnosis established clinically using a defined set of criteria incorporating the number and size of café-au-lait macules, presence of neurofibromas, and other systemic features including Lisch nodules and optic pathway glioma. Tuberous sclerosis complex presents with a characteristic cutaneous stigmata triad, facial angiofibromas (previously termed adenoma sebaceum), most often distributed symmetrically across the nasolabial folds, cheeks, and chin; the shagreen patch, a skin-colored to yellow-brown, cobblestoned, connective tissue nevus-type plaque most common on the lower back; and ash-leaf macules, hypopigmented, often oval or lance-shaped macules present from infancy and best visualized with Wood's lamp examination, together with periungual fibromas (Koenen tumors) that typically appear later in childhood or adolescence. Incontinentia pigmenti presents with a characteristic sequence of four overlapping clinical stages evolving over infancy and childhood: a vesicular/bullous stage present at or shortly after birth, following Blaschko's lines; a verrucous stage with linear, warty papules and plaques; a hyperpigmented, swirling, "marble cake"-patterned stage that is often the most clinically recognized; and a final atrophic, hypopigmented, linear streak stage that can persist into adulthood, with associated extracutaneous findings, dental, ophthalmologic, and neurologic, warranting multidisciplinary evaluation.

Clinical Presentation of Juvenile Xanthogranuloma, Xanthoma, Porphyria Cutanea Tarda, and Calcinosis Cutis

Juvenile xanthogranuloma presents in infancy as a solitary, or occasionally multiple, firm, yellow-orange papule or nodule, most common on the head, neck, or upper trunk, generally regressing spontaneously over several years. Xanthoma presents in several clinically distinct patterns correlating with the underlying lipid disturbance: xanthelasma, soft yellow plaques on the eyelids; tendinous xanthoma, firm nodules overlying tendons, particularly the Achilles tendon, associated with familial hypercholesterolemia; and eruptive xanthoma, a sudden crop of small, yellow-red papules, most common on the buttocks and extensor extremities, associated with marked hypertriglyceridemia and, distinctively, capable of resolving rapidly once the underlying triglyceride level is controlled. Porphyria cutanea tarda presents with photodistributed skin fragility, tense blisters, and erosions on sun-exposed skin, particularly the dorsal hands, together with milia formation during healing, hypertrichosis of the malar and temporal regions, and, in longstanding disease, sclerodermoid skin changes, a combination of fragility, blistering, and hypertrichosis this chapter notes is a distinctive presentation that should immediately raise suspicion for this diagnosis. Calcinosis cutis presents as firm, whitish-yellow papules, nodules, or plaques that can extrude a chalky white material when superficial or ulcerated, with the clinical distribution and associated findings, digital tip involvement in systemic sclerosis-associated dystrophic calcinosis, for example, often reflecting the specific underlying cause.

CLINICAL PEARL: Darier's sign, urtication of a mastocytosis lesion following gentle stroking, is a simple, specific bedside maneuver that reliably supports a clinical diagnosis of mastocytosis, while periorbital purpura following minor trauma ("pinch purpura") is a highly specific clinical clue to underlying systemic AL amyloidosis that should never be dismissed as ordinary bruising in an older patient. Flexural involvement is the single most useful bedside clue distinguishing X-linked ichthyosis from ichthyosis vulgaris, which characteristically spares these same sites.

Differential Diagnosis and Histologic Mimickers

Distinguishing the Epidermolysis Bullosa Subtypes From One Another

As introduced in the histopathologic features section above, the three major epidermolysis bullosa subtypes cannot be reliably distinguished by routine hematoxylin and eosin staining alone given their shared bland, minimally inflammatory blistering, making immunofluorescence antigen mapping, discussed in the ancillary studies section below, the essential diagnostic study for any suspected case, particularly given the substantially different prognostic and genetic counseling implications that follow an accurate subtype diagnosis; misclassifying severe generalized junctional epidermolysis bullosa as a milder subtype, for example, carries genuinely serious clinical consequence for both the affected infant's management and the family's genetic counseling.

Primary Cutaneous Amyloidosis Versus Systemic AL Amyloidosis

As introduced in the etiology section above, primary cutaneous amyloidosis and systemic AL amyloidosis both show Congo red-positive, apple-green birefringent deposits within the papillary dermis on polarized microscopy, a shared histologic finding that this chapter emphasizes must never be used alone to establish or exclude systemic disease, given that the fundamental distinction rests on distribution and clinical context rather than histology: primary cutaneous amyloidosis shows deposits confined to the papillary dermis in a patient without evidence of a plasma cell dyscrasia or systemic organ involvement, while systemic AL amyloidosis shows deposits additionally within vessel walls and, on systemic biopsy or imaging, other organs, confirmed by immunohistochemistry or mass spectrometry-based proteomic typing identifying immunoglobulin light chain as the amyloid subtype, discussed further in the ancillary studies section below, together with serum and urine protein electrophoresis and free light chain assay to identify the underlying plasma cell dyscrasia.

A 58-year-old patient presents with new-onset periorbital purpura following minor rubbing of the eyes, together with several weeks of fatigue and mild peripheral edema. Pattern assignment identifies eosinophilic, amorphous material within the papillary dermis and around dermal vessel walls, confirmed as amyloid by apple-green birefringence on Congo red staining under polarized light, with vessel wall involvement noted specifically given its atypical extent for an isolated primary cutaneous process. Differential narrowing weighs primary cutaneous amyloidosis against systemic AL amyloidosis given the vessel wall involvement, purpura, and systemic symptoms, and immunohistochemical typing for kappa and lambda light chain, together with serum and urine protein electrophoresis and free light chain assay, are pursued: the deposits show lambda light chain restriction, and serum free light chain assay confirms a markedly elevated lambda-to-kappa ratio. Given the vessel wall involvement, lambda light chain-restricted deposits, and confirmed serum paraproteinemia, a diagnosis of systemic AL amyloidosis is rendered, with the report explicitly flagging the finding for urgent hematology-oncology referral given this diagnosis's potential for life-threatening cardiac and renal involvement if untreated.

Scleromyxedema Versus Scleroderma and Scleredema

Scleromyxedema's sclerodermoid clinical appearance, waxy, indurated papules and plaques producing restricted mobility, can raise clinical concern for systemic sclerosis or scleredema, a differential resolved histologically by scleromyxedema's characteristic combination of diffuse dermal mucin deposition, fibroblast proliferation, and fibrosis, against systemic sclerosis's dermal sclerosis without significant mucin deposition and scleredema's mucin deposition without the fibroblast proliferation and papular clinical morphology of scleromyxedema, together with the serum protein electrophoresis findings discussed in the etiology section above that support scleromyxedema specifically given its strong paraproteinemia association.

Juvenile Xanthogranuloma Versus Xanthoma and Mastocytoma

As introduced in the histopathologic features section above, juvenile xanthogranuloma is distinguished from xanthoma primarily by the presence of Touton giant cells, absent in typical xanthoma, together with clinical context, juvenile xanthogranuloma presenting in infancy without an underlying lipid disturbance against xanthoma's association with a definable dyslipidemia and, generally, a later age of presentation. Juvenile xanthogranuloma's solitary, yellow-orange nodular clinical appearance can also raise consideration of solitary mastocytoma, discussed in the clinical presentation section above, a differential resolved by Darier's sign, positive in mastocytoma and absent in juvenile xanthogranuloma, together with tryptase and CD117 immunohistochemistry, positive in mastocytoma's mast cell infiltrate and negative in juvenile xanthogranuloma's histiocytic infiltrate, the latter instead highlighted by CD68 and Factor XIIIa, discussed further in the ancillary studies section below.

A 14-month-old infant presents with a solitary, firm, yellow-orange papule on the scalp, present for approximately two months and gradually enlarging. Pattern assignment identifies a dense dermal infiltrate of foamy histiocytes admixed with scattered Touton giant cells showing the characteristic wreath-like nuclear arrangement, without significant admixed mast cells or eosinophils. Differential narrowing weighs juvenile xanthogranuloma against solitary mastocytoma and xanthoma given the yellow-orange clinical color shared by all three, and CD68, Factor XIIIa, and CD117 immunohistochemistry are pursued: CD68 and Factor XIIIa are diffusely positive within the histiocytic infiltrate, while CD117 is negative, excluding a mast cell-rich process. Given the Touton giant cells, positive histiocytic markers, and negative mast cell markers, a diagnosis of juvenile xanthogranuloma is rendered, with the report reassuring the family regarding this diagnosis's expected spontaneous regression over the following several years and noting that no further evaluation is required in the absence of multiple lesions or ocular symptoms.

Porphyria Cutanea Tarda Versus Pseudoporphyria and Other Bullous Photodermatoses

Porphyria cutanea tarda's photodistributed blistering must be distinguished from pseudoporphyria, a clinically and histologically similar photodistributed blistering process associated with certain medications, most notably naproxen and other nonsteroidal anti-inflammatory drugs, and with hemodialysis, but occurring in the absence of any underlying porphyrin metabolic abnormality, a distinction resolved not by skin histology, which can appear essentially identical between the two, but by quantitative plasma or urine porphyrin analysis, discussed further in the ancillary studies section below, elevated in true porphyria cutanea tarda and normal in pseudoporphyria.

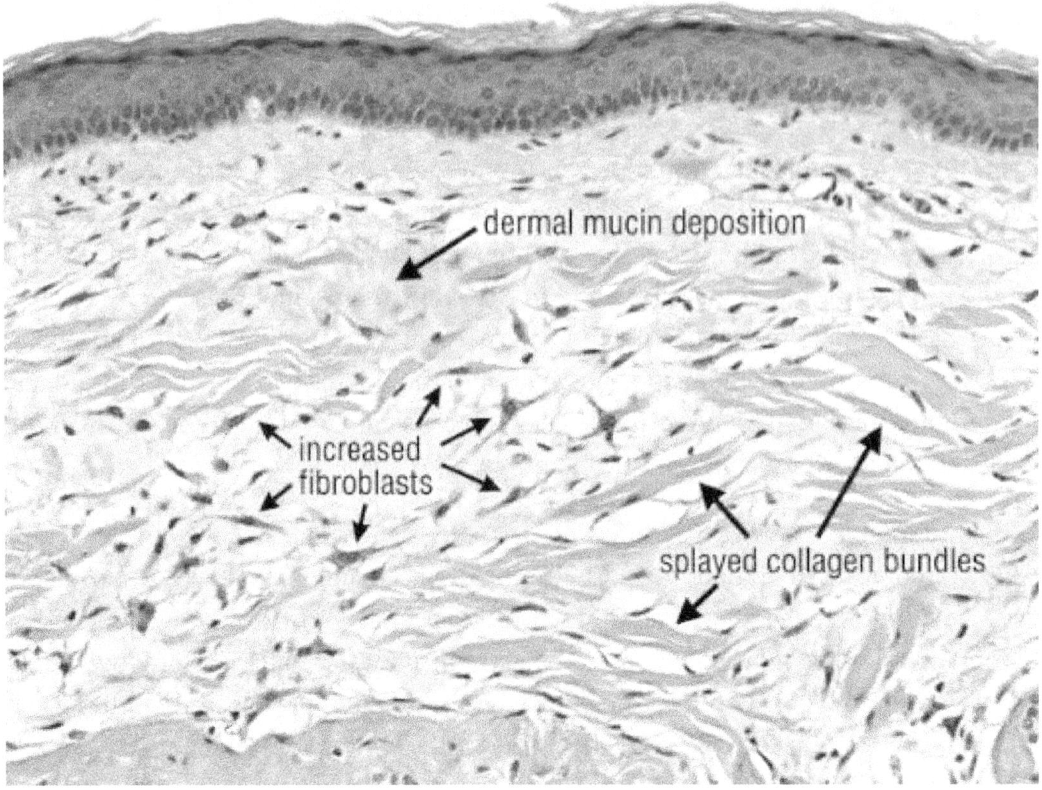

Ancillary Studies

This section details the specific confirmatory ancillary study appropriate to each entity discussed above, each chosen to resolve the specific diagnostic ambiguity that routine hematoxylin and eosin staining alone leaves unanswered for that entity.

Immunofluorescence Antigen Mapping and Electron Microscopy for Epidermolysis Bullosa

As demonstrated in the discussion above, immunofluorescence antigen mapping, applying a panel of antibodies against keratin 5/14, laminin 332, collagen XVII, and collagen VII to a perilesional skin biopsy and determining the precise level at which each antigen's staining is localized relative to the blister roof and floor, provides the practically decisive ancillary study for subtyping epidermolysis bullosa, absent or reduced staining for a specific protein localizing the defect and confirming the corresponding subtype. Transmission electron microscopy, historically the reference standard before antigen mapping became widely available, remains a valuable confirmatory study in ambiguous cases, directly visualizing the ultrastructural level of blister formation and the morphology of hemidesmosomes and anchoring fibrils. Targeted genetic testing for the causative gene provides definitive molecular confirmation and is essential for accurate genetic counseling, discussed further in the management implications section below.

Congo Red Polarization and Amyloid Typing

Congo red staining with apple-green birefringence under polarized light confirms the presence of amyloid but does not by itself distinguish primary cutaneous from systemic AL amyloidosis, discussed in the differential diagnosis section above; immunohistochemistry for kappa and lambda light chain restriction, and, where available, mass spectrometry-based proteomic typing, the current reference standard for definitive amyloid subtyping, together with serum and urine protein electrophoresis and serum free light chain assay to evaluate for an underlying plasma cell dyscrasia, are the essential ancillary studies whenever systemic disease is a genuine clinical consideration.

Mast Cell Tryptase and CD117 Immunohistochemistry, and KIT Mutation Analysis

Mast cell tryptase and CD117 (KIT) immunohistochemistry reliably highlight the dermal mast cell infiltrate of cutaneous mastocytosis, particularly valuable in adult-onset maculopapular cutaneous mastocytosis where the infiltrate can be subtle on routine hematoxylin and eosin staining, discussed in the histopathologic features section above. Serum tryptase level and, where systemic disease is suspected, bone marrow biopsy with KIT D816V mutation analysis are the appropriate ancillary studies for evaluating possible systemic mastocytosis in an adult patient with extensive or persistent cutaneous disease, discussed further in the management implications section below.

CD68 and Factor XIIIa Immunohistochemistry for Histiocytic Proliferations

As demonstrated in the worked case above, CD68 and Factor XIIIa immunohistochemistry confirm histiocytic lineage in juvenile xanthogranuloma and xanthoma, while CD1a and S100, characteristically negative in both entities, are applied specifically to exclude Langerhans cell histiocytosis whenever the clinical or histologic presentation raises that differential consideration, a distinction this chapter notes carries substantially greater clinical consequence than the juvenile xanthogranuloma versus xanthoma distinction given Langerhans cell histiocytosis's potential for systemic, multi-organ involvement.

Quantitative Porphyrin Analysis and Lipid Panel

Quantitative plasma or urine porphyrin analysis, showing an elevated uroporphyrin-to-coproporphyrin ratio, together with plasma porphyrin fluorescence scanning, confirms porphyria cutanea tarda and distinguishes it from pseudoporphyria, discussed in the differential diagnosis section above, while a fasting lipid panel is the essential ancillary study whenever xanthoma is diagnosed or suspected, given this finding's role as a cutaneous marker of an underlying, and potentially clinically significant, lipid disorder warranting its own independent management.

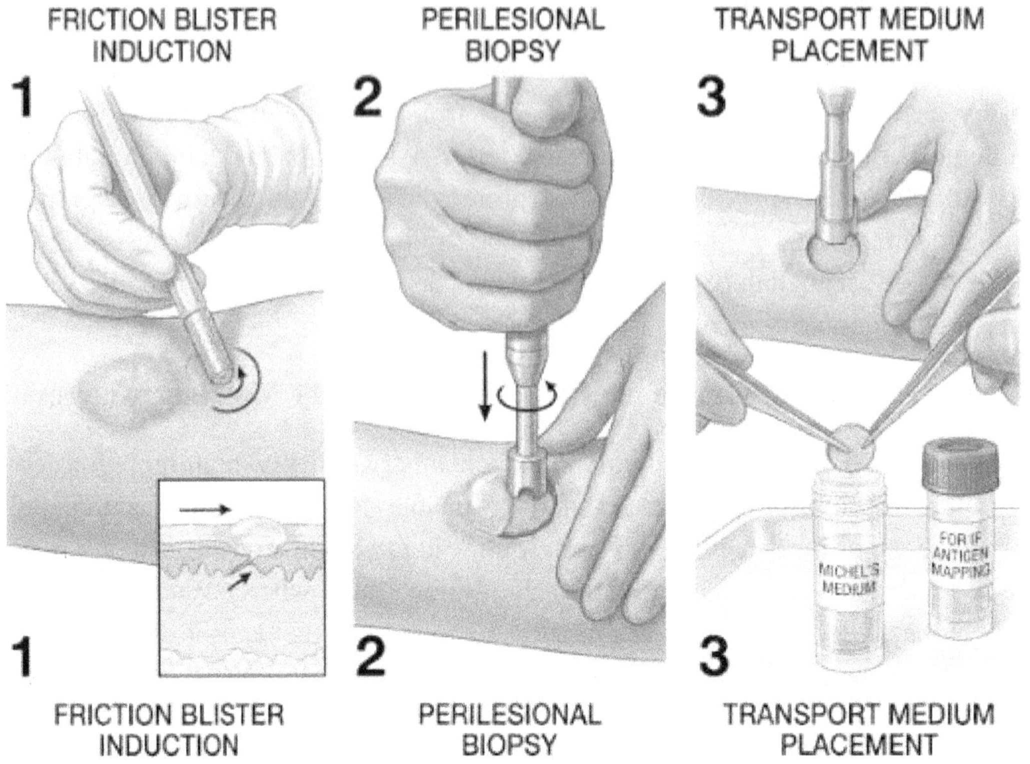

Management Implications

Management of Epidermolysis Bullosa and Genetic Counseling

Management of epidermolysis bullosa centers on meticulous wound care, blister prevention through friction avoidance, specialized non-adherent dressings, and prevention and treatment of secondary infection, together with nutritional support given the substantial protein loss and increased metabolic demand that widespread blistering produces, particularly in severe generalized subtypes. Genetic counseling, informed by the definitive molecular subtype confirmed through the antigen mapping and genetic testing discussed above, is essential for affected families given epidermolysis bullosa's varied inheritance patterns and recurrence risk, with emerging gene and cell-based therapies under active investigation for the most severe subtypes.

Management of Ichthyosis and Mastocytosis

Ichthyosis is managed with regular emollient application and, for more severe or extensive disease, keratolytic agents or topical or systemic retinoids to normalize epidermal desquamation, with management intensity generally correlating with disease severity across the spectrum from mild ichthyosis vulgaris to more extensive epidermolytic ichthyosis. Solitary mastocytoma and limited maculopapular cutaneous mastocytosis are managed conservatively with antihistamines for symptomatic relief and counseling regarding trigger avoidance, physical friction, temperature extremes, and specific medications known to provoke mast cell degranulation, given the expected spontaneous improvement of childhood-onset disease, while adult-onset or extensive disease warrants the systemic mastocytosis evaluation discussed in the ancillary studies section above and, where confirmed, referral to hematology for consideration of cytoreductive or targeted KIT-inhibitor therapy.

Management of Amyloidosis and Scleromyxedema

Primary cutaneous amyloidosis is managed symptomatically, topical corticosteroids and antihistamines for pruritus in lichen amyloidosis, given its benign, localized nature and the absence of any systemic disease requiring treatment, in direct contrast to systemic AL amyloidosis, which, as demonstrated in the worked case above, requires urgent hematology-oncology referral for plasma cell-directed chemotherapy or autologous stem cell transplantation given its potential for progressive, life-threatening cardiac and renal involvement. Scleromyxedema is managed with intravenous immunoglobulin as a generally preferred first-line systemic therapy, together with treatment directed at the underlying paraproteinemia in coordination with hematology, given this disorder's chronic course and potential for extracutaneous, including neurologic and cardiac, involvement in the related dermato-neuro syndrome.

Management of Neurofibromatosis Type 1, Tuberous Sclerosis Complex, and Incontinentia Pigmenti

Management across the genodermatoses in this chapter follows a common principle: definitive genetic and molecular confirmation, established through the ancillary studies discussed above, directly shapes both the immediate treatment pathway and the longer-term surveillance and counseling plan for the affected patient and family. Neurofibromatosis type 1 and tuberous sclerosis complex both warrant lifelong, multidisciplinary surveillance given their multi-organ hamartomatous and tumor predisposition, ophthalmologic, neurologic, and, for tuberous sclerosis complex, renal and cardiac surveillance in particular, with dermatologic management directed at symptomatic or cosmetically significant cutaneous lesions, laser therapy or topical mTOR inhibitor therapy for facial angiofibromas in tuberous sclerosis complex among the available options. Incontinentia pigmenti is managed supportively during the vesicular and verrucous stages, with careful attention to preventing secondary infection, together with early multidisciplinary ophthalmologic, dental, and neurologic evaluation given this disorder's potential extracutaneous involvement discussed in the clinical presentation section above.

Management of Juvenile Xanthogranuloma, Xanthoma, Porphyria Cutanea Tarda, and Calcinosis Cutis

Juvenile xanthogranuloma requires no treatment beyond observation given its expected spontaneous regression, though multiple lesions in an infant warrant ophthalmologic evaluation given a recognized, if uncommon, association with ocular juvenile xanthogranuloma and intraocular hemorrhage. Xanthoma is managed by addressing the underlying lipid disorder, dietary modification and lipid-lowering pharmacotherapy, with eruptive xanthoma in particular capable of rapid resolution once severe hypertriglyceridemia is controlled, discussed in the clinical presentation section above. Porphyria cutanea tarda is managed by identifying and addressing precipitating factors, alcohol cessation, hepatitis C treatment, and discontinuation of estrogen therapy where applicable, together with therapeutic phlebotomy to reduce hepatic iron stores or low-dose hydroxychloroquine to mobilize and eliminate excess porphyrins, both established, effective first-line therapies for this disorder. Calcinosis cutis is managed primarily by addressing the underlying cause, whether an inflammatory connective tissue disease or a metabolic derangement in calcium and phosphate homeostasis, with surgical excision, intralesional sodium thiosulfate, or other targeted therapy reserved for symptomatic, ulcerated, or functionally limiting deposits.

Documentation and Reporting Standards

The pathology report for suspected epidermolysis bullosa should explicitly state the level of blister formation identified and the results of any immunofluorescence antigen mapping performed, given the direct bearing of subtype confirmation on genetic counseling. The report for any dermal amyloid deposit should explicitly state whether vessel wall involvement is present and recommend correlation with serum and urine protein studies whenever primary cutaneous disease cannot be confidently distinguished from systemic disease on the biopsy findings alone, a conservative reporting practice this chapter endorses given the serious consequence of an unrecognized systemic AL amyloidosis diagnosis. Reports describing a foam cell-rich or histiocytic dermal infiltrate should explicitly note the presence or absence of Touton giant cells and the results of any CD68, Factor XIIIa, CD1a, or S100 immunohistochemistry performed, given this panel's direct role in distinguishing juvenile xanthogranuloma and xanthoma from the more clinically consequential Langerhans cell histiocytosis discussed in the ancillary studies section above.

Complications and Prognosis

Prognosis throughout this chapter is determined less by the presence of a deposit or defect itself than by its precise identity and systemic context, a theme this chapter has emphasized repeatedly given how frequently that context, rather than dermal histology alone, changes the clinical stakes. Recessive dystrophic epidermolysis bullosa carries a well-documented, substantially elevated lifetime risk of cutaneous squamous cell carcinoma arising within chronically scarred, ulcerated skin, a complication that this chapter notes represents the leading cause of mortality in adults with this subtype and warrants lifelong dermatologic surveillance with a low threshold for biopsy of any persistent or changing ulcerated area. Severe generalized junctional epidermolysis bullosa carries a poor prognosis in early infancy given the extent and severity of mucocutaneous involvement, while epidermolysis bullosa simplex generally carries a favorable long-term prognosis with improvement often noted over childhood. Systemic mastocytosis, when confirmed in an adult with extensive cutaneous disease, carries a variable prognosis depending on the specific World Health Organization subtype, ranging from an indolent course to, in a minority of cases, an aggressive or associated hematologic neoplasm-linked course, underscoring the importance of the systemic evaluation discussed above. Untreated systemic AL amyloidosis carries a poor prognosis, historically measured in months from diagnosis, driven substantially by cardiac involvement, a sobering natural history that stands in stark contrast to primary cutaneous amyloidosis's uniformly benign course and that this chapter emphasizes as the central reason this differential, developed in the worked case above, carries such outsized clinical consequence. Neurofibromatosis type 1 carries a lifetime risk of several tumor types beyond the neurofibromas discussed in Chapter 17, including optic pathway glioma and malignant peripheral nerve sheath tumor, warranting the lifelong surveillance discussed above, while tuberous sclerosis complex carries a variable prognosis driven substantially by the severity of associated central nervous system and renal involvement rather than by the cutaneous stigmata themselves.

Special Populations

Epidermolysis bullosa most often presents in the neonatal period, and any neonate with unexplained, widespread blistering warrants prompt dermatologic evaluation and biopsy given the time-sensitive nature of accurately distinguishing the epidermolysis bullosa subtypes for both immediate management and family counseling. Solitary mastocytoma and maculopapular cutaneous mastocytosis are predominantly pediatric presentations with a generally favorable, self-limited course, in contrast to adult-onset disease, which, as discussed above, carries a meaningfully higher association with systemic mastocytosis and therefore warrants a more thorough initial evaluation. Children presenting with multiple café-au-lait macules, particularly six or more exceeding the size thresholds used in the clinical diagnostic criteria, warrant referral for comprehensive neurofibromatosis type 1 evaluation even before other stigmata become apparent, given the value of early diagnosis for anticipatory surveillance, and any infant presenting with a blistering eruption following Blaschko's lines should prompt consideration of incontinentia pigmenti and, particularly in an affected female infant, examination of the mother for subtle signs of the same disorder given its dominant, though highly variable, inheritance pattern. Pregnant patients and women of reproductive age with porphyria cutanea tarda warrant particular attention to estrogen-containing medications and hormone therapy given their well-documented role as a disease-precipitating factor discussed in the etiology section above.

Patient Education and Counseling

Families of infants diagnosed with epidermolysis bullosa benefit from early referral to specialized multidisciplinary wound care and genetic counseling resources given this disease's lifelong, chronic course and the substantial caregiving burden it can impose, while patients diagnosed with primary cutaneous amyloidosis benefit from clear reassurance regarding this diagnosis's benign, localized nature once systemic disease has been appropriately excluded. Patients diagnosed with systemic AL amyloidosis or scleromyxedema benefit from prompt, clear counseling regarding the systemic evaluation and hematology-directed treatment pathway ahead, framed around the time-sensitive nature of early intervention for these diagnoses. Patients diagnosed with neurofibromatosis type 1 or tuberous sclerosis complex benefit from counseling regarding the lifelong, multidisciplinary surveillance these diagnoses warrant, framed constructively around anticipatory monitoring rather than any single feared complication, along with appropriate genetic counseling resources given both disorders' autosomal dominant inheritance pattern and the corresponding implications for future pregnancies and at-risk family members. Patients diagnosed with porphyria cutanea tarda benefit from clear, practical counseling regarding photoprotection and modification of the specific precipitating factors identified in their case, alcohol reduction, hepatitis C treatment referral, or discontinuation of estrogen therapy, framed around this disorder's generally excellent response to appropriately targeted treatment once the precipitating factor is addressed.

THE REACTION PATTERN RECOGNITION SYSTEM — The Genodermatosis and Deposition Disorder Level and Substance Pattern Family

---

The Pattern: Genodermatoses and deposition disorders organized by defective structural protein or deposited substance and its precise anatomic level, epidermal, junctional, or dermal, with ancillary confirmation required to distinguish superficially similar entities with dramatically different prognoses.

Histologic Signature: Intraepidermal, sub-basal, or sub-lamina densa cleft defines the epidermolysis bullosa subtype; absent granular layer defines ichthyosis vulgaris; epidermolytic hyperkeratosis defines epidermolytic ichthyosis; dermal mast cell infiltrate defines mastocytosis; Congo red-positive papillary dermal deposits define amyloidosis; diffuse dermal mucin with fibroblast proliferation defines scleromyxedema.

The Decision: Identify level or substance, then apply the specific confirmatory ancillary study, antigen mapping for epidermolysis bullosa, light chain typing and systemic workup for amyloid, tryptase/CD117 and KIT analysis for mastocytosis, or serum protein electrophoresis for scleromyxedema, before finalizing a prognostically accurate diagnosis.

Trap Logic: The three major epidermolysis bullosa subtypes appear similar without antigen mapping; primary cutaneous and systemic amyloidosis share histologically similar dermal deposits; scleromyxedema mimics scleroderma and scleredema clinically.

Pattern Anchor: Level or substance first, then the specific confirmatory ancillary study. Primary cutaneous versus systemic amyloidosis is never resolved by dermal histology alone; systemic workup is mandatory whenever this distinction is uncertain.

Summary and Key Concepts

Epidermolysis bullosa is classified by the precise level of blistering, intraepidermal in the simplex type, lamina lucida in the junctional type, and sub-lamina densa in the dystrophic type, distinguished definitively by immunofluorescence antigen mapping or electron microscopy given shared bland histology on routine staining.

Ichthyosis vulgaris (filaggrin), X-linked ichthyosis (steroid sulfatase), and epidermolytic ichthyosis (keratin 1/10) are distinguished by their granular layer histology, flexural involvement, and, for epidermolytic ichthyosis, characteristic epidermolytic hyperkeratosis.

Cutaneous mastocytosis is confirmed clinically by a positive Darier's sign and histologically by tryptase and CD117 immunohistochemistry, with adult-onset disease carrying a meaningfully higher systemic mastocytosis risk than childhood-onset disease.

Primary cutaneous amyloidosis and systemic AL amyloidosis share histologically similar Congo red-positive dermal deposits but carry dramatically different prognoses, distinguished by vessel wall involvement, light chain typing, and serum and urine protein studies rather than dermal histology alone.

Scleromyxedema shows diffuse dermal mucin deposition with fibroblast proliferation and is strongly associated with an underlying monoclonal gammopathy, distinguishing it from scleroderma and scleredema.

CHAPTER 20: SPECIAL SITES: NAIL, MUCOSAL, AND GENITAL DERMATOPATHOLOGY

Learning Objectives

1. Identify the histopathologic features of longitudinal melanonychia and apply the diagnostic criteria distinguishing benign nail matrix melanocytic activation from subungual melanoma.
2. Recognize the histopathologic features of oral lichen planus and oral epithelial dysplasia, and apply standardized dysplasia grading.
3. Distinguish differentiated (lichen sclerosus-associated) vulvar intraepithelial neoplasia from usual-type (human papillomavirus-associated) vulvar intraepithelial neoplasia by etiology, histopathology, and molecular profile.
4. Identify the histopathologic features of extramammary Paget disease and apply the immunohistochemical panel distinguishing primary cutaneous disease from disease secondary to an underlying visceral malignancy.
5. Recognize the diagnostic criteria for lichen sclerosus and its established association with squamous cell carcinoma risk at genital sites.
6. Apply site-specific biopsy and ancillary study techniques appropriately across the nail unit, oral mucosa, and anogenital skin.

Definition and Classification

Special Sites as a Distinct Diagnostic Domain

As the final core chapter of this textbook, this section closes the systematic organ-based and reaction-pattern-based progression established across the preceding nineteen chapters by addressing the sites most easily overlooked or misapplied when general cutaneous diagnostic criteria are extended to them without appropriate modification. This closing chapter addresses the nail unit, oral and other mucosal surfaces, and anogenital skin, three anatomically and histologically distinct compartments that, despite their differences, share a unifying diagnostic principle this chapter emphasizes throughout: site-specific anatomy fundamentally alters both the normal histologic baseline and the differential diagnosis at each location, such that criteria developed for glabrous or hair-bearing skin elsewhere in this book cannot be applied uncritically to these specialized sites without risking both overdiagnosis and, more consequentially, underdiagnosis of clinically significant disease. The nail unit's specialized matrix and bed epithelium, the oral mucosa's non-keratinized or parakeratinized squamous epithelium, and anogenital skin's combination of modified apocrine glands, specialized stroma, and frequent chronic inflammatory or human papillomavirus exposure each demand a site-specific diagnostic framework, developed in turn throughout this chapter.

Entities Covered in This Chapter

The table below summarizes each entity's key distinguishing feature and clinical significance as a quick-reference companion to the detailed discussion that follows. Nail unit entities include longitudinal melanonychia and subungual melanoma, and glomus tumor of the nail bed. Oral mucosal entities include oral lichen planus and oral epithelial dysplasia/leukoplakia. Anogenital entities include lichen sclerosus, differentiated and usual-type vulvar intraepithelial neoplasia, and extramammary Paget disease, each developed with particular emphasis on the specific differentials carrying the greatest diagnostic and clinical consequence at each site.

Entity	Site	Key Distinguishing Feature	Clinical Significance
Longitudinal melanonychia (benign)	Nail matrix	Melanocytic activation without significant atypia or increased density	Benign, requires monitoring
Subungual melanoma	Nail matrix	Increased melanocyte density with pagetoid spread and Hutchinson sign	Malignant, often delayed diagnosis
Glomus tumor	Nail bed	Uniform round cells around vascular channels, exquisite tenderness	Benign, symptomatic
Oral lichen planus	Oral mucosa	Band-like lymphocytic infiltrate, basal layer degeneration, Civatte bodies	Chronic, small malignant potential
Oral epithelial dysplasia/leukoplakia	Oral mucosa	Graded architectural and cytologic atypia	Premalignant, grade-dependent risk
Lichen sclerosus	Anogenital skin	Homogenized papillary dermis, basal vacuolar change	Chronic, SCC risk
Differentiated VIN	Vulva	Basal atypia with normal-appearing maturation, p53 mutant pattern	High-risk, lichen sclerosus-associated
Usual-type VIN	Vulva	Full-thickness atypia, HPV-associated, p16 block positive	HPV-driven, younger patients

Extramammary Paget disease	Anogenital/axillary apocrine skin	Pagetoid Paget cells within epidermis, mucin-positive	Primary cutaneous or secondary to internal malignancy
Onychomycosis	Nail plate	PAS/GMS-positive fungal hyphae within nail plate keratin	Benign, chronic, treatable
Zoon balanitis/vulvitis	Glans penis/vulva	Band-like plasma cell infiltrate, lozenge-shaped keratinocytes	Benign, chronic irritant
Oral melanotic macule	Oral mucosa	Basal melanin increase without melanocyte proliferation	Benign

Epidemiology of Special-Site Disease

The epidemiologic profile of each entity discussed in this chapter directly informs pretest clinical suspicion at the bedside. Onychomycosis is the most common nail disorder overall, increasing in prevalence with age and among patients with diabetes, peripheral vascular disease, or immunosuppression, and represents a substantially more common cause of nail dystrophy than any of the nail matrix pigmented lesions discussed in this chapter, a prevalence disparity this chapter notes is clinically important given onychomycosis's frequent role as a diagnostic distractor delaying recognition of a coexisting or underlying nail matrix neoplasm. Subungual melanoma, though rare in absolute terms, represents a disproportionately higher fraction of melanoma among patients with darkly pigmented skin, in whom cutaneous sun-exposed melanoma is comparatively uncommon, a demographic pattern directly paralleling the acral melanoma epidemiology discussed in Chapter 14. Lichen sclerosus shows a bimodal age distribution, prepubertal children and postmenopausal women representing the two peak incidence groups, while extramammary Paget disease is predominantly a disease of older adults, with secondary disease showing a higher relative frequency in perianal, as opposed to vulvar or scrotal, presentations given the greater proximity to colorectal mucosa.

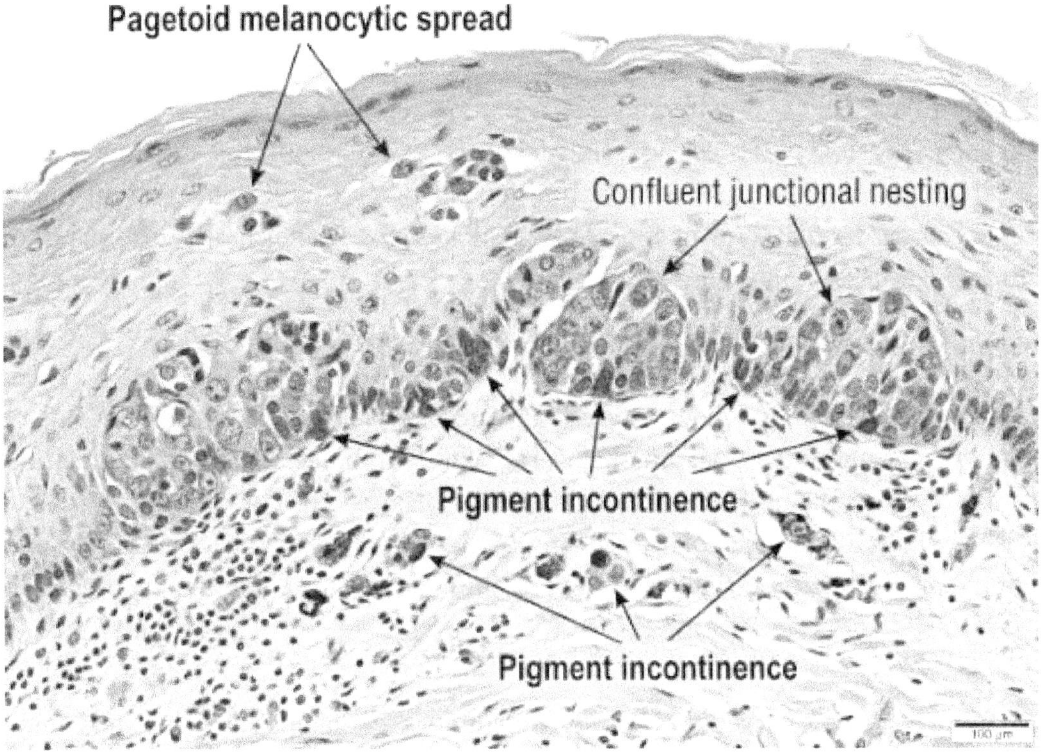

Etiology and Pathogenesis

Melanocyte Activation Versus Neoplastic Proliferation in the Nail Matrix

Longitudinal melanonychia most often reflects benign melanocytic activation, increased melanin production by a normal or near-normal density of nail matrix melanocytes, triggered by trauma, inflammatory nail disease, certain medications, or, in patients with darker constitutive pigmentation, physiologic ethnic variation, without the true neoplastic melanocytic proliferation that defines subungual melanoma, a fundamentally important etiologic distinction given the two entities' overlapping clinical appearance developed further in the differential diagnosis section below. Subungual melanoma arises through a genuine neoplastic transformation of nail matrix melanocytes, sharing molecular features with acral melanoma discussed in Chapter 14, including a comparatively low burden of ultraviolet-signature mutations and a higher frequency of KIT mutations relative to melanoma arising on sun-exposed skin, reflecting this site's minimal direct ultraviolet exposure.

HPV-Driven Versus Lichen Sclerosus-Associated Pathways in Vulvar Neoplasia

This distinction, developed in full below, exemplifies this chapter's recurring theme that etiology, rather than histologic severity alone, frequently determines an entity's true clinical significance at these special sites. Usual-type vulvar intraepithelial neoplasia arises through high-risk human papillomavirus infection, most often HPV-16, driving E6- and E7-mediated inactivation of p53 and retinoblastoma protein respectively, a viral oncogenic pathway that produces this entity's characteristic full-thickness epithelial atypia and its immunohistochemical p16 block-positive signature, discussed further in the ancillary studies section below, and that predominantly affects younger patients. Differentiated vulvar intraepithelial neoplasia, in contrast, arises independently of human papillomavirus infection, instead developing within a background of chronic lichen sclerosus or lichen simplex chronicus through accumulation of TP53 mutations, a p53-driven pathway that produces a comparatively subtle histologic appearance despite carrying a higher per-lesion risk of progression to invasive squamous cell carcinoma than usual-type vulvar intraepithelial neoplasia, a counterintuitive but well-established relationship this chapter emphasizes given its substantial clinical consequence, developed further in the differential diagnosis and management implications sections below.

Autoimmune and Fibrosing Mechanisms in Lichen Sclerosus

Lichen sclerosus is increasingly understood as an autoimmune-mediated process, supported by its association with other autoimmune disorders and by identification of circulating autoantibodies against extracellular matrix protein 1 in a substantial proportion of affected patients, driving the characteristic dermal sclerosis and basal layer vacuolar degeneration developed in the histopathologic features section below, though the precise inciting trigger for this autoimmune response remains incompletely defined.

Primary Apocrine Origin Versus Secondary Extension in Extramammary Paget Disease

Extramammary Paget disease arises through two distinct mechanisms carrying substantially different clinical implications: primary cutaneous extramammary Paget disease arises from an intraepidermal or intraepithelial adnexal (apocrine gland) origin without an associated underlying visceral malignancy, representing the majority of cases, while secondary extramammary Paget disease arises from pagetoid intraepithelial extension of an underlying visceral adenocarcinoma, most often anorectal, urothelial, or, at vulvar sites, a Bartholin gland or cervical primary, a mechanistic distinction that, discussed further in the ancillary studies section below, directly determines whether systemic oncologic workup is warranted.

Dermatophyte Invasion in Onychomycosis

This section addresses the remaining, more diagnostically straightforward entities in this chapter before returning to their specific histopathologic, clinical, and ancillary detail below. Onychomycosis arises most commonly from dermatophyte invasion of the nail plate, Trichophyton rubrum accounting for the substantial majority of cases, with non-dermatophyte molds and Candida species accounting for a smaller proportion, particularly at the fingernails and in immunosuppressed patients; the causative organism invades and digests nail plate keratin, producing the thickened, discolored, friable nail plate developed further in the clinical presentation section below, a comparatively simple, non-neoplastic pathogenesis that stands in useful contrast to the neoplastic and inflammatory processes discussed elsewhere in this chapter.

Chronic Friction and Irritation in Zoon Balanitis

This reactive pathogenesis is worth restating plainly given how easily this entity's alarming clinical appearance can be mistaken for a premalignant process, developed further below. Zoon balanitis (plasma cell balanitis), and its vulvar counterpart Zoon vulvitis, is understood to arise from chronic, low-grade friction and irritation of unprotected mucosal skin, occurring almost exclusively in uncircumcised men at the glans penis, with the resulting chronic inflammatory response producing the characteristic band-like plasma cell infiltrate developed in the histopathologic features section below, a reactive rather than neoplastic or infectious pathogenesis this chapter emphasizes distinguishes this entity fundamentally from the premalignant and malignant special-site entities discussed elsewhere in this chapter, despite some clinical overlap in appearance developed further in the differential diagnosis section below.

THE REACTION PATTERN RECOGNITION SYSTEM — Site-Specific Anatomy as the Universal Special Sites Anchor

The Pattern: Site-Specific Baseline Anatomy Combined with the Entity's Etiologic Driver, Trauma-Related Melanocyte Activation, HPV Infection, Autoimmune Sclerosis, or Adnexal Neoplasia, as the Framework for Classifying Every Special-Site Entity in This Chapter

Histologic Signature: Increased melanocyte density with pagetoid spread signals subungual melanoma against benign melanonychia's activation without density increase; full-thickness atypia with p16 block positivity signals usual-type vulvar intraepithelial neoplasia; basal atypia with preserved maturation and mutant-pattern p53 signals differentiated vulvar intraepithelial neoplasia; and pagetoid intraepidermal cells with cytoplasmic mucin signal extramammary Paget disease.

The Decision: Establish the specific anatomic site and its normal histologic baseline first, then apply site-specific criteria and escalate to immunohistochemistry, SOX10/Melan-A for nail matrix melanocytic lesions, p16/p53 for vulvar intraepithelial neoplasia subtyping, or CK7/GCDFP-15/CK20 for extramammary Paget disease, whenever routine morphology leaves genuine diagnostic uncertainty.

Trap Logic: Benign longitudinal melanonychia can mimic subungual melanoma clinically; differentiated vulvar intraepithelial neoplasia's subtle histology can be underdiagnosed despite carrying a higher per-lesion progression risk than the more overtly atypical usual-type; and primary and secondary extramammary Paget disease are histologically similar on hematoxylin and eosin staining alone.

Pattern Anchor: Site-specific baseline anatomy first, then the entity's etiologic driver. Subtle histologic atypia at a special site, particularly differentiated vulvar intraepithelial neoplasia, must never be dismissed as reactive change without correlation with the full clinical and immunohistochemical picture.

Histopathologic Features and Diagnostic Criteria

Diagnostic Features of Benign Melanonychia, Subungual Melanoma, and Glomus Tumor

Benign longitudinal melanonychia shows an increase in melanin pigment within nail matrix keratinocytes and melanophages in the underlying stroma, with melanocyte density at or only mildly above the expected baseline for this site, without significant cytologic atypia, confluent junctional nesting, or pagetoid upward migration of melanocytes into the overlying epithelium. Subungual melanoma shows an increased density of melanocytes along the nail matrix basal layer, frequently with confluent, back-to-back nesting, cytologic atypia, and pagetoid spread, individual atypical melanocytes migrating upward into the epithelium in a pattern directly analogous to the melanoma in situ pattern discussed in Chapter 14, a density and architectural distinction this chapter emphasizes as the essential criterion separating this entity from benign melanocytic activation, developed further in the differential diagnosis section below. Glomus tumor of the nail bed shows a well-circumscribed proliferation of uniform, round, epithelioid glomus cells with round nuclei and scant cytoplasm arranged around thin-walled vascular channels, a bland, monotonous cytology that stands in useful diagnostic contrast to the entities discussed elsewhere in this chapter given its purely benign, non-atypical appearance.

Diagnostic Features of Oral Lichen Planus and Oral Epithelial Dysplasia

Oral lichen planus shows a band-like lymphocytic infiltrate at the epithelial-connective tissue interface with basal layer vacuolar degeneration and scattered apoptotic keratinocytes (Civatte bodies), a histologic pattern directly analogous to cutaneous lichen planus but showing a less pronounced sawtooth epidermal architecture given oral mucosa's non-keratinized or parakeratinized epithelial structure. Oral epithelial dysplasia is graded, analogous to cervical and other squamous mucosal dysplasia grading systems, as mild, moderate, or severe based on the proportion of full epithelial thickness showing architectural disorganization and cytologic atypia, nuclear pleomorphism, increased nuclear-to-cytoplasmic ratio, and abnormal mitotic figures, with severe dysplasia showing atypia extending through the full or near-full thickness of the epithelium, a grade this chapter notes carries a substantially higher risk of progression to invasive squamous cell carcinoma than mild dysplasia, discussed further in the complications and prognosis section below.

Diagnostic Features of Onychomycosis, Zoon Balanitis, and Oral Melanotic Macule

Onychomycosis shows periodic acid-Schiff or Gomori methenamine silver-positive fungal hyphae within the nail plate keratin, best visualized with these special stains given fungal elements' frequently subtle appearance on routine hematoxylin and eosin staining alone, together with compact orthokeratosis and, at times, a subungual hyperkeratotic debris accumulation. Zoon balanitis shows a dense, band-like infiltrate of plasma cells within the superficial dermis, together with characteristic lozenge-shaped (diamond-shaped) keratinocytes within an attenuated, often spongiotic epidermis, and extravasated erythrocytes with hemosiderin deposition, a distinctive combination of plasma cell-rich infiltrate and lozenge keratinocytes this chapter emphasizes as the diagnostic histologic signature of this entity. Oral melanotic macule shows increased melanin pigmentation within basal keratinocytes without an increase in melanocyte number or density, directly analogous to a simple lentigo, without the atypia, increased density, or pagetoid spread that would suggest a melanocytic neoplasm.

Clinical Presentation and Clinicopathologic Correlation

Clinical Presentation of Nail Unit Pigmented Lesions

Longitudinal melanonychia presents as a longitudinal, pigmented band extending from the proximal nail fold to the free edge of the nail plate, and the ABCDEF criteria provide a structured clinical framework for assessing malignant potential: Age (peak incidence fifth through seventh decades) and African, Asian, or Native American ethnicity; Band width exceeding three millimeters or irregular, variegated coloration; Change in the band's size or morphology over time; Digit most commonly involved (thumb, great toe, or index finger); Extension of pigment onto the surrounding proximal or lateral nail fold (Hutchinson sign), a specific and highly concerning clinical finding directly correlating with the pagetoid epidermal spread described in the histopathologic features section above; and Family or personal history of melanoma, criteria this chapter emphasizes should prompt biopsy of the nail matrix whenever multiple criteria are present rather than reassurance and observation alone.

Clinical Presentation of Oral Mucosal Disease

Oral lichen planus presents most classically as bilateral, reticulated white striae (Wickham striae) on the buccal mucosa, though erosive and atrophic variants presenting with painful ulceration and erythema also occur and carry a somewhat higher, though still modest, malignant transformation risk than the reticular variant. Oral leukoplakia presents as a white patch or plaque that cannot be scraped off or attributed to another identifiable cause, a clinical diagnosis of exclusion that, given its purely descriptive definition, requires biopsy for histologic dysplasia grading to determine malignant potential, discussed above, while erythroplakia, a red, velvety patch, carries a substantially higher likelihood of harboring severe dysplasia or invasive carcinoma at the time of biopsy than leukoplakia, a clinical distinction this chapter emphasizes should lower the threshold for prompt biopsy whenever an oral mucosal lesion shows any erythematous component.

Clinical Presentation of Anogenital Disease

Lichen sclerosus presents with well-demarcated, ivory-white, atrophic plaques classically in a figure-eight (hourglass) distribution encompassing the vulva and perianal skin, with progressive architectural change, labial resorption, clitoral hood adhesion, and introital narrowing, in longstanding disease, together with pruritus and, in more advanced disease, pain with intercourse or defecation. In male patients, lichen sclerosus (historically termed balanitis xerotica obliterans at this site) presents with ivory-white, sclerotic involvement of the glans and foreskin, frequently producing phimosis, progressive inability to retract the foreskin, that not uncommonly prompts the circumcision through which this diagnosis is first histologically confirmed, together with a comparable squamous cell carcinoma risk to that discussed for vulvar disease below, making male genital lichen sclerosus every bit as clinically significant a diagnosis as its more extensively studied vulvar counterpart. Differentiated and usual-type vulvar intraepithelial neoplasia both present as a vulvar plaque, papule, or erosion, though differentiated vulvar intraepithelial neoplasia typically presents as a comparatively subtle, ill-defined, gray-white or erythematous plaque arising within a background of lichen sclerosus, while usual-type vulvar intraepithelial neoplasia more often presents as a discrete, well-demarcated, sometimes multifocal, pigmented or warty papule or plaque, a clinical distinction that, while useful, this chapter emphasizes must always be confirmed histologically given the substantially different management and malignant potential of each. Extramammary Paget disease presents as a slowly enlarging, well-demarcated, eczematous, erythematous plaque with a moist, weeping, or scaly surface, most common on the vulva, perianal skin, or scrotum, a presentation frequently mistaken for and treated as chronic eczema or a candidal intertrigo before biopsy is ultimately performed, a diagnostic delay this chapter notes is a well-documented and clinically consequential pattern for this specific entity.

Clinical Presentation of Onychomycosis, Zoon Balanitis, and Oral Melanotic Macule

Onychomycosis presents in several recognized clinical patterns: distal lateral subungual onychomycosis, the most common pattern, showing subungual hyperkeratosis, onycholysis, and yellow-white discoloration beginning at the distal or lateral nail edge; white superficial onychomycosis, showing well-demarcated white patches on the nail plate surface; and proximal subungual onychomycosis, involving the proximal nail fold, a comparatively uncommon pattern this chapter notes should prompt consideration of underlying immunosuppression, including HIV infection, when identified. Zoon balanitis presents as a well-demarcated, glistening, orange-red to brown patch or plaque on the glans penis, often described as having a "cayenne pepper" stippled quality reflecting the extravasated erythrocytes described in the histopathologic features section above, a presentation that, given its persistent, non-healing appearance, is frequently mistaken clinically for erythroplasia of Queyrat, discussed in Chapter 15, or another premalignant process. Oral melanotic macule presents as a solitary, well-demarcated, uniformly tan-brown macule, most common on the lower lip or gingiva, generally stable over time without the growth or color change that would raise concern for a melanocytic neoplasm.

CLINICAL PEARL: The ABCDEF criteria and Hutchinson sign provide a structured, reproducible framework for assessing longitudinal melanonychia at the bedside, while any persistent, treatment-resistant eczematous or lichenified anogenital plaque, particularly one that fails a reasonable trial of topical therapy, warrants biopsy to exclude extramammary Paget disease or vulvar intraepithelial neoplasia rather than continued empiric treatment. Progressive phimosis in an adult male should always prompt consideration of underlying genital lichen sclerosus rather than being attributed to simple, unexplained foreskin tightening.

Differential Diagnosis and Histologic Mimickers

Benign Longitudinal Melanonychia Versus Subungual Melanoma

As introduced in the histopathologic features section above, distinguishing benign longitudinal melanonychia from subungual melanoma rests on melanocyte density, architectural pattern, confluent versus discrete nesting, and pagetoid spread, criteria this chapter emphasizes require careful, deliberate assessment given both the nail matrix's comparatively thin, technically challenging biopsy specimens and the well-documented tendency for subungual melanoma diagnosis to be delayed, often attributed initially to trauma or a benign nevus, a delay directly contributing to this entity's comparatively poor prognosis relative to melanoma at other sites, discussed further in the complications and prognosis section below.

A 61-year-old patient presents with a 6-millimeter-wide, irregularly pigmented longitudinal band on the right thumbnail, present for approximately eight months and slowly widening, with pigment now visible extending onto the proximal nail fold. Pattern assignment identifies an increased density of melanocytes along the nail matrix basal layer with confluent junctional nesting and scattered melanocytes showing pagetoid upward migration into the overlying nail matrix epithelium, together with moderate cytologic atypia. Differential narrowing weighs benign melanocytic activation against subungual melanoma given the band's width, the Hutchinson sign, and the density and architectural findings on histology, and SOX10 and Melan-A immunohistochemistry are pursued to more precisely delineate melanocyte density and confirm the pagetoid spread pattern. Given the increased melanocyte density, confluent nesting, pagetoid spread, and clinical Hutchinson sign, a diagnosis of subungual melanoma in situ is rendered, with the report recommending complete surgical excision with margin assessment and explicit clinical correlation given this entity's recognized potential for underestimation of invasive depth on a limited nail matrix biopsy.

Differentiated Versus Usual-Type Vulvar Intraepithelial Neoplasia

As introduced in the etiology section above, differentiated vulvar intraepithelial neoplasia shows a comparatively subtle histologic appearance, basal layer atypia, enlarged nuclei with prominent nucleoli and abnormal basal mitotic figures, with preserved, near-normal maturation and keratinization in the upper epithelial layers, a subtlety this chapter emphasizes carries genuine risk of underdiagnosis as reactive or inflammatory change, particularly given this entity's typical background of lichen sclerosus, itself already associated with basal layer changes. Usual-type vulvar intraepithelial neoplasia, in contrast, shows more readily apparent full-thickness architectural disorganization and cytologic atypia, koilocytic change, and increased mitotic activity extending through the epithelium, a more overtly abnormal appearance that, paradoxically, this chapter notes is generally easier to recognize despite differentiated vulvar intraepithelial neoplasia's higher per-lesion progression risk to invasive carcinoma.

A 68-year-old patient with a longstanding history of biopsy-confirmed vulvar lichen sclerosus presents with a new, ill-defined, gray-white plaque arising within a background of chronic sclerotic change. Pattern assignment identifies basal layer keratinocyte atypia with enlarged, hyperchromatic nuclei and prominent nucleoli, abnormal mitotic figures confined to the basal and immediately suprabasal layers, and preserved, near-normal maturation and keratinization throughout the remaining epithelial thickness, without koilocytic change. Differential narrowing weighs reactive atypia associated with lichen sclerosus against differentiated vulvar intraepithelial neoplasia given the basal atypia and abnormal mitoses, and p53 and p16 immunohistochemistry are pursued: p53 shows a mutant expression pattern (strong, diffuse basal overexpression), while p16 is negative (patchy, non-block-positive pattern). Given the basal atypia, abnormal mitoses, mutant p53 pattern, and negative p16, a diagnosis of differentiated vulvar intraepithelial neoplasia is rendered, with the report explicitly flagging this diagnosis's higher per-lesion progression risk relative to usual-type disease and recommending close dermatologic and gynecologic surveillance given the ongoing lichen sclerosus background.

Glomus Tumor Versus Other Causes of Subungual Pain and Nail Bed Nodularity

Glomus tumor's exquisite point tenderness and characteristic cold-induced pain, discussed further in the clinical presentation section below, together with its bland, monotonous glomus cell cytology described above, generally distinguish it readily from the pigmented and dysplastic entities discussed elsewhere in this chapter, though a subungual glomus tumor without a clinically apparent bluish-red discoloration can occasionally be mistaken for a subungual exostosis or a simple traumatic hematoma before imaging or biopsy clarifies the diagnosis, underscoring the value of a careful cold-sensitivity history in any patient presenting with unexplained, localized nail bed pain.

Extramammary Paget Disease Versus Pagetoid Squamous Cell Carcinoma In Situ and Superficial Spreading Melanoma

Extramammary Paget disease's pagetoid intraepidermal cell population must be distinguished from pagetoid (Bowenoid) squamous cell carcinoma in situ and from superficial spreading melanoma in situ, both of which can show a superficially similar pagetoid growth pattern; this differential is resolved by cytoplasmic mucin content, present in Paget cells and absent in squamous and melanocytic lesions, together with the immunohistochemical panel discussed in the ancillary studies section below, CK7 positive and mucicarmine or periodic acid-Schiff-positive in extramammary Paget disease, p63 and high molecular weight cytokeratin positive in squamous cell carcinoma in situ, and SOX10/Melan-A positive in melanoma in situ.

Zoon Balanitis Versus Erythroplasia of Queyrat and Extramammary Paget Disease

As introduced in the clinical presentation section above, Zoon balanitis's persistent, glistening, erythematous glans plaque frequently prompts biopsy to exclude erythroplasia of Queyrat (penile squamous cell carcinoma in situ, discussed in Chapter 15) and, less commonly, extramammary Paget disease, a differential resolved decisively by histology: Zoon balanitis shows the band-like plasma cell infiltrate and lozenge keratinocytes described above without epithelial dysplasia, while erythroplasia of Queyrat shows full-thickness keratinocytic atypia analogous to Bowen disease, and extramammary Paget disease shows the pagetoid, mucin-positive Paget cells described earlier in this chapter, three histologically distinct findings this chapter emphasizes should never be conflated given their dramatically different management pathways, observation or topical therapy for Zoon balanitis against the malignancy-directed management appropriate for the other two.

A 54-year-old uncircumcised patient presents with a persistent, glistening, orange-red patch on the glans penis, present for approximately five months and unresponsive to a trial of topical antifungal therapy. Pattern assignment identifies a dense, band-like plasma cell infiltrate within the superficial dermis, scattered lozenge-shaped keratinocytes within a mildly spongiotic and attenuated epidermis, and extravasated erythrocytes with hemosiderin-laden macrophages, without epithelial dysplasia, koilocytic change, or pagetoid intraepidermal cells. Differential narrowing weighs erythroplasia of Queyrat and extramammary Paget disease against Zoon balanitis given the persistent, non-healing clinical appearance, and the absence of epithelial dysplasia and pagetoid cells, together with the characteristic plasma cell-rich infiltrate and lozenge keratinocytes, supports the benign diagnosis; CK7 and mucicarmine staining are performed to definitively exclude extramammary Paget disease and return negative. Given the absence of dysplasia or pagetoid Paget cells and the characteristic plasma cell infiltrate, a diagnosis of Zoon balanitis is rendered, with the report reassuring the referring clinician regarding this diagnosis's benign, chronic irritant nature and recommending topical corticosteroid therapy or circumcision for definitive, recurrence-resistant management.

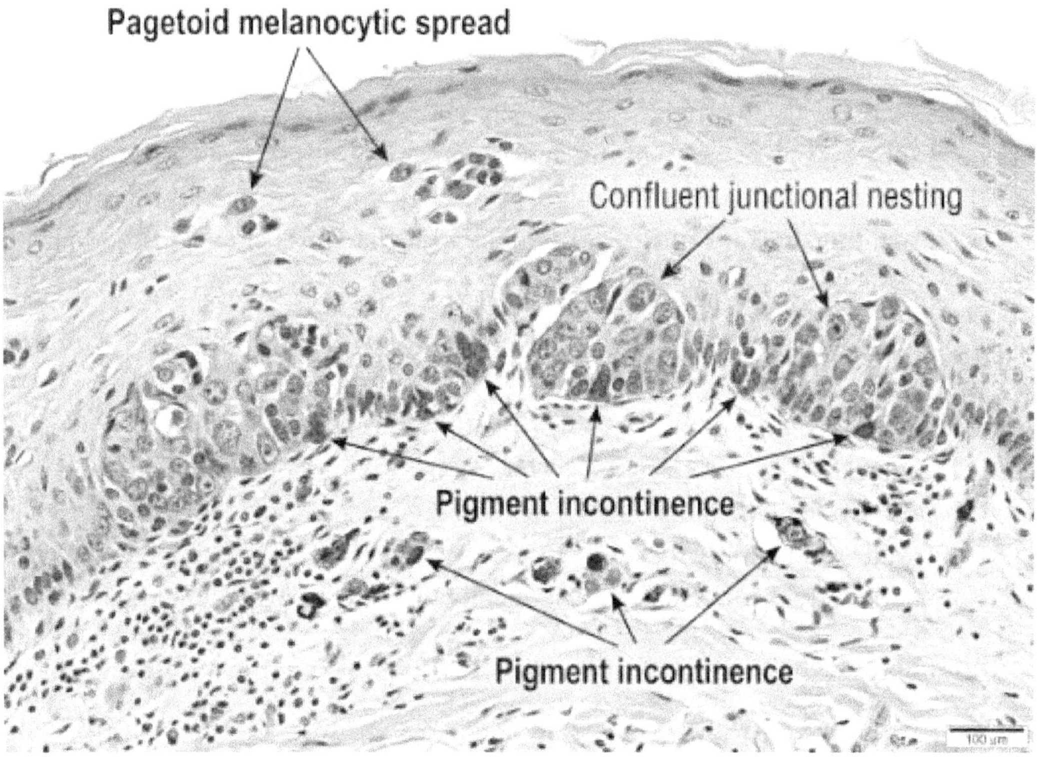

Oral Melanotic Macule Versus Early Oral Mucosal Melanoma

Oral mucosal melanoma, a rare but aggressive melanoma subtype most common on the hard palate and gingiva, can present in its earliest, radial growth phase as a flat, pigmented macule closely resembling the entirely benign oral melanotic macule described in the histopathologic features section above, a differential this chapter emphasizes carries substantial clinical consequence given oral mucosal melanoma's characteristically poor prognosis and the value of detection at its earliest, most treatable stage; the distinguishing features favor melanoma: an increased density of melanocytes along the basal layer, cytologic atypia, confluent nesting, and pagetoid spread, directly analogous to the criteria applied to subungual melanoma earlier in this chapter, against oral melanotic macule's simple basal melanin increase without melanocyte proliferation.

A 49-year-old patient presents with an incidentally noted, irregularly pigmented, 8-millimeter macule on the hard palate, of uncertain duration. Pattern assignment identifies an increased density of melanocytes along the basal layer of the oral mucosal epithelium with focal confluent nesting and rare melanocytes showing pagetoid upward migration, together with mild cytologic atypia. Differential narrowing weighs oral melanotic macule against early oral mucosal melanoma given the irregular pigmentation and the increased melanocyte density with pagetoid spread, and SOX10 and Melan-A immunohistochemistry are pursued to confirm the extent and pattern of the melanocytic proliferation, both showing a markedly increased melanocyte density with a pagetoid distribution pattern consistent with the routine staining impression. Given the increased melanocyte density, confluent nesting, and pagetoid spread, a diagnosis of oral mucosal melanoma in situ (radial growth phase) is rendered, with the report recommending complete surgical excision with wide margins and prompt multidisciplinary head and neck oncologic referral given this entity's characteristically aggressive behavior once invasive growth is established, underscoring the substantial clinical value of recognizing this diagnosis at its earliest, in situ stage.

Ancillary Studies

SOX10 and Melan-A Immunohistochemistry for Nail Matrix Melanocytic Lesions

As demonstrated in the worked case above, SOX10 and Melan-A immunohistochemistry allow precise quantification of melanocyte density and clearer visualization of architectural pattern and pagetoid spread than hematoxylin and eosin staining alone, an application this chapter notes is particularly valuable in the nail matrix given this site's comparatively subtle baseline melanocyte population and the correspondingly narrow margin for confidently distinguishing benign activation from early melanoma.

p16 and p53 Immunohistochemistry for Vulvar Intraepithelial Neoplasia Subtyping

As demonstrated in the worked case above, p16 immunohistochemistry showing diffuse, block-positive staining confirms high-risk human papillomavirus-driven usual-type vulvar intraepithelial neoplasia, while p53 immunohistochemistry showing a mutant expression pattern, either strong diffuse basal overexpression or, alternatively, complete absence of staining reflecting a null mutation, both interpreted as abnormal, supports a diagnosis of differentiated vulvar intraepithelial neoplasia, this reciprocal, largely mutually exclusive staining pattern providing the practically decisive ancillary distinction between these two etiologically and prognostically distinct entities whenever histology alone leaves genuine uncertainty.

CK7, GCDFP-15, and CK20 Immunohistochemistry for Extramammary Paget Disease

CK7 immunohistochemistry shows diffuse positivity in essentially all extramammary Paget disease regardless of primary versus secondary origin, functioning primarily to confirm the diagnosis and exclude the pagetoid mimickers discussed in the differential diagnosis section above, while GCDFP-15 and CK20 together help distinguish primary cutaneous disease, generally GCDFP-15 positive and CK20 negative, reflecting apocrine origin, from secondary disease extending from an underlying gastrointestinal or urothelial malignancy, which more often shows CK20 positivity and, when a specific primary is suspected, site-specific markers, GATA3 for urothelial origin or CDX2 for colorectal origin among the additional markers applied, an immunohistochemical distinction this chapter emphasizes directly determines whether systemic oncologic staging workup, discussed further in the management implications section below, is warranted.

PAS/GMS Staining and Fungal Culture for Onychomycosis

As demonstrated in the histopathologic features discussion above, periodic acid-Schiff or Gomori methenamine silver staining reliably identifies fungal hyphae within the nail plate, providing a rapid histologic confirmation of onychomycosis, while fungal culture or polymerase chain reaction-based species identification, though slower, provides organism-specific identification that can guide antifungal selection, particularly relevant for the non-dermatophyte mold and Candida-associated cases discussed in the etiology section above.

CD138 and Kappa/Lambda Immunohistochemistry for Zoon Balanitis

As demonstrated in the worked case above, CD138 immunohistochemistry confirms the plasma cell lineage of Zoon balanitis's characteristic infiltrate, while kappa and lambda light chain immunohistochemistry or in situ hybridization confirm polyclonality, excluding a clonal plasma cell process, an ancillary confirmation this chapter notes is rarely necessary given this entity's generally distinctive combined histologic and clinical presentation but remains available whenever genuine diagnostic uncertainty persists.

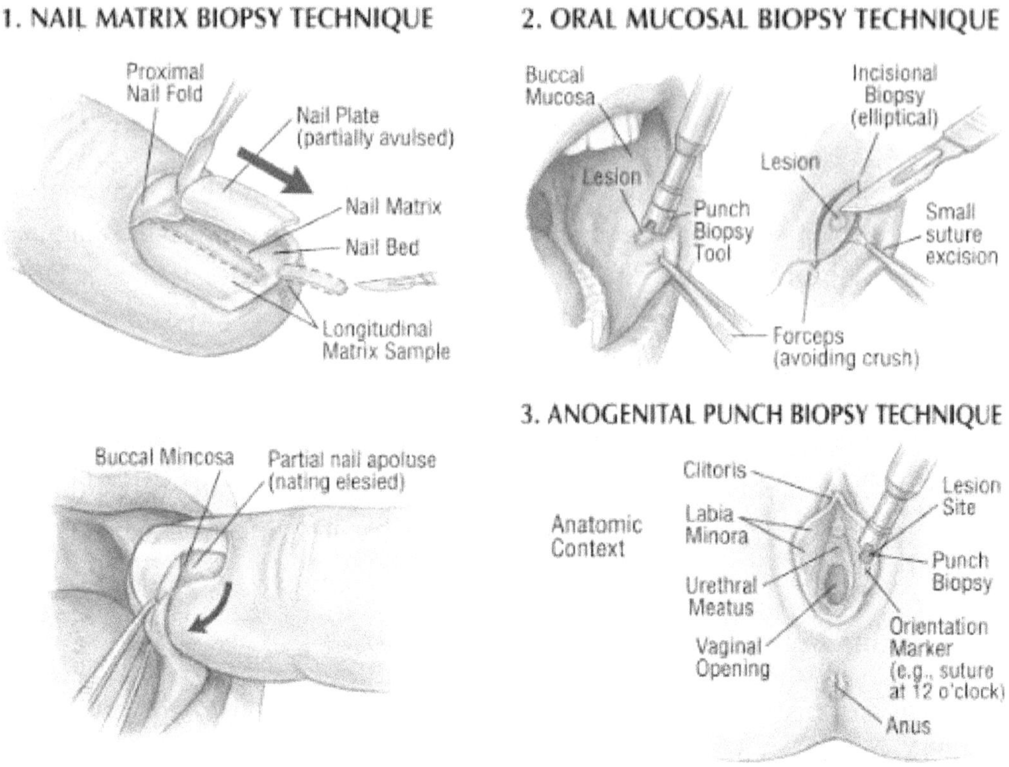

Management Implications

Management of Nail Unit and Oral Mucosal Disease

Benign longitudinal melanonychia meeting few ABCDEF criteria and without Hutchinson sign is generally managed with clinical monitoring and dermoscopic follow-up, while subungual melanoma, once confirmed, is managed with wide surgical excision, often requiring digit amputation for invasive disease given the nail unit's limited soft tissue reservoir for adequate margin control, together with sentinel lymph node biopsy consideration for tumors with sufficient depth, analogous to the staging approach discussed for cutaneous melanoma in Chapter 14. Glomus tumor of the nail bed is managed with simple surgical excision, generally curative given this tumor's uniformly benign behavior, with excision itself frequently providing the definitive diagnostic confirmation given how strongly this tumor's exquisite, characteristic point tenderness and cold sensitivity narrow the clinical differential even before histologic confirmation is obtained. Oral lichen planus is managed with topical corticosteroids for symptomatic disease, together with longitudinal surveillance given its small but genuine malignant transformation risk, particularly for the erosive variant, while oral epithelial dysplasia is managed according to grade, close observation with repeat biopsy for mild dysplasia, and complete excision for moderate to severe dysplasia given the substantially higher progression risk this grade carries.

Management of Lichen Sclerosus and Vulvar Intraepithelial Neoplasia

Lichen sclerosus is managed with high-potency topical corticosteroids as first-line therapy, which effectively controls symptoms and, importantly, reduces the associated squamous cell carcinoma risk when used consistently, together with longitudinal surveillance given this disorder's chronic, relapsing course and its well-established association with vulvar and, less commonly, penile squamous cell carcinoma. Differentiated vulvar intraepithelial neoplasia, given its higher per-lesion progression risk discussed above, is managed with complete surgical excision rather than the topical or ablative approaches sometimes appropriate for usual-type disease, together with continued lichen sclerosus management and close surveillance of the surrounding field given this entity's tendency to arise multifocally within a chronically diseased background. Usual-type vulvar intraepithelial neoplasia is managed with excision, ablative therapy, or topical imiquimod depending on lesion extent and patient factors, with human papillomavirus vaccination status and partner considerations forming part of the broader counseling discussion.

Management of Extramammary Paget Disease

Primary cutaneous extramammary Paget disease is managed with wide local excision or Mohs micrographic surgery given this entity's characteristic subclinical extension well beyond its apparent clinical margin, a pattern this chapter notes parallels dermatofibrosarcoma protuberans and angiosarcoma discussed in Chapter 17, with topical imiquimod an emerging option for select superficial or recurrent disease. Secondary extramammary Paget disease, once confirmed by the immunohistochemical panel discussed above, requires prompt referral for identification and treatment of the underlying visceral malignancy, with prognosis in this setting determined substantially by the underlying malignancy's stage and behavior rather than by the cutaneous Paget disease itself, making the primary-versus-secondary distinction, and the systemic workup, colonoscopy, cystoscopy, and pelvic imaging where clinically indicated, that follows a secondary diagnosis, the single most consequential management decision point in this specific entity.

Management of Onychomycosis, Zoon Balanitis, and Oral Melanotic Macule

Onychomycosis is managed with oral antifungal therapy, terbinafine the generally preferred first-line agent given its superior mycologic cure rate relative to topical therapy alone, with topical antifungal lacquers reserved for milder, distal disease or for patients in whom systemic therapy is contraindicated, together with confirmation of the diagnosis by the histologic or culture-based methods discussed above before committing a patient to a prolonged systemic treatment course. Zoon balanitis, as demonstrated in the worked case above, is managed with topical corticosteroid or calcineurin inhibitor therapy, with circumcision offering definitive, recurrence-resistant management by removing the chronic friction and moisture retention that drives this condition's pathogenesis, discussed in the etiology section above. Oral melanotic macule requires no treatment once its benign nature is confirmed, either clinically in a stable, characteristic-appearing lesion or histologically when biopsy is performed given diagnostic uncertainty or patient preference.

Documentation and Reporting Standards

The pathology report for a nail matrix melanocytic lesion should explicitly document melanocyte density, architectural pattern, and the presence or absence of pagetoid spread, together with the immunohistochemical findings when performed, given the genuinely narrow diagnostic margin at this site. The report for vulvar intraepithelial neoplasia should explicitly state the subtype, differentiated or usual-type, and the p16/p53 immunohistochemical results supporting that subtype, given the direct bearing of this distinction on management intensity discussed above. The report for extramammary Paget disease should explicitly state the CK7, GCDFP-15, and CK20 immunohistochemical findings and their interpretation regarding primary versus secondary origin, recommending systemic oncologic correlation whenever a secondary origin cannot be confidently excluded. The report for oral epithelial dysplasia should explicitly state the dysplasia grade using standardized terminology, mild, moderate, or severe, given this grade's direct bearing on the management pathway discussed above, and the report for any oral pigmented lesion biopsied to exclude melanoma should explicitly document melanocyte density and the presence or absence of pagetoid spread, mirroring the reporting standard applied to nail matrix melanocytic lesions given the two sites' shared underlying diagnostic logic developed throughout this chapter.

Complications and Prognosis

Oral lichen planus, particularly the erosive variant, carries a small but well-documented lifetime risk of malignant transformation to oral squamous cell carcinoma, a risk that, while modest in absolute terms, warrants the longitudinal surveillance discussed in the management implications section above rather than a one-time diagnosis and discharge from care. Subungual melanoma carries a comparatively poor prognosis relative to melanoma at other cutaneous sites, reflecting both this entity's well-documented tendency toward delayed diagnosis, discussed in the differential diagnosis section above, and, independently, a greater average Breslow depth at diagnosis. Severe oral epithelial dysplasia and erythroplakia both carry a substantial risk of progression to invasive squamous cell carcinoma if untreated, underscoring the importance of the grade-based management approach discussed above. Lichen sclerosus carries a lifetime squamous cell carcinoma risk concentrated in patients with poorly controlled or long-untreated disease, a risk this chapter emphasizes is meaningfully reduced, though not eliminated, by consistent topical corticosteroid therapy, while differentiated vulvar intraepithelial neoplasia carries a substantially higher and more rapid progression risk to invasive carcinoma than usual-type disease, developed throughout this chapter. Primary extramammary Paget disease carries a generally favorable prognosis when completely excised, though local recurrence is well-documented given this tumor's characteristic subclinical extension, while secondary extramammary Paget disease's prognosis is governed by the underlying visceral malignancy. Onychomycosis, while not independently life-threatening, carries a meaningfully elevated risk of secondary bacterial cellulitis, particularly in patients with diabetes or peripheral vascular disease, given the nail plate's compromised barrier function, an under-recognized complication this chapter notes warrants more consistent treatment in this specific population than onychomycosis's benign reputation might otherwise suggest. Zoon balanitis carries an excellent prognosis and no malignant potential once distinguished from its histologic and clinical mimickers discussed above, and oral mucosal melanoma, in contrast, carries one of the poorest prognoses of any melanoma subtype discussed in this book, reflecting both its aggressive intrinsic biology and its characteristic delayed diagnosis given the oral cavity's comparatively limited routine visual surveillance relative to sun-exposed skin.

Special Populations

Longitudinal melanonychia in a pediatric patient is more often benign than in an adult, reflecting a lower baseline incidence of subungual melanoma in this population, though the same ABCDEF assessment framework and threshold for biopsy when multiple concerning criteria are present remain appropriate practice regardless of age. Lichen sclerosus can affect prepubertal children, presenting with figure-eight vulvar or perianal involvement that can be mistaken for evidence of abuse, an important special-population consideration this chapter notes warrants careful, informed clinical evaluation, and childhood-onset lichen sclerosus shows a recognized potential for spontaneous improvement around puberty, distinct from the chronic, persistent course typical of adult-onset disease. Multiple pigmented oral macules in a child or young adult should prompt consideration of Peutz-Jeghers syndrome, a hereditary polyposis syndrome presenting with characteristic perioral and oral mucosal lentigines, a special-population pattern-recognition point this chapter notes distinguishes syndromic multifocal oral pigmentation from the solitary, sporadic oral melanotic macule discussed above. Diabetic and immunosuppressed patients with onychomycosis warrant more proactive treatment and monitoring given their elevated secondary cellulitis risk discussed in the complications and prognosis section above, and proximal subungual onychomycosis identified in a young or otherwise healthy-appearing patient should prompt consideration of underlying HIV infection or another immunosuppressed state given this pattern's recognized association, discussed in the clinical presentation section above.

Patient Education and Counseling

Patients diagnosed with benign longitudinal melanonychia benefit from clear counseling regarding the specific monitoring plan and the clinical findings that would prompt repeat biopsy, while patients diagnosed with subungual melanoma benefit from counseling that directly acknowledges this diagnosis's often-delayed recognition and frames the treatment pathway ahead around the best achievable outcome from the current diagnosis forward. Patients diagnosed with lichen sclerosus benefit from clear counseling regarding this disorder's chronic nature, the importance of consistent topical therapy in reducing malignancy risk, and the value of longitudinal surveillance, framed to encourage sustained treatment adherence rather than treatment abandonment once symptoms improve. Patients diagnosed with extramammary Paget disease benefit from clear counseling regarding the systemic workup that follows a secondary diagnosis and, for primary disease, realistic expectations regarding local recurrence risk and the value of continued surveillance following excision. Patients diagnosed with Zoon balanitis benefit from clear, reassuring counseling regarding this diagnosis's entirely benign, chronic irritant nature once the malignant and premalignant mimickers discussed above have been excluded, an important point of reassurance given how alarming this diagnosis's persistent, non-healing clinical appearance can understandably feel to an affected patient. Patients diagnosed with onychomycosis benefit from realistic counseling regarding the multi-month treatment course typically required for visible nail plate clearance given the nail's slow growth rate, together with counseling regarding the medication-specific monitoring, periodic liver function testing for prolonged oral terbinafine courses among the relevant considerations, appropriate to the systemic antifungal regimen selected.

THE REACTION PATTERN RECOGNITION SYSTEM — The Special Sites Anatomy and Etiology Pattern Family

The Pattern: Nail, mucosal, and anogenital entities organized by site-specific baseline anatomy and etiologic driver, trauma-related melanocyte activation, HPV infection, autoimmune sclerosis, or adnexal neoplasia, with site-specific criteria required at every level of this chapter's differential diagnoses.

Histologic Signature: Increased melanocyte density with pagetoid spread defines subungual melanoma; band-like lymphocytic infiltrate with Civatte bodies defines oral lichen planus; basal atypia with preserved maturation and mutant p53 defines differentiated vulvar intraepithelial neoplasia; pagetoid mucin-positive cells define extramammary Paget disease.

The Decision: Establish site-specific baseline anatomy, then apply site-specific criteria, escalating to SOX10/Melan-A, p16/p53, or CK7/GCDFP-15/CK20 immunohistochemistry whenever routine morphology leaves genuine diagnostic uncertainty at these historically underrecognized special sites.

Trap Logic: Benign melanonychia mimics subungual melanoma; differentiated vulvar intraepithelial neoplasia's subtle histology risks underdiagnosis despite higher progression risk than usual-type disease; primary and secondary extramammary Paget disease appear histologically similar without immunohistochemical distinction.

Pattern Anchor: Site-specific baseline anatomy first, then etiologic driver. Subtle special-site atypia, particularly differentiated vulvar intraepithelial neoplasia, must never be dismissed as reactive change without full clinical and immunohistochemical correlation.

Summary and Key Concepts

Nail, mucosal, and anogenital sites each demand site-specific diagnostic criteria given their distinct baseline anatomy, with the nail matrix's comparatively subtle melanocyte population requiring careful density and architectural assessment to distinguish benign melanonychia from subungual melanoma.

Oral lichen planus and oral epithelial dysplasia are distinguished by their characteristic band-like lymphocytic infiltrate and graded architectural/cytologic atypia respectively, with dysplasia grade directly determining malignant transformation risk.

Differentiated (lichen sclerosus-associated, p53-mutant) and usual-type (HPV-driven, p16 block-positive) vulvar intraepithelial neoplasia carry distinct etiologies and, counterintuitively, differentiated disease's subtler histology carries a higher per-lesion progression risk to invasive carcinoma.

Lichen sclerosus is managed with high-potency topical corticosteroids, which reduce its well-established squamous cell carcinoma risk, making consistent treatment adherence and longitudinal surveillance essential.

Extramammary Paget disease requires CK7, GCDFP-15, and CK20 immunohistochemistry to distinguish primary cutaneous disease from disease secondary to an underlying visceral malignancy, a distinction that directly determines whether systemic oncologic workup is warranted.

Onychomycosis, Zoon balanitis, and oral melanotic macule round out this chapter's special-site entities as generally benign, non-malignant processes whose principal diagnostic value lies in confidently distinguishing them from their more consequential mimickers discussed throughout this chapter.

THE REACTION PATTERN MASTER ATLAS

The Reaction Pattern Master Atlas consolidates the Pattern Anchor, the single definitive clinical decision point, distinguishing threshold, or diagnostic rule, from every chapter of this textbook into one indexed, cross-referenced navigator. Organized by diagnostic category and listed in the order each pattern family is developed across the twenty preceding chapters, this Atlas is designed as a rapid bedside and sign-out reference: locate the relevant pattern family, review its Pattern Anchor, and turn to the cited chapter for the full Rhythm Layer development, worked cases, and ancillary study detail supporting that anchor. This Atlas contains no questions, drills, item banks, or answer keys of any kind; it is a pure, structured reference index built entirely from the reaction-pattern logic this book has applied chapter by chapter.

Foundational Diagnostic Framework

Chapter 1 — Foundations of Histologic Pattern Recognition

Pattern Anchor: Before diagnosing any epidermal, dermal, or follicular abnormality, confirm biopsy site, patient age, and baseline pigmentation; site- and age-appropriate normal variation is the most common source of false-positive overcalls in foundational dermatopathology.

Chapter 2 — Ancillary Study Decision Points

Pattern Anchor: Every ancillary test answers a specific, narrow question; before ordering or interpreting one, state the question it is being asked to answer, and read the result only against that question.

Chapter 3 — The Pattern-Based Method Itself

Pattern Anchor: A reaction pattern is a starting hypothesis to be actively tested against its mimickers, not a final answer reached the moment a plausible match is recognized.

Inflammatory and Reactive Pattern Family

Chapter 4 — The Spongiotic Pattern Family

Pattern Anchor: Eosinophil-rich spongiosis in an elderly patient is pemphigoid until clinically excluded; treatment-refractory spongiotic dermatitis warrants consideration of mycosis fungoides; a neutrophil-rich or sandwich-sign spongiotic pattern warrants a PAS-D stain before an eczematous diagnosis is finalized.

Chapter 5 — The Psoriasiform Pattern Family

Pattern Anchor: Before finalizing a psoriasis diagnosis, actively look for what psoriasis should not have: checkerboard cornification (pityriasis rubra pilaris), fungal hyphae (tinea), or atypical epidermotropic lymphocytes (mycosis fungoides). Each absence, confirmed rather than assumed, strengthens the diagnosis.

Chapter 6 — The Interface Pattern Family

Pattern Anchor: Junctional obscuration sorts lichenoid from vacuolar interface; within each family, the specific mimickers are resolved more by clinical context, medication history, transplant timing, and distribution, than by histology alone, more so than in almost any other reaction pattern in this book.

Chapter 7 — The Vesiculobullous Pattern Family

Pattern Anchor: A vesiculobullous biopsy is incomplete without a paired perilesional specimen for direct immunofluorescence; routine histology establishes the level of split, but immunofluorescence establishes the specific diagnosis in nearly every case in this chapter.

Chapter 8 — The Granulomatous Pattern Family

Pattern Anchor: Never diagnose sarcoidosis before fungal and acid-fast special stains have been performed and reported as negative. This single discipline prevents the most consequential error this pattern family can produce: treating unrecognized infection with immunosuppression.

Chapter 9 — The Vasculopathic and Vasculitic Pattern Family

Pattern Anchor: Fibrinoid necrosis of the vessel wall means vasculitis and immunosuppression; an occluded lumen with an intact wall means vasculopathy and a coagulation or calcification workup. Get the wall assessment right first, because it redirects the entire subsequent evaluation.

Chapter 10 — The Panniculitis Pattern Family

Pattern Anchor: Deep tissue first, compartment second, vasculitis status third, specific histologic clue last. Never diagnose lupus panniculitis without explicitly excluding adipocyte rimming by atypical lymphocytes at high power, and never diagnose infectious panniculitis or lipodermatosclerosis without correlating necrosis pattern against organism stains, culture, and the venous stasis background respectively.

Chapter 11 — The Connective Tissue Disease Pattern Family

Pattern Anchor: Interface points toward lupus erythematosus or dermatomyositis and requires clinical-serologic distinction; sclerosis points toward morphea or systemic sclerosis and requires distribution-serologic distinction. Biopsy to fascia depth when eosinophilic fasciitis is a consideration, and never assume mucin-rich sclerosis is morphea without excluding scleredema and scleromyxedema first.

Chapter 12 — The Infectious Dermatoses Pattern Family

Pattern Anchor: Match the inflammatory pattern and any cytopathic change to organism class before ordering special stains; actively exclude dermatophyte infection with PAS-D staining whenever an annular, scaly, treatment-resistant eruption is biopsied; never let a single negative special stain level override strong clinical suspicion for fungal or parasitic infection; treat neonatal, disseminated, and necrotizing presentations as diagnostic emergencies.

Melanocytic and Pigmented Lesion Patterns

Chapter 13 — The Melanocytic Nevus and Simulator Pattern Family

Pattern Anchor: Symmetric, matures, uniform: benign, regardless of how alarming individual cytologic features appear in isolation. When these criteria are not clearly met, use ancillary studies and descriptive, uncertainty-acknowledging diagnosis rather than forcing a definitive call.

Chapter 14 — The Melanoma Diagnostic and Staging Pattern Family

Pattern Anchor: Asymmetric, fails to mature, atypical: melanoma. Breslow depth, ulceration, and mitotic rate, measured precisely and reported completely, directly determine surgical margins, sentinel lymph node biopsy eligibility, and systemic therapy pathway. When morphology alone leaves genuine uncertainty, escalate to ancillary studies and multidisciplinary review rather than a forced unilateral call.

Epithelial and Adnexal Neoplasm Patterns

Chapter 15 — The Keratinocytic Neoplasm Staging Pattern Family

Pattern Anchor: No atypia: benign. Lower-third atypia: actinic keratosis. Full-thickness atypia without invasion: in situ. Invasion present: malignant. Peripheral palisading with retraction: basal cell carcinoma, an entirely distinct basaloid lineage from the keratinocytic atypia axis governing the rest of this chapter. Verrucous carcinoma and Marjolin ulcer require deliberate deep sampling and clinical context, respectively, given their deceptively bland or confounded presentations.

Chapter 16 — The Adnexal Neoplasm Differentiation Pattern Family

Pattern Anchor: Line of differentiation first, then organization versus destruction. A recurrent chalazion, a painful dermal nodule, or a sebaceous neoplasm outside the eyelid each warrant the specific ancillary workup and syndrome consideration detailed in this chapter.

Mesenchymal, Lymphoid, and Systemic Deposition Patterns

Chapter 17 — The Mesenchymal Tumor Differentiation and Depth Pattern Family

Pattern Anchor: Line of differentiation first, then depth and circumscription versus infiltration. Atypical fibroxanthoma and pleomorphic dermal sarcoma are exclusion diagnoses; a negative pancytokeratin, S100/SOX10, and desmin panel is mandatory before either diagnosis is rendered.

Chapter 18 — The Cutaneous Lymphoma Clonality and Stage Pattern Family

Pattern Anchor: Lineage first, then epidermotropism, atypia, and depth. Clonality studies support but never independently establish a lymphoma diagnosis; integration with morphology and clinical course is mandatory in every case.

Chapter 19 — The Genodermatosis and Deposition Disorder Level and Substance Pattern Family

Pattern Anchor: Level or substance first, then the specific confirmatory ancillary study. Primary cutaneous versus systemic amyloidosis is never resolved by dermal histology alone; systemic workup is mandatory whenever this distinction is uncertain.

Special Site Patterns

Chapter 20 — The Special Sites Anatomy and Etiology Pattern Family

Pattern Anchor: Site-specific baseline anatomy first, then etiologic driver. Subtle special-site atypia, particularly differentiated vulvar intraepithelial neoplasia, must never be dismissed as reactive change without full clinical and immunohistochemical correlation.

Cross-Reference Index by Diagnostic Decision Type

This closing index groups every Pattern Anchor above by the type of decisive diagnostic move it represents, allowing rapid lookup not only by chapter but by the specific kind of diagnostic uncertainty the reader is currently facing at the microscope or bedside.

Decision Type	Governing Pattern Anchor(s)	Chapter
Exclude infection before immunosuppression	Sarcoidosis versus infectious granuloma; organism-class matching	8, 12
Assess vessel wall integrity first	Fibrinoid necrosis versus occluded lumen with intact wall	9
Confirm architectural symmetry and maturation	Benign nevus versus melanoma axis	13, 14
Apply an atypia-based staging axis	Actinic keratosis through invasive squamous cell carcinoma	15
Apply an exclusion immunohistochemical panel	Atypical fibroxanthoma/pleomorphic dermal sarcoma; oral/nail melanocytic lesions	17, 20
Distinguish primary from systemic/secondary disease	Amyloidosis; extramammary Paget disease	19, 20
Require ancillary confirmation before finalizing	Direct immunofluorescence; clonality studies; antigen mapping	7, 18, 19

This Atlas is intended as a living reference within the reader's own practice: return to it whenever a case presents genuine diagnostic ambiguity, use it to confirm that the full pattern-based method, hypothesis, active mimicker testing, and, where indicated, ancillary confirmation, has been applied before a diagnosis is finalized, and consult the cited chapter for the complete clinical, histologic, and evidentiary development behind each anchor summarized here.

CONCLUSION

This textbook was built around a single, deliberate premise: that dermatopathology is best taught not as an inventory of diagnoses to be memorized but as a discipline of pattern recognition disciplined by active testing against mimickers. Chapter 3 introduced that method explicitly, and every chapter that followed, from the inflammatory reaction patterns of Chapters 4 through 12 through the neoplastic and special-site chapters that completed this book, applied it in the same disciplined sequence: recognize the candidate pattern, test it deliberately against its closest mimickers, and escalate to the specific ancillary study that resolves genuine uncertainty rather than accepting a plausible first impression as a final answer. That sequence, more than any single diagnostic criterion in any single chapter, is what this book has tried to teach.

The Reaction Pattern Recognition System, threaded through every chapter as the Rhythm Layer and consolidated at the end of this book in The Reaction Pattern Master Atlas, was built to make that method visible and reusable rather than implicit. Each Pattern, Histologic Signature, Decision, Trap Logic, and Pattern Anchor was written to function as a complete, self-contained diagnostic unit, one the reader can return to at the microscope, in a multidisciplinary tumor board, or during sign-out, without needing to reread the surrounding chapter in full. The Master Atlas exists specifically so that reuse is fast: twenty Pattern Anchors, cross-referenced by chapter and by decision type, standing as a single-page-per-family index to the diagnostic logic this entire book was written to instill.

That logic rests on a few convictions worth restating plainly at the close of this book. Site, age, and clinical context are not footnotes to histology; they are load-bearing components of the diagnosis itself, as true in the interpretation of a nail matrix melanocytic proliferation as in the reading of a spongiotic dermatitis. Ancillary studies, immunohistochemistry, molecular testing, direct immunofluorescence, culture, and special stains, exist to answer specific, narrow questions, and their value lies in being ordered and read against that specific question rather than applied indiscriminately. And the differentials that carry the greatest clinical consequence in this specialty, dermatofibroma against dermatofibrosarcoma protuberans, atypical fibroxanthoma against pleomorphic dermal sarcoma, primary against secondary extramammary Paget disease, differentiated against usual-type vulvar intraepithelial neoplasia, are rarely the differentials that announce themselves as difficult at first glance. Recognizing which decision points in this specialty are quietly high-stakes, and treating them with the corresponding diagnostic rigor, is itself a skill this book has tried to build alongside the histologic knowledge on every page.

Dermatopathology continues to evolve, in its molecular classification of mesenchymal and lymphoid neoplasms, in its immunohistochemical panels, and in its integration with clinical genomics, and no textbook, including this one, is a substitute for staying current with the specialty's evolving evidence base and society guidelines over the course of a career. What this book has tried to offer instead is a durable diagnostic architecture, the pattern-based method of Chapter 3, applied consistently across twenty chapters and consolidated in the Master Atlas, that remains useful precisely because it teaches a way of thinking rather than a static list of facts. New entities will be described, molecular markers will be refined, and classification schemes will be revised; the discipline of testing a pattern against its mimickers before committing to a diagnosis will not go out of date.

KEY POINT: Every diagnosis in this book, and every diagnosis the reader will render after closing it, is strongest when it follows the same sequence: recognize the pattern, test it against its mimickers, and let clinical and ancillary correlation, not the most familiar-looking answer, decide the close call.

This book was written for the medical student encountering dermatopathology for the first time, the resident building diagnostic confidence case by case, and the practicing clinician who returns to a reference for the differential that genuinely matters at that moment, and it was written with the conviction that all three deserve the same rigor, the same clinical reasoning made explicit rather than assumed, and the same refusal to let a superficially reassuring pattern stand in for a properly tested one. The chapters close here, but the method they taught, and the Atlas built to keep it within reach, are meant to travel with the reader well beyond this book's final page.

www.ingramcontent.com/pod-product-compliance
Lightning Source LLC
LaVergne TN
LVHW062034101126
852251LV00025B/328